D1556247

John W. McLean

Dental Ceramics
Proceedings of the First International
Symposium on Ceramics

Dental Ceramics

Proceedings of the First International Symposium on Ceramics

Edited by
John W. McLean

Quintessence Publishing Co., Inc.   1983
Chicago, Berlin, London, Rio de Janeiro, Tokyo

© 1983 by Quintessence Publishing Co., Inc., Chicago, Illinois

All rights reserved.

This book or any part thereof must not be reproduced by any means or in any form without the written permission of the publisher.

Lithography: Industrie- und Presseklischee, Berlin
Composition: Thormann & Goetsch, Berlin
Printing: Thormann & Goetsch, Berlin
Binding: Lüderitz & Bauer – GmbH, Berlin

Printed in Germany

ISBN 0-86715-112-9

Lecturers in Alphabetical Sequence

Kenneth Anusavice, Ph.D., D.M.D.
Professor and Chairman
Department of Dental Biomaterials
College of Dentistry
University of Florida, Gainesville, Florida

Raymond L. Bertolotti, Ph.D., D.D.S.
Associate Clinical Professor, Biomaterials Science
School of Dentistry
Department of Restorative Dentistry
University of California, San Francisco

Dr. David Binns
British Ceramic Research Association
Stoke-on-Trent, England

Dr. Frank J. J. Clarke, B.Sc., D.I.C., Ph.D., F.Inst.P.
Division of Electrical Science Metrology
National Physical Laboratory
Middlesex, England

William L. Comcowich, D.D.S.
Clinical Instructor
Department of Fixed Prosthodontics
University of Colorado Dental School

Professor Sumiya Hobo, D.D.S., M.S.D., D.D.Sc.
Tohoku Dental University
Visiting Professor, University of California at Los Angeles School of Dentistry

Professor Derek W. Jones, B.Sc., Ph.D., F.I. Ceram.
Professor and Head Division of Dental Biomaterials Science
Faculty of Dentistry
Dalhousie University
Halifax, Nova Scotia, Canada

John W. McLean, O.B.E.
D.Sc., M.D.S. (University of London), F.D.S. R.C.S. (England)
Consulting Professor in Fixed Prosthodontics and Biomaterials
Louisiana State University Medical Center School of Dentistry

Lloyd Miller, D.M.D., F.I.C.D., F.A.C.D.
Clinical Professor
Tufts University School of Dental Medicine
Graduate and Postgraduate Prosthodontics

Jack D. Preston, D.D.S.
Chairman and Professor
Department of Fixed Prosthodontics
Harrington Professor, Esthetic Dentistry
University of Southern California School of Dentistry

Professor Peter Schärer, D.M.D., M.S.
Head, Department of Crown and Bridge Prosthodontics
Dental School, University of Zurich, Switzerland

David E. Southan, M.D.S., Ph.D. (Sydney), F.D.S. R.C.S. (England), F.R.A.C.D.S., F.I.C.D.
Department of Prosthetic Dentistry
University of Sydney, Australia

Mr. Joseph Tuccillo
President, Argen Precious Metals, Inc., New York

Peter A. Weiss, D.M.D.
Associate Professor
Department of Post-Graduate Prosthodontics
Henry M. Goldman School of Dentistry, Boston University

Foreword

Any international symposium will be criticized in that it has not covered everything that the audience desires. *The First International Symposium on Dental Ceramics* is no exception. This meeting was limited to the science and clinical art of dental ceramics, but in the second meeting to be held in London in 1984, a wide coverage of laboratory procedures is planned specifically for the technician.

It is natural for both dentist and technician to be more impressed with practical subjects rather than scientific ones. However, as a clinician and editor of this book, I believe that we can go round and round on the same clinical circuit until a scientific development allows us to enter a new clinical channel. Accurate scientific reports are also the only way we can assess our materials and, indeed, the manufacturer's claims. For example, far too many alloys are marketed for porcelain bonding without the manufacturer even stating their constituents. We are in much greater need of definite recommendations for shade matching and Dr. *Clarke,* in the final section of this book, sets out the scientist's view on how difficult it is to measure the colour of teeth and to develop colour measuring instruments.

I believe that the contents of this book represent a significant contribution to original thought and deserve our attention even where we may not comprehend all the detail. The authors are recognized authorities in their field and the quality of their presentations needs no further embellishment. The reader will find authoritative statements on the composition of porcelain, how it can be strengthened, why it breaks, the problems of porcelain bonding and the causes of failure. Modern ideas on occlusion are excellently presented and the design of preparations and metal substructures is critically analysed. The reader will find a detailed assessment of modern dental alloys for porcelain bonding and the quality of the illustrations show the high standard of aesthetics that is now obtainable. The bibliography is also one of the most comprehensive ever presented and should assist any serious student of ceramics. If the reader is prepared to examine in detail each chapter, he will find an immense amount of information which is of direct clinical use. For the dental scientist it is hoped that he will find an accurate presentation of the state of our art.

John W. McLean,
38 Devonshire Street,
London, W1N 1LD

Table of Contents

The Future for Dental Porcelain

John W. McLean

The standard of aesthetics in dental porcelain has now reached a stage where the development of new porcelains and metals meet ever increasing demands on their optical and physical properties. There is little doubt that more and more dental ceramists are becoming aware of the importance of maintaining depth of translucency in their crowns if they are to be undetectable from their human counterparts. The building of colour in depth is receiving increasing attention and refinements in placing gingival, body and enamel porcelains have reached a high standard of sophistication. The future for dental porcelain is therefore circumscribed by these exacting aesthetic requirements. To achieve translucency in enamel porcelains it is essential that a high proportion of glassy material is used and for this reason any advances in the composition of dental porcelain rely heavily on modern glass technology. Current dental porcelains are, essentially, felspathic glasses in which the addition of fluxes such as B_2O_3, K_2O, Na_2O and CaO lower the firing temperature and can, where necessary, increase the thermal expansion to that of the gold or base-metal alloys.

Dental porcelains, being essentially glass powders, rely upon their densification by low temperature sintering in which the original glassy grains retain much of their original shape. The fired porcelain is a brittle solid with low impact strength and a very limited capability for distributing localized stresses. It is therefore weak in tension but strong in compression. It is hardly surprising that the chief complaint from dentists is the tendency for these materials to chip or fracture in service. In particular, the reproduction of occlusal surfaces in dental porcelain presents a great technological challenge. The first priority in any future porcelain research should be that of strengthening dental porcelain without sacrificing aesthetics.

Strengthening Dental Porcelain

In order to strengthen dental porcelain it must either be supported by a high strength ceramic or metal, or the porcelain itself must be made stronger. Current and future research, which will be discussed in more depth later in this symposium, would appear to centre around five approaches to strengthening dental porcelain (*Binns,* 1977; *McLean,* 1969).

1. Enamelling of metals.
2. Dispersion strengthening of glasses.
3. Enamelling of high strength crystalline ceramics.
4. Controlled crystallisation of glasses (castable glass-ceramics).
5. Production of pre-stressed surface layers in dental porcelain via ion-exchange.

Enamelling of Metals

The fused porcelain-to-gold crown is now the most widely-used restoration in fixed prosthodontics. The alloys used for the construction of metal-ceramic crowns and fixed bridgework must meet many more requirements than the traditional gold alloys used in dentistry. They must match the veneer porcelain in thermal expansion, in order to minimize stresses forming at the interface, and possess adequate mechanical properties such as high yield strength, high modulus of elasticity, hardness, and high-temperature strength. A large number of metal-ceramic systems have now been developed for use in dentistry and they may be classified as follows.

Noble-Metal Alloy Systems

High gold

1. Gold-platinum-palladium alloys.
2. Gold-platinum-tantalum alloys.

Low gold

3. Gold-palladium-silver alloys.
4. Gold-palladium alloys.

Gold-free

5. Palladium-silver alloys.
6. Palladium-indium-tin-cobalt alloys.
7. Palladium-tin-gallium alloys.

Base-Metal Alloy Systems

Nickel-chromium alloys.
Cobalt-chromium alloys (rarely used in ceramic bonding).

The current gold-platinum-palladium alloys are well tried and clinically tested and set the standard for much of our future work. The only reason, at the present time, for wishing to replace them is their high cost and also lack of fit, due to metal creep, when firing the porcelain. Alloys containing 84–85 % gold are too near the porcelain firing temperatures of 900° C to 950° C. The high-gold alloys are easy to cast and since the addition of base-metals such as indium and tin can be carefully controlled, oxide production is not excessive. The tin and indium oxides appear to form a solid solution with the porcelain at the interface, bringing the metal into atomic contact with the porcelain. The strength of the gold alloys is adequate for most clinical situations, when used in correct section, but for bridges involving two or more pontics, or

Table 1   Gold-Palladium Alloy. From US Patent No. 4, 123, 262 (*Cascone*, 1978)

Composition		Mechanical Properties	
Gold	51.5%	Ultimate tensile strength	758 MPa
Palladium	38.5%	Yield strength	579 MPa
Indium	8.5%	Elongation percent	10
Gallium	1.5%	Brinell Hardness	214

in cases of multi-splinting of periodontally involved teeth, improvements in yield strength and modulus of elasticity are desirable.

One of the more promising developments in the gold-alloy systems has been the introduction of the gold-palladium alloys (*Cascone*, 1978) in which silver has been omitted. A typical composition and mechanical properties of these alloys is given in Table 1. The higher melting temperature of the gold-palladium alloys reduces the risk of metal creep on firing the porcelain and the alloys also possess good mechanical properties (Table 1). Major improvements in the mechanical properties of the noble-metal alloys are unlikely in the future since the possible permutation of alloy constituents is now well documented. Future research may be better concentrated on producing improved porcelains for metal bonding since this area has been comparatively neglected. Bonding to the palladium alloys could then be improved and offer a cheaper alternative to gold.

New Porcelains for Metal Bonding

Distortion of metal-ceramic crowns and fixed partial dentures can be a problem to the clinician. Distortion is a result of changes in the metal as well as contraction of the fired porcelain. The greatest distortion appears to occur in the degassing and final glaze stage (*Bridger* and *Nicholls*, 1981) and is reversible, since the framework will rebound elastically if the porcelain is removed chemically. A study measuring alloy and pre-solder creep ratio and porcelain viscous flow ratio as a function of temperature showed that, while the nickel-chromium alloys investigated remained "elastic" during porcelain fusion, most precious-metal alloys exhibited creep in significant clinical amounts (*Bertolotti*, 1981). The relative stiffness ratios of the fused material was shown to affect the rate of high temperature deformation in both the porcelain and the alloys. Such behaviour precludes the existence of a uniform "porcelain-softening temperature".

A further problem with the base-metal

alloys is that they readily oxidise. The nickel-chromium alloys contain approximately 20% chromium in order to protect the alloy against corrosion and tarnish. At high temperatures, chromium oxide can form in quite thick layers and will produce a weak layer of a dark green oxide (*McLean* and *Sced,* 1973). Controlling the thickness of the oxide layer is a major problem for the ceramist since it has also been shown that if chromium or nickel are combined in the porcelain, they reduce the thermal expansion of the porcelain, thus incurring the danger of a high degree of residual stress at the bond (*McLean* and *Sced,* 1973). It has been argued that a lowering of expansion may improve the strength of the bond (*Moffa* et al., 1973) by inducing greater compressive stresses. It is the author's opinion that the ideal state should be one in which minimal stresses occur at the bond. However, due to the complex geometry of metal copings and framework, this is very difficult to achieve. The significance of metal design, alloy constituents, and porcelain compatibility will be discussed in depth at this symposium.

Reduction of chromium oxide formation can be achieved by the addition of beryllium to the alloy since a layer of beryllium oxide inhibits excessive chromium oxide formation. Unfortunately, beryllium is a highly toxic metal and must be used under the most stringent safety precautions in the dental laboratory. The problems of oxidation in ceramic bonding alloys will be further discussed in this symposium and at this stage it is sufficient to say that the two major problems in bonding porcelain to metal are:

1. Deformation of metal during firing of the porcelain.
2. Controlling oxidation of the nickel-chromium alloys.

Reduction of the firing temperature of the porcelain might reduce the risk of excessive oxide production in chromium-containing alloys. In addition, the sag resistance of noble-metal alloys would be improved since their melting temperatures are fairly close to that of the regular metal-bonding porcelains (ca. 150° C). A porcelain firing at 800° C would therefore be a desirable objective providing other properties such as hydrolytic stability are not affected (*McLean,* 1978; *Karino,* 1976).

Work on producing lower-firing temperature porcelains has shown that when porcelains contain at least 10% of leucite ($K_2O \cdot Al_2O_3 \cdot 4SiO_2$) as a crystalline phase, it is possible to produce low-firing temperature porcelains with matching thermal expansions to that of gold or nickel-chromium alloys. Leucite is a very high expansion phase (20×10^{-6} °C) and its crystallization in dental porcelain may be brought about by suitable formulation of the dental porcelain and the correct heat treatment. Increasing the K_2O (potash) content of the porcelain will move the composition into the leucite field and increase the tendency to crystallize, particularly in the presence of nucleating agents such as TiO_2. However, when the K_2O content rises above 16%, it is difficult to obtain leucite crystallization (*Karino,* 1976). Further work revealed that the silica, alumina, potash ratio in the glass frit should not be less than SiO_2

56%, Al_2O_3 13% and K_2O 6% if crystallization of leucite is to occur. Low-firing temperatures could not be achieved if the silica and alumina content is more than 62% and 16% respectively.

Ideal compositions for a dental porcelain firing at 800° C are given in Table 2. The glass frits for making these porcelains are prepared as finely divided powders and then sintered at 700° C for 3 hours to allow the crystallization of leucite to take place. It is claimed that the thermal expansion of the frit may be raised from $11 \times 10^{-6 \circ}$ C to 12.5 to $10 \times 10^{-6 \circ}$ C (*Karino, 1976*). A commercial porcelain, Cera 8*, recently marketed in Japan, is based on this work and has yet to be evaluated clinically. Its chemical and physical properties are given in Table 3.

* Cera 8 Porcelain. Towa-Giken Co., Osaka, Japan.

Table 2   Composition of Low-Fusing Porcelain

	Opaque Wt.%	Dentine Wt.%	Enamel Wt.%
SiO_2	42.0	57.8	57.8
Al_2O_3	10.7	14.6	14.6
Na_2O	7.5	8.7	8.7
K_2O	10.7	14.6	14.6
B_2O_3	2.1	2.7	2.7
MgO	0.5	0.5	0.4
ZrO_2	21.2	0.4	0.1
SnO_2	3.2	0.4	0.1
Trace Elements	2.1	0.3	1.0

Courtesy of Karino, S.

Table 3   Chemical and Physical Properties of CERA 8 Low-Fusing Porcelain
Tested according to B.S.5612

Type	Flexural Strength (MPa)	Standard Deviation	Chemical Solubility Wt.Loss (%)	Thermal Expansion 20–350° C
Opaque	87.6	11.5	0.15	12.2×10^{-6}
Dentine	79.0	16.7	0.13	11.6×10^{-6}
Enamel	77.7	12.7	0.13	12.4×10^{-6}
Range of Values for Commercial Porcelains	51–95		0.01–0.07	$11.7–14.2 \times 10^{-6}$

One of the major problems with all low-firing porcelains is hydrolytic stability and it will be noted that the chemical solubility of Cera 8 is higher than the current metal-ceramic porcelains. However, no studies have yet been undertaken to establish clinically how resistant porcelain should be to oral fluids before the safety margin is exceeded. Preliminary work with these new low-firing porcelains indicates that they are worthy of further investigation.

Clinical Technique for Low-fusing Porcelains

Cera 8 porcelain consists of opaque porcelains firing at 800° C and body and enamel porcelains firing at 790° C. The construction of a metal-ceramic crown should follow the standard procedure for the current metal-ceramic porcelains.

Opaque application

The opaque is applied by standard procedure using the brush technique described by *McLean* (1980). Two thin applications of opaque provide better covering power on the metal coping, and multi-blending of colours (gingival, body and incisal) are recommended.

Recommended firing schedule
Opaque

500° C $\xrightarrow{\text{in vacuo}}$ 780° C at 50° C per minute
780° C $\xrightarrow{\text{in air}}$ 800° C

Application of Veneer Porcelains

Gingival, body and enamel porcelains are applied using the brush technique and colour is built in depth as shown in Figs. 1 a and b for the body porcelains and Figs. 2a to c for the enamel porcelains.

Recommended firing schedule
Dentine and Enamels
500° C $\xrightarrow{\text{in vacuo}}$ 770° C at 50° C per minute
770° C $\xrightarrow{\text{in air}}$ 790° C

The above firing schedule will produce a high biscuit finish (Fig. 3a) which allows grinding and shaping of the crown with clean diamond stones (Fig. 3b).

Glazing

Staining must be done using special low temperature stain.

Recommended glazing schedule
500° C $\xrightarrow{\text{in air}}$ 790° C

The completed crowns using the Cera 8 porcelain are shown in Figs. 4a and b.

Future Development

Low-fusing porcelains firing at 800° C do not allow post-ceramic soldering using current soldering techniques. Firing of these porcelains also requires greater care with regard to firing temperatures and vacuum pressures. High vacuum pressures will tend to cause bloating in the glass veneer and high temperatures increase the risk of the porcelain becoming too glassy. Future development of these porcelains will need to take into

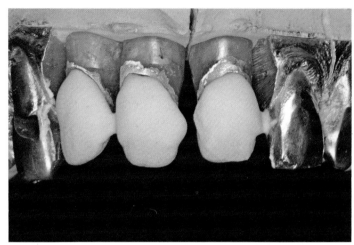

Fig.1a   Gingival dentines applied to low-fusing opaques.

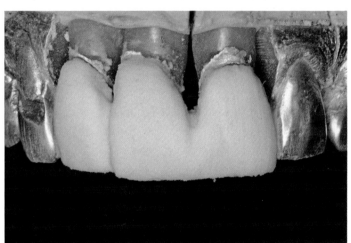

Fig.1b Body dentines completed and teeth built to full contour.

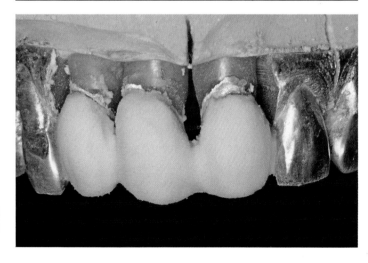

Fig.2a   Body porcelains carved back to provide enamel blend lines.

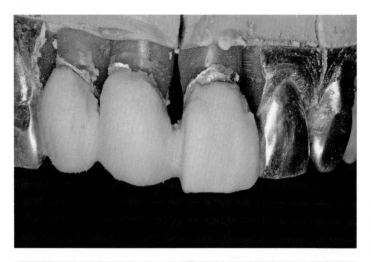

Fig. 2b Enamel porcelains applied to maxillary left central and characterised by using inlaid clear porcelain and stain.

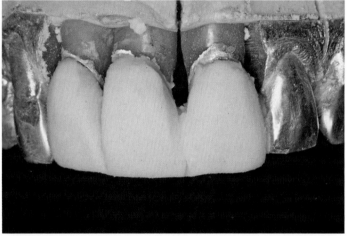

Fig. 2c Completion of enamel build-up.

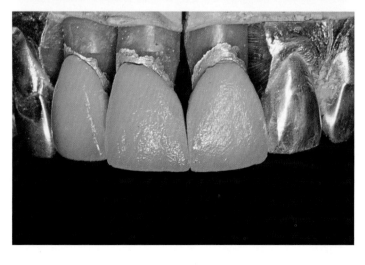

Fig. 3a Cera 8 crowns fired to high biscuit at 790° C.

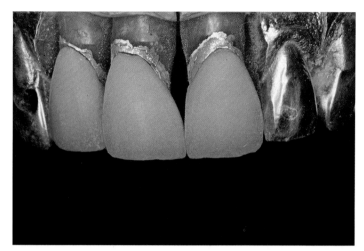

Fig. 3b   Cera 8 crowns after surface characterisation with diamond stones.

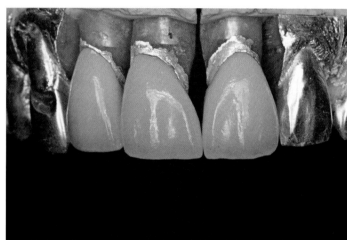

Fig. 4a   Cera 8 crowns after glazing at 790°C in air. The porcelain is very translucent but showing a slightly glassy appearance.

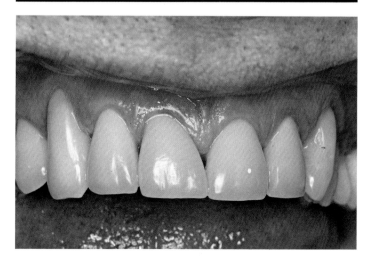

Fig. 4b   Completed crowns on 12, 11, 21 after cementation.

account the above factors. However, the advantages of low temperature firing on oxide production and metal creep, together with the potential for using lower melting temperature metals, is one of great significance.

Dispersion Strengthening of Glasses

The elimination of metal substructures in fixed prosthodontics is desirable, not only for aesthetic reasons but also because of the high cost of production. The replacement of metal copings with a higher strength ceramic is once again receiving attention.

It is well-known that the strength and elasticity of glass can be increased by physical interaction with an included phase of high elasticity (*Binns*, 1962; *Hasselman* and *Fulrath*, 1966). Dispersion strengthening of glass utilizes this principle whereby ceramic crystals of high strength and elasticity are fused in a glassy matrix to form crystal-glass composites. These composites form a constant strain system and fracture has an equal chance of starting in either phase. In the absence of thermal expansion differences, the strength and elasticity will increase, approximately, in proportion to the amount of the crystal phase. The choice of ceramic crystals is fairly wide but for dental use there are several limiting aspects:

1. Bonding with dental porcelain veneers.
2. Fusion temperature suitable for dental furnaces.
3. Colour and surface texture.
4. Marginal fit and stability after firing.
5. Ease of manufacture in a dental laboratory.

Research in 1963 by *McLean* and *Hughes* indicated that when fused alumina crystals of 99.5% purity and with a size range of 20 to 30 μm (specific surface area 1153 cm^2/g) were incorporated in a specially prepared borosilicate glass containing a high combined alumina content, the fired product would produce strength figures approximately double that of regular felspathic porcelain. The transverse strength of these new "Aluminous Porcelains" was found to be in excess of 20,000 p.s.i. (140 MPa) and with a light transmission of up to 20% on 1mm thick discs (*McLean* and *Hughes,* 1965). The subsequent commercialisation of these porcelains established the principle of using high strength core porcelains for the construction of dental ceramic crowns (Fig. 5, *McLean,* 1965).

The strength of aluminous porcelain jacket crowns was limited by the inherent brittleness of all ceramics. Invariably, fractures in dental porcelain originate from microcracks, often less than 0.1 μm wide, which are present on the surface and act as stress concentrators. Microcracks on the fit surface of the porcelain crown are generally regarded as the most dangerous. *Southan* and *Jorgensen* (1972) studied crowns made by the platinum foil technique and concluded that "polymorphic pore strata" almost invariably occurred at the internal surface of crowns due to poor condensation and lack of wetting of the platinum foil by the liquid glass phase during porcelain sintering.

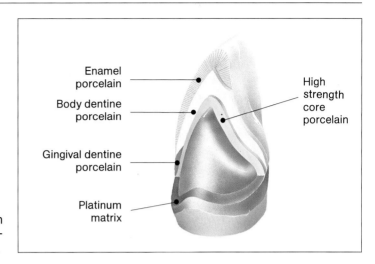

Enamel porcelain

High strength core porcelain

Body dentine porcelain

Gingival dentine porcelain

Platinum matrix

Fig. 5 Diagram of the use of high strength core porcelains for reinforcing porcelain veneer crowns.

Electroplating Technique for Bonding Porcelain

In order to further improve the strength of aluminous porcelain jacket crowns, an attempt was made to eliminate surface flaws on the fit surface by deliberately bonding the platinum foil to the inner surface of the crown. This procedure appeared to eliminate open surface defects from which tensile failure may originate, and was achieved by coating the surface of the platinum foil with up to 0.2 μm of tin. An electroplating technique was found to be the simplest method and on subsequent oxidation of the tin, it was found that aluminous core porcelain could be firmly bonded to the oxidised platinum surface (*McLean* and *Sced,* 1976). Testing of discs of coated and uncoated platinum foil/aluminous porcelain combinations showed that an increase in bi-axial flexural strength of approximately 80% could be expected from the tin oxide bonded porcelain (Table 6, *Sced* et al., 1977). *Minassian* (1978) tested porcelain crowns using the twin-foil platinum bonded technique and found that there was a statistically significant increase in fracture strength from 184 N for standard aluminous porcelain crowns to 286 N for the bonded platinum crowns (Table 4).

Rojers (1979) has developed an electroformed pure gold coping for jacket crowns. The gold coping is electroformed on a "Hydrocal" die using a conductive silver paint to metallize the surface. Surface treatment of the gold with a flash coating of electrodeposited tin then ensures "wetting" of the fused porcelain to produce a strong porcelain jacket crown. The current VMK 68 porcelain was used in these experiments because of its matching thermal expansion to gold. Because of the close approximation of the melting temperature of pure gold and VMK 68 porcelain, great care is required in firing the crown, in order to avoid distortion by metal creep of the gold coping. This technique may be more easily used with CERA 8 low-fusing porcelain.

Table 4 Strength of Platinum Bonded Aluminous Porcelain Jacket Crowns

Die No.	Platinum Bonded Crowns Fracture Load (N)	Aluminous Porcelain Standard Crowns Fracture Load (N)	
		1st set	2nd set
1	274.5	197.5	191.5
2	310.0	171.5	165.0
3	300.5	175.0	175.0
4	280.8	222.0	187.5
5	300.5	215.0	177.5
6	320.0	175.0	175.0
7	258.5	172.5	159.5
8	272.5	178.5	185.0
9	261.5	183.5	202.5
10	288.5	173.0	209.5
Mean	286.8N	184.5N	
S.D.	20.5	17.6	

From Minassian, R. M.D.S. Thesis, University of Bristol.

Table 5 High Strength Ceramics

Ceramic	Flexural Strength MPa
Fine-grained alumina	420–520
Partially-stabilized zirconia	640
Hot-pressed silicon nitride	800–900
Hot-pressed silicon carbide	400–750
Dental porcelain	51–95
Aluminous porcelain	125–135

High Strength Ceramics

The replacement of metal with high strength ceramics could offer great possibilities in dentistry. However, the choice of ceramic materials that are suitable for use in clinical practice is very limited. The major types of high strength ceramics which might be used in dental restorations are shown in Table 5. Partially stabilized zirconia and hot-pressed silicon nitride and carbide are not suitable because of problems of shaping, forming and sintering. In addition, the application of veneer porcelains to these materials is not very practical because of colour differences and incompatibility of thermal expansions.

The only high strength ceramic that has been used practically in dentistry is alu-

Table 6   Flexural Strengths of High-Alumina and Alumina-Glass Composites Compared with Tin-Oxide Bonded Platinum Discs and Regular Porcelain

Material	Bi-axial flexural strength MPa	
	Range	Mean
Felspathic porcelain	46.4– 66.7	56.5
Aluminous Porcelain Vitadur N	69.1–115.3	92.2
Platinum-bonded aluminous porcelain Vita-Pt	139.9–171.5	155.7
High-Alumina/Aluminous porcelain composite	326.4–364.9	345.6
High-Alumina 98 % purity	517.0–575.1	546.0

mina, and techniques for using sintered high-alumina have been described by *McLean* (1966). By using a plasticised alumina dough, a high alumina ceramic of 97 % purity could be fired onto a platinum matrix. The alumina dough or putty was moulded by hand to form a coping with a design similar to that used in a metal-ceramic crown. The alumina ceramic was then sintered at 1650° C in an air-fired furnace. Due to the negligible glass phase in high-alumina, it was found that very little pyroplastic flow occured and, during sintering, the "green" coping would not slump and flow onto the platinum matrix. High-alumina will either fissure or contract and tends to distort the platinum matrix. With our present powder technology it is impossible to reduce the volume porosity of an alumina powder bed much below 35 to 40% and shrinkages similar to dental porcelain are encountered if the ceramic body is to be sintered to high density. It is for this reason that sintered high alumina profiles were introduced for the construction of pontics and all-ceramic bridgework (*McLean,* 1967).

Future Research

Alumina ceramics continue to be the most promising materials for future development. In considering high alumina ceramics there is always a question as to what is "high" alumina? Referring to the alumina-silica phase diagram by *Bowen* and *Grieg* with corrections by *Schaier*, there is a division between phases of free corondum and those containing various amounts of it at the mullite line ($3Al_2O_3 - 2SiO_2$). Those compositions containing more alumina than the amount required by the mullite formula (72 %) are termed high alumina ceramics. Anything below this should be referred to as alumina porcelains (*Blodgett,* 1961).

The author attempted the construction of small fixed bridges in high alumina in 1965 using a 75% alumina body of the following formulation:–

	Wt. %
Alumina	65
Ball clay	20–21
Nepheline syenite	10
Lithium fluxes	4–5

The 75 % alumina ceramic could be fired at 1310° C and flexural strength figures in excess of 215 MPa were obtained (*McLean,* 1966). The material could be moulded in the form of a dough and no problems were found in shaping the green ceramic on a platinum matrix. However, although the pyroplasticity of the 75 % alumina body was better than the 98 % bodies, the problem of controlling firing shrinkage still arose. The fabrication of single crowns presented no great problem providing a two-bake technique was used similar to the conventional jacket crown technique. However, even short span bridges were difficult to construct due to the shrinkage across the pontic areas. Finally, the strength figures for this material were still too low to allow the use of 2.5 mm cross-sectional connectors and work was abandoned in favour of strengthening the aluminous porcelains by elimination of surface flaws (*McLean* and *Sced,* 1973).

The technique of baking aluminous porcelain onto tin-oxide coated platinum foil, as previously described, can provide strength figures of over 80 % above that of non-coated platinum foil crowns. Aluminous porcelains are also being manufactured with flexural strengths of 50 to 60 % above that of regular felspathic porcelain. Experimental aluminous porcelains have also been made that are twice as strong as regular porcelain (*McLean,* 1966). Even higher figures can be obtained when aluminous porcelain is baked onto high-alumina to form a laminate of equal thickness. The potential for all these systems is compared with regular dental porcelain in Table 6, and results from clinical testing show that for anterior crowns, bi-axial flexural strengths of around 140 to 150 MPa are adequate. The incidence of fracture for these crowns is given in Table 7 and of a total of 418 incisor crowns inserted, a failure rate of 2.1 % might be regarded as acceptable. In the case of the canine teeth it is interesting to note that an even lower incidence of 1.3% occurred. However, for posterior restorations, due to high tensile stresses developing in the central fossae of the molar teeth, it would appear that higher strengths are needed. A failure rate of 15.2 % over 7 years cannot be regarded as acceptable. Due to the early failures of the platinum bonded molar crowns, greater care was taken in designing the preparation and alumina core. By flattening the occlusal table, reducing the cusp form, and thickening the core at the central fossa and periphery, it was found that

Table 7 Results of Clinical Testing of Bonded Platinum Aluminous Porcelain Crowns

Year	Total No. Crowns	Molars	Pre-molars	Ca-nines	Incisors	No. of Failures* Molars	No. of Failures* Pre-molars	No. of Failures* Ca-nines	No. of Failures* Inci-sors
1974	93	13	21	9	50	3	3	–	–
1975	112	26	20	11	55	5	1	–	2
1976	102	11	19	9	63	1	1	–	2
1977	109	1	18	14	76	–	–	–	1
1978	121	8	27	17	69	–	2	1	2
1979	82	–	11	10	61	–	1	–	2
1980	60	–	9	7	44	–	–	–	–
Total	679	59	125	77	418	9	8	1	9
					Failure per cent	15.2	6.4	1.3	2.1

* Failure includes chipping or complete fracture

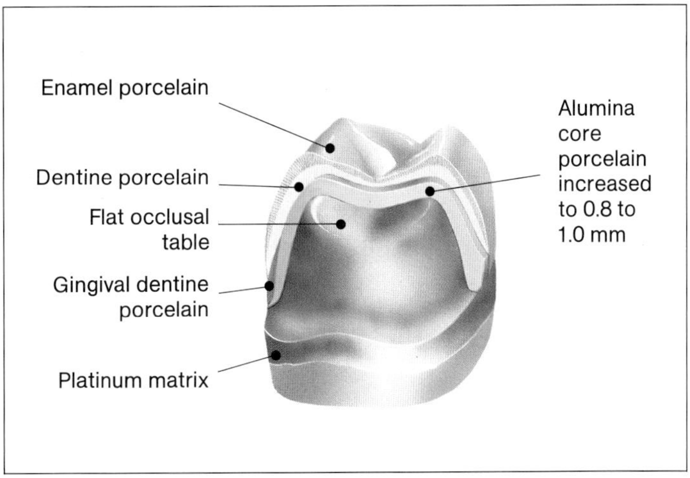

Fig. 6 Design of preparation and aluminous porcelain coping for a molar platinum bonded alumina crown. Occlusal table must be flattened and central fossa reinforced with the maximum section of core porcelain.

Enamel porcelain

Dentine porcelain

Flat occlusal table

Gingival dentine porcelain

Platinum matrix

Alumina core porcelain increased to 0.8 to 1.0 mm

resistance to fracture was improved (Fig. 6). Pre-molar crowns were more successful and, of the eight failures, three of these were due to chipping of marginal ridges. Again this problem could be overcome by designing the core porcelain to reinforce the marginal ridges as in a metal substructure. In general practice the margin of safety for the platinum bonded posterior crown is not great enough to recommend its universal use. The bi-axial flexural strength required is difficult to quantify but if we accept that figures of 140 to 150 MPa are insufficient and that the strength of cast metal-ceramic crowns is now proven to be adequate in most clinical situations, then clearly we need to be close to the range of strengths for high-gold alloys. Yield strengths of around 450 MPa to 550 MPa for the average high-gold ceramic bonding alloy are close to the flexural strengths of high-alumina (ca. 500 MPa). If the inherent brittleness of ceramics is also taken into account and we accept that an average occlusal thickness on a molar crown is 1.0 to 1.5mm, then a pure ceramic coping must possess a flexural strength close to that of high-alumina (Table 6).

Non-Shrink Ceramics

The introduction of the new "Cerastore"* crown is of considerable interest. The Cerastore ceramic is used as the reinforcing core material in a similar way to

* Coors Biomedical, Lakewood, Colorado.

the aluminous porcelain crown. However, unlike aluminous porcelain, the "green" ceramic, on firing, does not shrink. The raw ceramic contains aluminium oxide and magnesium oxide which, on firing, react to form magnesium aluminate spinel ($MgAl_2O_4$). Because magnesium aluminate spinel occupies a greater volume than does the combination of magnesium oxide and aluminium oxide reacting to form the spinel, there is a resultant volume increase sufficient, it is claimed, to compensate for firing shrinkage (*Starling* et al., 1981).

The preferred batch formulation for this shrink-free ceramic is given in Table 8. The calcium stearate and Accrawax are used as a binder and lubricant during the compaction operation. On firing to a temperature of just over 1300° C, the magnesia and some of the alumina combine to form the spinel. The barium glass frit, including silica from the silicone resin, combine to form the glass phase. The crystalline content of the ceramic is claimed to be between 70% and 95% by weight of the body, the remainder being the interstitial glass.

The ceramic coping is made by forming a wax pattern on an epoxy die, coated with a release agent, which is invested in a stone plaster mould. Using the traditional "lost wax" process, the wax is evacuated via a sprue-way and the ceramic mixture transfer moulded at a temperature of 150° C. At this temperature the silicone resin will soften. On cooling, the green ceramic is removed from the investment and die and will have a chalk-like consistency. In this condition the sprue and any flash is removed and the green ceramic

Table 8   Formula for Shrink-free Ceramic

from European Patent Application No. 80304485.8

Riley, E. J. and *Sozio, R. B.* (1980) and *Starling et al.* (1981)

U.S. Pat. No. 4,265,669

Material	Weight grams	Weight (%)
Al_2O_3 (particle size 0.4 to 10 μm average 2.5 μm)	100	43.29
Al_2O_3 (−325 mesh, Tyler)	40	17.32
BaO–SiO_2–Al_2O_3 glass frit (53 % BaO, 42 % SiO_2, 5 % Al_2O_3)	30	12.99
MgO (−200 mesh, Tyler)	20	8.66
Edgar plastic kaolin	9	3.90
Calcium stearate	2	.86
Accrawax C (Steryl amide wax, melting temperature 290° F)	2	.86
Silicone resin (General Electric SR 350 upwards of 60 % by weight SiO)	28	12.12

fired to final density. The recommended firing schedule is as follows:

Room temperature → 500° C
160° C/hour
Hold for 16 hours
500° C → 650° C
150° C/hour
Hold for 8 hours
650° C → 1315° C
420° C/hour
Remove from furnace

The fired ceramic has a density of about 2.80 g/cc, a flexural strength of about 125 MPa, a compressive strength in excess of 450 MPa, and a low coefficient of thermal expansion below 8×10^{-6}° C. The comparatively low flexural strength figures do not allow its use in fixed partial dentures (see Table 5).

The "Cerestore" coping is replaced on the master die and a suitable aluminous veneer porcelain is used to complete the crown shape. At this stage of its development the "Cerastore" crown would appear to be no stronger than aluminous porcelain and for this reason it has yet to be proven as a universal material for crowning all the posterior teeth. However, there must be great potential for a non-shrinking ceramic, since the major problem encountered by all technicians when fabricating dental porcelain is controlling firing shrinkage.

Glass Ceramics

Controlled crystallisation of glass was developed by Stookey at the Corning Glass Works in the United States, and new and unique properties were ob-

29

Table 9 Glass Ceramics

Composition	Catalyst	Use
$Li_2O-Al_2O_3-SiO_2$	Metal, Metal Phosphate or TiO_2	Photosensitive−Low expansion
$MgO-Al_2O_3-SiO_2$	TiO_2 or P_2O_5	Low dielectric loss−high resistivity
$Li_2O-MgO-SiO_2$	Metal phosphate	High thermal expansion
$Li_2O-ZnO-SiO_2$	Metal phosphate or Cu, Au, Ag	High mechanical strength

served in these glass ceramics. Not only was the strength of these materials markedly improved but very high thermal shock resistance was imparted.

Controlled crystallisation of glass depends upon the fact that glass, at ordinary temperatures, is a super-cooled liquid which does not crystallise on cooling from a melt. It can be made to crystallise by heating to a suitable temperature with crystal seed or nuclei present. The glass is then converted to a dense mass of very tiny interlocking crystals. Titanium dioxide is an effective nucleating agent and the starting glass must be homogeneous with qualities like optical glass. Spodumene is a suitable glass, compounded from the oxides of lithium, aluminium and silicon, and has been used extensively to make "Pyroceram" cooking ware. Normally the ware is heated to a temperature where the glass shows the first signs of softening. After myriads of nuclei have been formed in this way, the glass is slowly heated to higher temper-atures where tiny spodumene crystals grow on the nuclei, converting the transparent glass to an opaque white mass composed chiefly of spodumene crystals. Typical compositions for glass ceramics are given in Table 9 where it may be seen that formulations can be produced for various industrial usages.

MacCulloch (1968) reported on experiments with lithia, zinc oxide, silica, in which metal phosphates were used as nucleating agents. The glass was transparent and amber in colour in the glassy state but became translucent and tooth-like after crystallisation or "ceraming" for one hour at 600° C. At this stage, modulus of rupture figures in excess of 124 MPa (18,000 p.s.i.) were obtained, a flexural strength similar to the Coors "Cerastore" ceramic. It will be appreciated that glass ceramics can only be cast in a single colour and as yet no techniques are known for producing layered structures as in a jacket crown or metal-ceramic restoration. In an attempt to solve this problem, *MacCulloch* made the vitreous glass photosensitive by using silver as a nucleating agent. On cooling, the bars responded to ultra-violet light so that by differentially irradiating the surface, the glass, on heating to the ceraming temperature, could be made to crystallise at different rates, thus creating a polychromatic effect. Further characterisation was accomplished by applying printed transfers containing tooth pigments to the surface which on ceraming could produce gingival effects, crack lines, or even facsimile gold fillings.

MacCulloch showed that the glass ceramic could be centrifugally cast when molten, resulting in improved fit of crowns and inlays. The margins of cast glass do not produce the ragged edges of the conventional felspathic porcelains, resulting in very well adapted margins. The strength of the current glass-ceramics is not adequate for the construction of fixed partial dentures and, even assuming translucent materials could be produced with flexural strengths of 300 MPa, it is doubtful whether long span bridges would resist fracture in the connector areas. The most promising use for these materials would be in the construction of artificial posterior teeth or for single crown or inlay construction. Posterior teeth do not demand the high aesthetic standard of the incisor region and a single shade tooth might be acceptable for the public health services in place of the gold alloys. The major problem with all ceramic restorations is that they must be constructed with sufficient cross-section to develop strength. Frequently, even with aluminous porcelain,

the dentist is expecting a 0.5 mm section of ceramic to perform like metal. Such an expectation cannot be fulfilled with current ceramic technology.

Summary

Progress in dental ceramics is limited by the inherent problems of clinical dentistry—space, colour and occlusal forces.

Porcelain veneer crowns have to be accommodated in spaces of 1 to 2 mm and in order to simulate human enamel they must be translucent and of the correct surface texture. Occlusal forces in point contact can be very high and often their direction can produce the most undesirable tensile stresses in a ceramic. Fractures in the central fossae of molars or crescent-shaped fractures in the incisors are but two examples. Unfortunately, the strength of ceramics can never be determined reliably from "average" strengths and we must expect wide variations, particularly in flexural strengths. The margin of safety required in ceramics is, therefore, always greater than other materials such as metals if we accept the variables in dental technology. For this reason, the dental ceramist has a major part to play in optimising both his design of substructures and the subsequent baking of the porcelain. We need very high strengths in ceramics if a clinical safety factor is to be achieved, particularly over long periods where the effect of moisture and static fatigue can play a major part.

Dr. Jones will demonstrate that all dental

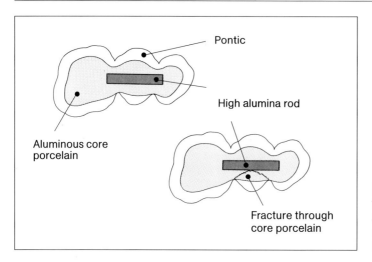

Fig. 7 Diagram showing the potential site of fracture in the occlusal table of an all-porcelain bridge made with alumina reinforced rods.

ceramics tend to fail at the same critical strain, of the order of 0.1%. For this reason any increase in strength and also toughness can only be achieved by an increase in the elastic modulus. At the present time, alumina-reinforced ceramics offer the best possibilities for achieving the above objectives, but due to their low thermal expansion they are incompatible with most metals except platinum. For this reason alumina porcelains can only be used for the construction of individual crowns except where pre-formed high-alumina reinforcement is used. However, bridges made with high-alumina profiles have very limited application since there is no means, as yet, of reinforcing occlusal tables with an alumina ceramic with a flexural strength of 500 MPa, this being the minimal strength required in fixed partial dentures (Fig. 7).

Aluminous porcelain bonded to platinum by the tin-oxide coating process might be extended further if aluminous porcelains with higher strength were produced. This could be achieved by developing very fine-grained alumina porcelains which were pre-sintered or even vacuum hot-pressed prior to supplying them as fine-ground powders to the dental technician. Manufacturers are reluctant to experiment in this area for good commercial reasons. The cast metal-ceramic technique is now well-established and commercial laboratories often do not wish to stock two types of porcelain. In addition, many dentists have lost the facility for preparing accurate shoulder preparations which are demanded by the all-ceramic restoration. The porcelain fused-to-metal crown is therefore firmly entrenched. On the debit side there is little doubt that dentistry has paid a price for this so-called rationalisation. Some laboratories no longer appear capable of making a porcelain jacket crown and have lost their critical appraisal of what an all-porcelain restoration can achieve. *Dr. Southan* will be evaluating the porcelain jacket crown technique later in this symposium and illustrating the importance of high light transmission on aesthetics in dental crown work. The "Metal-Ceramic Smile" is now so prevalent that many students have lost their critical appreciation of what constitutes near-perfection. It is therefore important that research on high strength ceramics continues since our ultimate goal must be to return to the use of ceramic materials which permit the maximum amount of light transmission through the body of the tooth.

These comments should, in no way, detract from the tremendous progress made in the metal-ceramic technique. However, in order to improve this system we must have the aesthetic standard set by the all-porcelain restoration. The aesthetics of porcelain veneer crowns reinforced with metal can only be improved by either making the metal thinner or improving the colour systems in dental porcelain. The base-metal alloys can only be reduced in thickness by a small amount if safety margins are not to be exceeded. However, in the case of individual crowns, the development of thinner copings or swaged metal foil linings must have great potential. The use of low-fusing porcelains (800° C) could open up a new field in the use of modified gold alloys where lower firing temperatures would be of great benefit.

The development of improved colour systems will be reviewed by Dr. *Clarke* and suggestions made for rationalising our present methods of shade matching and colour measurement. Translating this into practice will require the formulation of new porcelain colours. The aesthetics of the metal-ceramic crown can be improved by the use of primary and secondary dentine colours (*McLean, 1977*). Intermediate dentino-enamels may then be used to increase the translucency of facial surfaces. If we consider the present colour systems, most technicians find problems in obtaining depth of enamel translucency without moving to the grey side (low value). This is due to over-translucent enamel porcelains which because of their high light transmission can only be used in thin section. A thicker section enamel would need to be intermediate in colour and translucency between the body or secondary dentine and the enamel; hence the term dentino-enamel. The highly translucent enamels could then be used to build individual characterisation in the approximal and incisal tip of the tooth. The basic colour system illustrated in Figure 8 consists of:–

1. The primary dentine covering the opaque and extending over the gingival area to provide the "neck effect". The primary dentine should be more opaque and higher in chroma than the secondary dentine and acts as a reflective colour base for the whole crown.
2. The secondary or body dentine. This material should be of standard body colours and would be used as an intermediate layer to increase light diffusion and provide the characterisation to the body of the tooth. The secondary dentine should therefore be shaped to give different layering effects for the enamels.

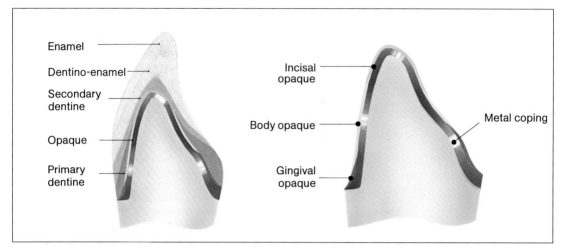

Enamel

Dentino-enamel

Secondary dentine

Opaque

Primary dentine

Incisal opaque

Body opaque

Gingival opaque

Metal coping

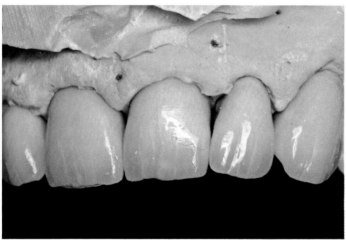

Fig. 8 Diagram illustrating the use of primary and secondary dentine porcelains and the layering of dentino-enamel and translucent enamel porcelains.

Fig. 9a Anterior VMK 68 crowns made using dentino-enamels and the incremental sectional technique for building enamel defects and cracks. (Crowns constructed by *Michael Kedge*.)

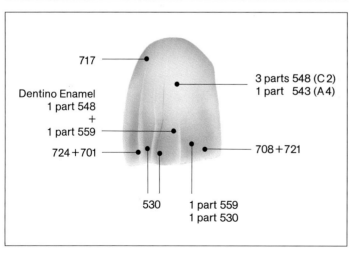

717

Dentino Enamel
1 part 548
+
1 part 559

724 + 701

3 parts 548 (C 2)
1 part 543 (A 4)

708 + 721

530

1 part 559
1 part 530

Fig. 9b Diagram of the colours used to produce the central incisor crown in Figure 9a.

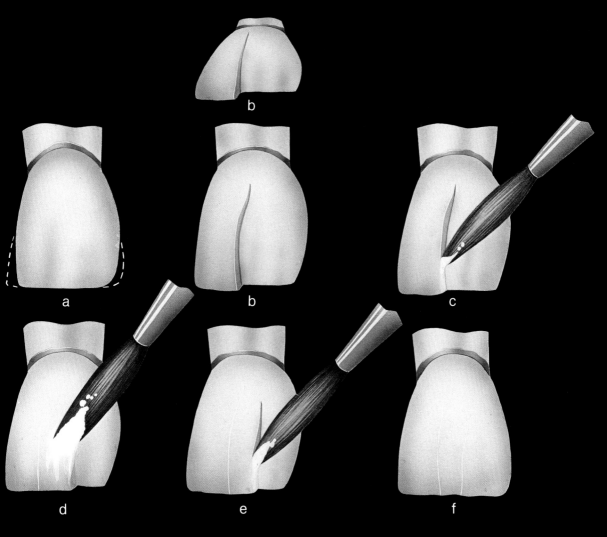

Fig. 9 c   Segmental technique for building enamel crack lines.
a) Dentino-enamel build-up completed just short of full contour.
b) Enamel porcelain applied to mesial incisal edge and an irregular wall created simulating the crack line.
c) Stain painted very lightly down lateral aspect of wall and covered with a further segment of enamel or clear porcelain. Clear porcelain mixed with enamel used segmentally can enhance the three-dimensional effect.
d) Completion of lateral segment of enamel porcelain with a further crack line developed.
e) Stain painted down second lateral wall.
f) Completion of enamel porcelain build-up now produces a three-dimensional effect.

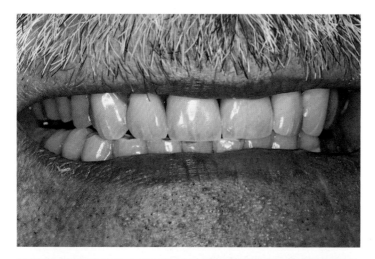

Fig.10a Anterior view of VMK 68 crowns made for 13, 12, 11, 21, 22, 23 using dentino-enamels. Note the low value and absence of high-spots. (Crowns constructed by *Michael Kedge*.)

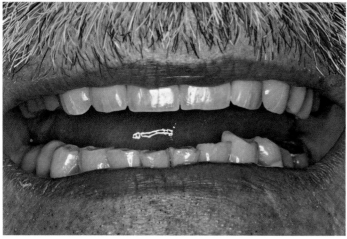

Fig.10b Anterior view of maxillary VMK 68 crowns blending with natural lower incisors. The enamel porcelains using the incremental sectional technique show excellent light break-up.

3. Dentino-enamel. As its name implies, this is a cross between dentine and enamel and is used to give depth of translucency to the facial surface. It can be modified with standard enamels or, as in Figure 8, the highly translucent enamels are used to characterise the incisal edge. Dentino-enamel should be used in thicker section.

4. Enamel. These are the most translucent porcelains and should be used sparingly to provide approximal and incisal effects which are normally present in human teeth.

5. Opalescent Enamel. It is desirable to include two or three enamel porcelains giving an opalescent effect. These enamels should preferably be of different refractive index to the regular enamel. Crowns made using this system are illustrated on the working cast

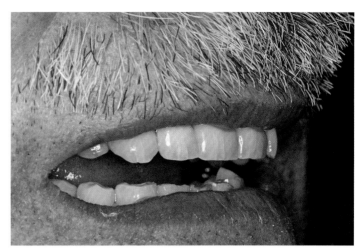

Fig.10c   Right lateral view of the VMK 68 maxillary crowns.

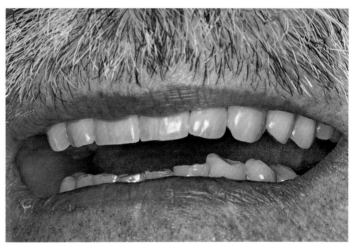

Fig.10d   Left lateral view.

in Figures 9a to c, and after cementation in Figures 10a to d.

Future improvements in the aesthetics of anterior metal-ceramic crowns will depend upon more sophisticated techniques of layering of coloured porcelain and the break-up of enamel porcelain colours using internal staining and enamels of varying degrees of translucency and opalescence. Essentially a light beam entering the facial surface of porcelain must at no time meet a barrier of sudden change in diffuse light transmission (*McLean,* 1977). Even when the light strikes the opaque surface, the latter should be masked with a primary dentine which should act as a diffusion zone or barrier to prevent high reflection off the opaque. Equally a sudden change from the translucent enamel to the body dentine can produce an area of high value or

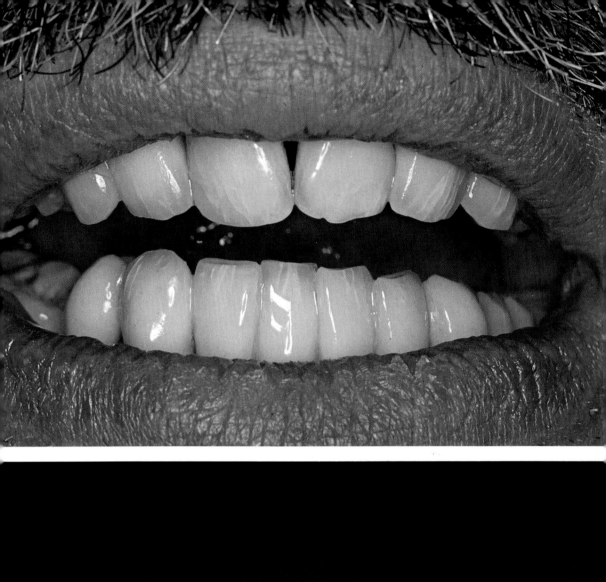
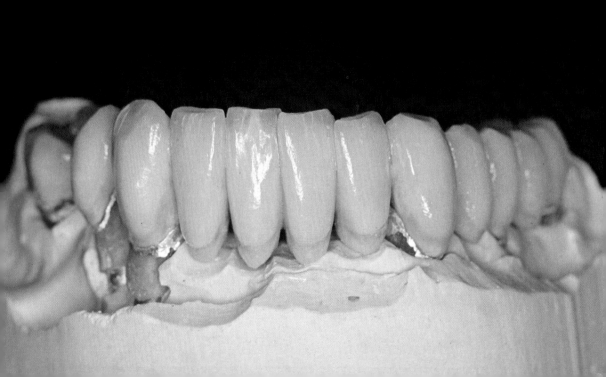

the typical "high spot", hence the use of secondary dentine and dentino-enamel porcelains. Characterisation of the incisal enamel using the incremental sectional technique, illustrated in Figure 9c, will enable the technician to produce teeth that can defy detection from their human counterparts (*Geller,* 1980) as illustrated in Figures 11a and b.

Acknowledgements

I am indebted to *Michael Kedge* for his help and encouragement in producing the section on colour systems in metal-ceramic porcelains: to *Willi Geller* for his original contribution to the development of new systems of building enamel colours in porcelain, and to my daughter, *Diana,* for interpreting our ideas in the colour illustrations and diagrams.

Fig. 11a   Rehabilitation in VMK 68 porcelain using the incremental sectional technique. Patient has congenitally missing maxillary lateral incisors. Canines converted to lateral incisors to match patients natural central incisors, 14 and 24 converted to canine teeth and mandibular bridge inserted to replace lost incisor teeth. Note the reproduction of the enamel defects in the lateral incisors to match the patients maxillary incisors.

Fig. 11b   Mandibular rehabilitation seated on plaster cast with silver dies showing use of dentino-enamels.

References

Bertolotti, R. L. (1981): Thermally assisted deformation in ceramometal systems. I.A.D.R. Program and Abstracts No. 833.

Binns, D. B. (1962): Some physical properties of two-phase crystal-glass solids. I. The Science of Ceramics, Vol. I, pp 315–334. London: Academic Press.

Binns, D. B. (1977): The Physical and Chemical Properties of Dental Porcelain. In: Dental Porcelain: The State of the Art. U. Southern California. Ed. Yamada, H. N. and Grenoble, P. B.

Blodgett, W. E. (1961): High strength alumina porcelains. Amer. Ceram. Soc. Bulletin 40: 74.

Bridger, D. V. and Nicholls, J. I. (1981): Distortion of ceramometal fixed partial dentures during the firing cycle. J. Prosthet. Dent. 45: 507.

Cascone, P. J. (1978): Dental Gold Alloy. U.S. Patent No. 4, 123, 262.

Geller (1980): Private Communication.

Hasselman, D. P. H. and Fulrath, R. M. (1966): Proposed fracture theory of a dispersion-strengthened glass matrix. J. Amer. Ceram. Soc. 49: 68.

Karino, S. (1976): Dental Glaze. Japanese Patent Application No. 53–31716.

MacCulloch, W. T. (1968): Advances in dental ceramics. Brit. dent. J. 125: 361.

Minassian, R. (1978): An investigation into some factors affecting the strength of porcelain jacket crowns. MDS Thesis, University of Bristol.

McLean, J. W. (1965): A higher strength porcelain for crown and bridge work. Brit. Dent. J. 123: 267.

McLean, J. W. and Hughes, T. H. (1965): The reinforcement of dental porcelain with ceramic oxides. Brit. dent. J. 119: 251.

McLean, J. W. (1966): The development of ceramic oxide reinforced dental porcelains with an apprais-al of their physical and clinical properties. MDS Thesis, University of London.

McLean, J. W. (1967): High alumina ceramics for bridge pontic construction. Brit. Dent. J. 123: 571.

McLean, J. W. (1969): Dental Porcelain. N.B.S. Special Publication, Dental Materials Research, Proc. 50th Ann. Symposium, pp. 77–83.

McLean, J. W. and Sced, I. R. (1973): The base-metal alloy/porcelain bond. Trans. Brit. Ceram. Soc. 5: 235.

McLean, J. W. and Sced, I. R. (1976): The Bonded Alumina Crown. I. The bonding of platinum to aluminous dental porcelain using tin-oxide coatings. Austral. Dent. J. 21: 119.

McLean, J. W. (1978): The future of restorative materials. J. Prosthet. Dent. 42: 154.

McLean, J. W. (1980): The Science and Art of Dental Ceramics Vol. II. Chicago: Quintessence Publishing Co.

Moffa, J. P., Lugassy, A. A., Gucker, A. D. and Gettleman, L. (1973): An evaluation of non-precious alloys for use with porcelain veneers. J. Prosthet. Dent. 30: 424.

Rogers, O. W. (1979): The dental application of electroformed pure gold. I. Porcelain jacket crown technique. Austral. Dent. J. 24: 163.

Sced, I. R., McLean, J. W. and Hotz, P. (1977): The strengthening of aluminous porcelain with bonded platinum foils. J. Dent. Res. 36: 1067.

Southan, D. and Jorgensen, K. D. (1972): Faulty porcelain jacket crowns. Austral. Dent. J. 17: 436.

Starling, L. B., Stephan, J. E. and Stroud, R. D. (1981): Shrink-free ceramic and method and raw batch for the manufacture thereof. U.S. Patent No. 4, 265, 669.

The Chemical and Physical Properties of Dental Porcelain

David Binns

Introduction –
The Historical Development of Present-Day Dental Porcelain

The satisfactory replacement of tooth structure lost as a result of caries or accidental damage requires a material with a wide range of specific properties. It should have adequate strength, hardness at least equal to that of dental enamel, and should be readily formable into the required shapes; it should be biocompatible, resistant to the oral environment and capable of supplying the range of colour and translucency required to simulate natural dentition. If these requirements were put as a problem to a materials scientist he would have to say that of available materials only a ceramic could fulfil all the conditions. However, the use of dental porcelain as a prosthetic material was not introduced by such a process of analysis, and the compositions of present-day porcelains have been arrived at by a long process of development from available materials.

The first use of porcelain by Chemant at the end of the 18th century to form "incorruptible teeth of mineral paste" was dictated by the need for biological and chemical inertness. The material used for such early tooth replacements was the basic triaxial porcelain, the constituents of which were kaolinite ($Al_2O_3.SiO_2.2H_2O$), potash feldspar ($K_2O.Al_2O_3.6SiO_2$) and quartz (SiO_2), giving a composition in the mullite field of the $K_2O-Al_2O_3-SiO_2$ phase diagram. After firing, such a composition contains mullite and residual quartz, the refractive indices of which are substantially above that of the feldspathic glass matrix. As a result of these differences in refractive index, as well as residual porosity, the level of attainable translucency is small compared with that of dentine and enamel. Hence, although it was found that the colour of natural teeth could be matched by adding stains to porcelain, satisfactory simulation was not possible. The translucency required was attained by the virtual elimination of clay, thus removing the composition from the mullite field, and reducing the quartz content. These changes resulted in the high-firing dental porcelain which is still used in the manufacture of denture teeth,

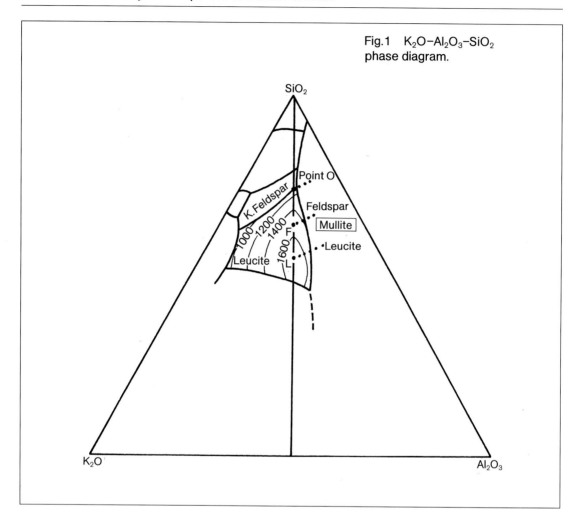

Fig.1 $K_2O-Al_2O_3-SiO_2$ phase diagram.

the compositional range of which is (*Claus,* 1980):

Potash feldspar	70–80%
Quartz	10–30
Kaolin	0– 3

It can be seen from the $K_2O-Al_2O_3-SiO_2$ phase diagram shown in Figure 1 that feldspar lies in the primary phase field of leucite ($K_2O.Al_2O_3.4SiO_2$). It melts incon-

gruently, i.e. when it is heated to 1150°C a melt of composition indicated by point 0 on the diagram is formed, together with crystalline leucite. As the temperature increases leucite dissolves in the melt, the composition of which moves along the line OF, until at 1530°C the feldspar is completely molten. It will be seen also that with quartz solution in molten feldspar its liquidus temperature falls, to reach 1300°C with 20% quartz. When porcelain powders were made from such compositions it was the common practice to prefrit the constituents to facilitate reaction and reduce the content of residual free quartz which has a deleterious effect on strength, thermal shock resistance and translucency. From the phase diagram it might be expected that on cooling a feldspar melt, leucite would crystallize out. However, commercial potash feldspars contain appreciable proportions of albite ($Na_2O.Al_2O_3.6SiO_2$) and free quartz, so that their K_2O contents are well below the theoretical proportion of 16.9%; *Hermansson* and *Carlsson* (1978) showed that alumino-silicate glasses containing up to 12% K_2O could not be crystallized by prolonged heating, even in the presence of TiO_2 as nucleating agent. Prefritted feldspar-based dental porcelains are, therefore, substantially glassy and their designation as porcelain is somewhat of a misnomer. Alkali feldspar melts have high viscosities; viscosity measurements have shown also that in alkali silicate and alkali alumino-silicate melts the rate of change of viscosity with temperature is low. This feature is of importance in conferring favourable firing properties. However the firing temperature of such feldspathic porcelain powders is about 1250°C, and progressive compositional changes have been made to bring firing temperatures down to 1100°C, 1000°C, then to the current level of 900–980°C. Consideration of the $K_2O-Al_2O_3-SiO_2$ phase diagram indicates that the liquidus temperature of compositions along the feldspar–quartz join will be lowered by decreasing the Al_2O_3 content. Melting temperatures can

also be lowered by increasing the Na_2O content and introducing bivalent glass modifiers such as the alkaline earth oxides and ZnO; the choice of fluxing oxides is to some extent limited by considerations of toxicity. The glass-forming oxide B_2O_3 also has a pronounced effect on the softening point of silicate glasses. Progressive changes on the lines suggested have been used to reduce the firing temperature of dental porcelain powders; typical compositions of materials firing at different temperatures are shown in Table 1.

Table 1 Typical Chemical Compositions (%) of Jacket-Crown Porcelains

	Firing Temperature (°C)		
	1250/ 1300	1060/ 1100	900/ 980
SiO_2	70.6	63.7	67.3
Al_2O_3	17.2	19.5	10.8
CaO			2.2
Na_2O	2.8	2.2	4.6
K_2O	9.4	8.2	7.9
B_2O_3		6.0	6.8

Dental porcelains within the composition range of Table 1 have been used since the 1880s in the construction of jacket-crown restorations. During the early 20th century attempts were made to extend the range of application by

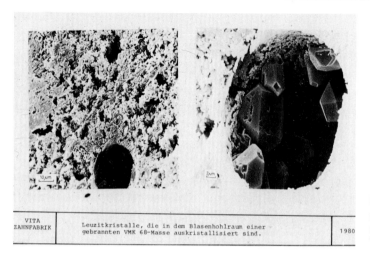

| VITA ZAHNFABRIK | Leuzitkristalle, die in dem Blasenhohlraum einer gebrannten VMK 68-Masse auskristallisiert sind. | 1980 |

Fig. 2 Scanning electron micrographs showing leucite crystals in dental porcelain (by courtesy of Vita Zahnfabrik).

using metal reinforcement of porcelain. These efforts, however, met with little success because of lack of thermal expansion compatibility between metal and porcelain. Current low-firing jacket-crown porcelains have thermal expansion coefficients in the range $5.5–7.5.10^{-6}/°C$, which would indicate compatibility with Pt and Pt-Ir alloys. However, the casting alloys which could be used in dental restorations, such as the Au–Ag–Pd system and the base-metal Ni–Cr alloys, all have thermal expansion coefficients in the range $13.5–15.5.10^{-6}/°C$. To reach such a range in a purely glassy system, whilst maintaining other desirable properties, would be very unlikely. However, in 1962, *Weinstein* et al (1962) described the production of porcelain-metal restorations on dental alloy frameworks using porcelain powders containing 11–15% K_2O; thermal expansion was controlled by mixing feldspar-based compositions and high-K_2O frits. Work carried out at the Osaka Munic-

ipal Technical Research Institute and described by *Hoshikawa* and *Akagi* (1972) showed that such thermal expansions resulted from the crystallization of leucite, the thermal expansion coefficient of which is of the order of 27.10^{-6}. Glasses in the $Na_2O–K_2O–Al_2O_3–SiO_2$ system containing 8–17% K_2O were subjected to heat treatments at temperatures from 700–1200°C. It was found that leucite crystallized out in glasses containing not less than 11% K_2O, and the results showed that 15–25% leucite was needed to increase the base glass thermal expansion coefficient from $10.7.10^{-6}$ to the $13–15.10^{-6}$ range required for porcelain-metal bonding; for a base glass of dental porcelain composition the proportion would probably be about 35–45%. The proportion of leucite is governed by the K_2O content and the temperature and time of heat treatment. The basic change required to produce a porcelain of the thermal expansion necessary for metal bonding is to increase the K_2O content to the required level; an average composition is given below:

SiO_2	63.2%
Al_2O_3	17.5
CaO	0.8
Na_2O	5.7
K_2O	11.7
B_2O_3	1.0

It is necessary, of course, to ensure that the porcelain spends sufficient time in the crystallization range to develop the required leucite content. Figure 2 shows scanning electron micrographs of a section of a metal-bonding dental porcelain. Groups of 2–3 µm leucite crystals can be seen in the porcelain surface and, in a cavity, crystals that have grown to 8–12 µm. Excessive crystal growth could have a harmful effect on both strength and thermal expansion. Large thermal mismatch in such crystal-glass composites gives rise to stresses in both phases. When the inclusions exceed a critical size, cracks are formed, generally in the glassy matrix, which act as stress raisers and reduce strength; the resultant reduction of coupling between the phases will also lower thermal expansion. The tendency towards crystal growth does not seem to be excessive in normal metal-bonding porcelains, but the production of fine crystals, and rapid crystallization, could be facilitated by adding small amounts of suitable nucleating agents. Comparison of jacket-crown and metal-bonding porcelain enamels shows that the leucite crystals in the latter have a negligible effect on translucency. The scattering of light by inclusions in a trans-

parent matrix depends upon the difference in refractive index between the phases; Figure 3 shows an experimental curve of translucency against R.I. difference for composites of a crystal phase with different glasses. The R.I. of leucite is 1.508–1.509 and that of the porcelain matrix ~1.495. The difference in R.I.'s is therefore less than 1% of that of the matrix so that the crystal inclusions are unlikely to have any appreciable effect on the light transmission of the porcelain. It is an interesting observation that the development of a satisfactory metal-bonding porcelain was made possible by the presence in the $K_2O–Al_2O_3–SiO_2$ field of an unusually high thermal expansion phase of suitable R.I.

Apart from the reduction in firing temperature and the introduction of porcelains for bonding to metals the most significant recent advance in dental porcelain has been the development of higher strength aluminous porcelain (*McLean* and *Hughes*, 1965). It had been known for some time that a glassy matrix could be strengthened by the incorporation in it of a high elasticity, high strength, crystalline phase (*Binns*, 1962). Consideration of possible materials indicated the suitability of alumina for the purpose because of its availability, high elasticity and strength, and compatibility in terms of thermal expansion and colour. It was found possible to incorporate 40–50% Al_2O_3 in core porcelain, the proportion in dentine and enamel being limited by the effect on translucency. To obtain the full reinforcing effect, the Al_2O_3 must be effectively wetted by the glassy matrix and it is essential, therefore, to incorpo-

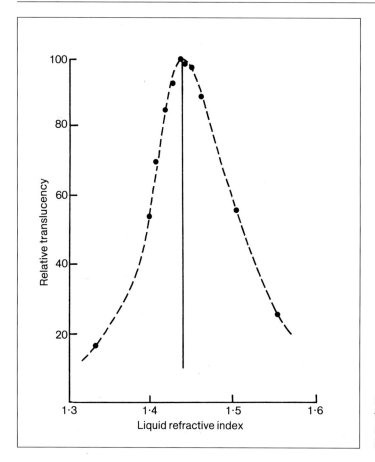

Fig.3 Variation of translucency for a crystalline phase immersed in liquids of different refractive indices.

rate it at high temperature. The increase in strength found with the incorporation of Al_2O_3 depends on effective firing and also on the method of measurement, but the reported increases range from 50–100%.

It is unlikely that the development of dental porcelain has ceased with the compositions shown in Table 1. Consideration of phase diagrams, and the effects of various ions on glass melting temperatures and viscosities, indicates ways in which firing temperatures can be lowered. It is not surprising, therefore, that the development of more fusible compositions is being actively pursued. However, desirable properties such as adequate firing range and resistance to chemical attack must be maintained, and it is likely that there is a correlation between melting temperature and chemical solubility; progress in reducing firing temperature will then have to be balanced against increasing solubility. Although there is no doubt that current dental porcelains are very stable in the mouth there is no information on which a limit of solubility could be based.

The Production of Dental Porcelain Powders

The original source of dental porcelain was potash feldspar, which still forms a major constituent of modern materials. The use, as raw material, of a natural mineral led to a search for feldspars containing minimum proportions of impurity oxides, notably Fe_2O_3 and TiO_2, which form colour centres in the fused materials. Hand-sorting and beneficiation procedures such as froth flotation may also be used. Table 2 gives analyses of some suitable feldspars.

It might be thought that high translucency and neutral colour could be obtained repeatably by the use of pure chemicals as raw materials. However, it is found that the mixing of a major part of the porcelain composition on an atomic scale provided by the use of feldspar has considerable advantage in lowering the fusion temperature and increasing homogeneity.

In the production of ceramic glazes and enamels the normal practice is to frit some or all of the constituents, which involves melting and quenching the resultant glasses; this process facilitates the subsequent grinding to produce powders. Because of the high viscosity of dental porcelain, very high temperatures would be needed to produce pourable glasses, so that the normal procedure is to melt in a container coated with a wash of refractory powder and remove the

Table 2 Chemical Compositions (%) of High-Purity Potash Feldspars

Source	Idaho	Sweden	Morocco	Morocco	Portugal
SiO_2	65.1	69.2	64.5	64.4	64.3
TiO_2	<0.01	<0.01	<0.01	<0.01	<0.01
Al_2O_3	18.8	16.7	18.9	18.7	19.2
Fe_2O_3	<0.01	0.06	<0.01	<0.01	0.03
CaO	0.05	0.10	0.05	0.02	0.05
MgO	<0.02	<0.02	<0.02	<0.02	<0.02
Na_2O	3.46	2.73	1.91	1.45	2.99
K_2O	11.8	10.9	13.7	14.4	12.5
P_2O_5	0.19		0.38	0.37	0.37
Loss	0.17	0.21	0.37	0.28	

melt after cooling. It is a common practice to produce glasses of different softening points which are mixed to provide the final porcelain powder. The chief purpose of this is to lengthen the softening range but it is also thought to make the porcelain less glassy in appearance and to improve thermal shock resistance. Throughout the production process great care is necessary to avoid contamination, which may have a disastrous effect on colour. The most critical stage is that of milling; since abrasion cannot be entirely prevented, grinding media and the linings of cylinder and pan mills must be chosen to have the minimum effect on colour.

The development discussed in the previous section was concerned with the production of base porcelain compositions, i.e. translucent glasses with nearly neutral colour. These, however, need considerable modification before they can be used in the building up of restorations; a range of different shades must be produced, and light transmission from the high opacity of metal bonding opaques to the high translucency of incisal porcelains. The light scattering or opacifying effect of an inclusion in a glass depends on its particle size and refractive index, the nearer the particle size to the wavelength of light and the greater the difference in refractive index between glass and inclusion the greater the opacity. Crystal phases of the tetravalent metal oxides TiO_2, SnO_2, ZrO_2, CeO_2, together with Zircon ($ZrO_2.SiO_2$) have particularly high refractive indices and are used in total amounts up to 8–10% in metal-bonding opaques. To produce a range of shades, ceramic and glass stains such as: chrome-tin, chrome-alumina, manganese-alumina (pink); praseodymium-zircon, vanadium-zirconia (yellow); cobalt aluminate, cobalt silicate (blue) can be used. To produce grey shades, absorption bands in different parts of the spectrum are needed. For this purpose several different stains may be used, or a more complex stain such as cobalt and nickel in zircon or tin oxide; the antimony-tin oxide complex may also be used to give a grey colour. Additions must also be made to simulate the fluorescence of natural teeth, which will, however, be considered later in discussing the aesthetic properties of dental porcelain. These opacifying and colouring oxides have high densities and if they are to perform their function they must be present as fine particles. These two properties will cause segregation if the oxides are merely mixed with base porcelain powders; they are, therefore, normally fritted into base porcelain to produce highly coloured component powders.

Condensation and Firing of Dental Porcelain

The first stage of forming a porcelain restoration is the mixing of powder with sufficient liquid to form a paste of creamy consistency, when the proportion of liquid is sufficient to fill the voids between particles and provide a film between them; the excess of liquid allows relative movement of particles and deformation of the powder-liquid mass. In this state the suspension can be applied to the platinum matrix or metal coping before the process of removing excess liquid by brush or tissue begins. As this happens the individual particles move closer together under the action of the surface tension of the liquid. At this stage some vibration is necessary to reorient and displace particles to reach the maximum packing. Although in the past the most common liquid used has been distilled water, so-called modelling fluids are increasingly used, particularly in the porcelain-metal technique, where thin even layers of opaque are necessary for effective masking of metal copings. The chief functions of these liquids are:

1. To encourage the relative movement of the porcelain grains and to facilitate the application of thin layers.
2. To increase the cohesion of damp or dry porcelain layers.

Such liquids are water-based and common constituents are long-chain secondary alcohols, the binding effect of which will increase with molecular weight. The objective of porcelain condensation is to approach as nearly as possible to the maximum density for the powder used, which depends on its particle shape and size distribution. For uniform spheres it has been found experimentally that the maximum packing is 60–64% of the solid density (*McGeary,* 1961) and *Budworth* (1969) has provided a theoretical basis for a maximum random close-packing density of 61%. The efficiency of packing is reduced for particles of irregular shape, particularly with fine particles, but packing densities can be increased by mixing particles of different sizes. If gap grading of spherical particles is used, in which successively finer fractions of monodisperse particles are added, it is possible to obtain powder beds of over 90% theoretical density for ternary mixes (*McGeary*). However, such densities can only be achieved by dry vibration compaction at specific frequencies, the fractions being added in sequence; the mixed powders, if disturbed, would be liable to segregation and the behaviour in suspension in a fluid would not allow the building-up process used in the preparation of a dental restoration. Dental porcelain powder gradings are continuous, and modern vacuum-firing powders cover a particle size range from 2–75 µm diameter, with median diameters from 20–30 µm. When condensed by a process of vibration and excess-fluid removal such powders exhibit linear shrinkages of 11–15% and volume shrinkages of 30–38%. Air firing necessitates the use of powders with substantially smaller proportions of the finer fractions, as can be seen from the particle size distributions shown in Figure 4. The air-firing porcelain grading produces a more open large-pored powder bed which facilitates the escape of air before the structure becomes sealed; it will, however, have higher shrinkage. If fired in air the vacuum-firing grading would give a larger proportion of the fine bubbles which have a pronounced effect on translucency. A recent development in metal-bonding porcelains has been the introduction of paint-on opaques to facilitate the appli-

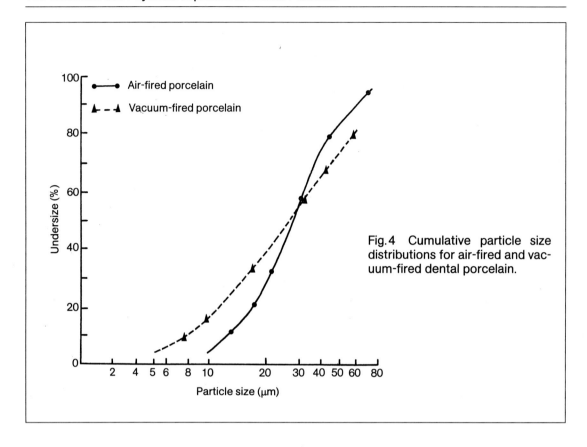

Fig. 4 Cumulative particle size distributions for air-fired and vacuum-fired dental porcelain.

cation of thin even layers. The particle size distribution of one such material is compared with that of the corresponding normal opaque in Figure 5, which shows differential curves of weight frequency against particle size. It will be seen that the size distribution of the paint-on material has been made bimodal by the addition of ~5% of ultra-fine (<1 μm) powder. Such an addition results in a marked reduction in shrinkage.

It has been seen that modern dental porcelains are substantially glassy, since even in metal-bonding porcelains the crystalline leucite is completely immersed in a glassy matrix. In the sintering of glass powder compacts it has been found that densification occurs by viscous flow, the driving force being the surface tension of the glass (*Frenkel*, 1945). If contraction is taken as an index of sintering it is found that for glass powder compacts:

$$\frac{d}{dt} \cdot \frac{\Delta L}{L_o} = \frac{\gamma}{2r\eta} \quad\text{—— (1) (\textit{Cutler}, 1969)}$$

where

$\dfrac{\Delta L}{L_o}$ is the fractional shrinkage

t is the time

γ is the surface tension

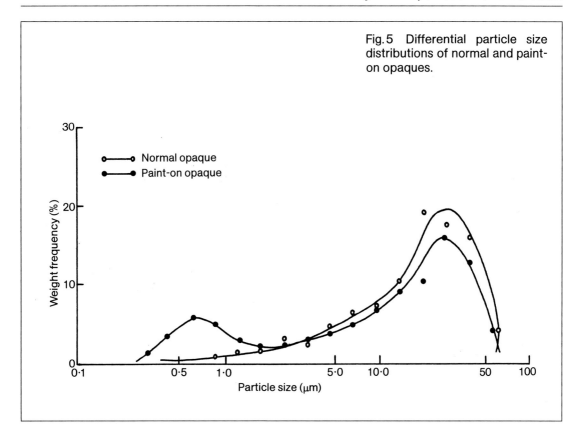

Fig. 5 Differential particle size distributions of normal and paint-on opaques.

η is the viscosity
r is the particle radius

i.e. the rate of sintering is proportional to the surface tension and inversely proportional to the viscosity and particle size. In the viscous sintering process, two well-defined stages can be distinguished. In the first, lenses are formed at points of contact between grains and increase in size by bulk viscous flow as the particles approach more closely. At some stage the continuous pore structure becomes sealed off into a number of pore spaces which rapidly become spherical voids under the influence of surface tension.

The *Frenkel* theory of viscous sintering was initially developed from a contacting-sphere model and it was expected that the equation developed would only be valid over a limited contraction range; shrinkage isotherms for crystalline systems are seldom linear for more than the first 3–4% linear shrinkage. However, experiment has shown that for glasses the contraction rate is constant up to quite large contractions. According to *Frenkel* a spherical cavity of radius r is subject to a pressure deficiency of $\frac{\gamma}{r}$, which will cause viscous flow of the surrounding material and tend to reduce the pore size; *Kuczynski* and *Zaplatynski* (1956) have shown that when glass capillaries are heated the inner radius (r) tends to close at a uniform rate by viscous flow:

$$r_0 - r = \frac{\gamma t}{2\eta} \quad \text{(2)}$$

Equations (1) and (2) show that throughout the sintering process the rate of densification is dependent on the surface tension and viscosity of the glass and, in the early stages, on the powder particle size. The surface tension of glass is relatively insensitive to composition and temperature, and observed values cover a relatively narrow range. Sintering is, therefore, primarily governed by viscosity, which is very dependent on glass composition and changes rapidly with temperature. The wider size gradings of recent dental porcelains, apart from improving packing and reducing shrinkage will have had some effect on sintering rates. The particle shape of powders, which is affected by the mode of crushing, has been shown by *Cutler* and *Henrichsen* (1968) to have a marked effect on sintering, angular particles densifying more rapidly than round ones because of the effect of the smaller radii of curvature of grains at the point of contact.

If sintering takes place at atmospheric pressure spherical voids will contract until the increased gas pressure balances the external pressure due to surface tension, when the rate of densification will become very slow. Under such conditions voids in crystalline solids continue to shrink by the diffusion of vacancies; grain boundaries, which are absent in glasses, acting as vacancy sinks. However *Vines* et al (1958) showed that pores in dental porcelain can be virtually eliminated by firing in vacuum or in a diffusible atmosphere, such as helium, hydrogen or water vapour, and low gas pressures have been used in the firing of dental porcelain since the 1940s. The use of vacuum in sintering is only of advantage until the pore structure becomes sealed. After that stage the optimum firing treatment would involve the application of atmospheric or higher pressure. When pressure has been used in the later stages of firing and cooling, care has to be taken to avoid subsequent heating at low pressure, which might cause the expansion of residual pores.

The introduction of vacuum firing had a substantial effect on the properties of dental porcelain in two respects. The immediate effect was to make possible the attainment of higher translucency and necessitate changes in opacifier content. Indirectly, also, it made possible the addition of finer fractions to powder gradings with consequent improved packing, lower shrinkage and improved working properties. It might be expected that vacuum firing would also increase strength, but the evidence is not conclusive that static strength is increased by the elimination of residual spherical pores. However *Kulp* et al (1961) gave evidence of increased impact strength and lower service breakages with vacuum firing.

The softening, or decrease in viscosity, responsible for the sintering of glass powders can also have undesirable effects such as the bulk deformation

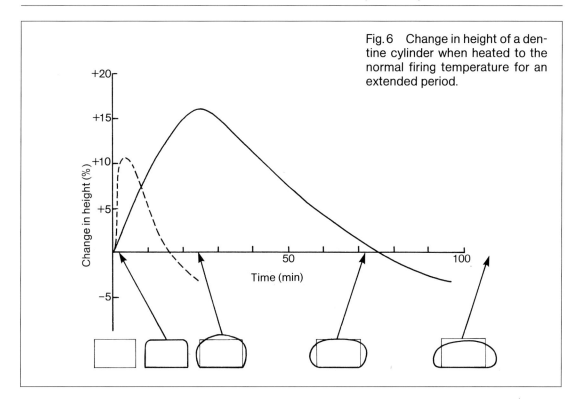

Fig. 6   Change in height of a dentine cylinder when heated to the normal firing temperature for an extended period.

responsible for changes in geometry of the sintered solid. A dental restoration at its maximum firing temperature could deform under various forces such as the intrinsic force of surface tension and external forces, such as gravity or mechanical loading due to framework distortion or thermal stresses. There is no doubt that in a specimen of the dimensions of a restoration the most important of these effects is surface tension, so that loss of detail and rounding of edges will be observed before slumping and dimensional changes resulting from it. The rate at which detail is lost will be a function of

$\dfrac{\gamma}{\eta\rho}$ where γ is the surface tension, η the

viscosity and ρ the radius of curvature of the surface detail. Comparison with the relationships governing viscous sintering shows that the processes are essentially similar and might be difficult to separate. However, two factors allow the production of dense restorations with satisfactory surface detail and maintainance of shape:

1. The radii of contacts between particles and of residual pores (r) are considerably less than those of surface details (ρ) so that densification can proceed at higher values of η than bulk deformation.

2. The rate of change of η with temperature is low for the alkali alumino-silicate

53

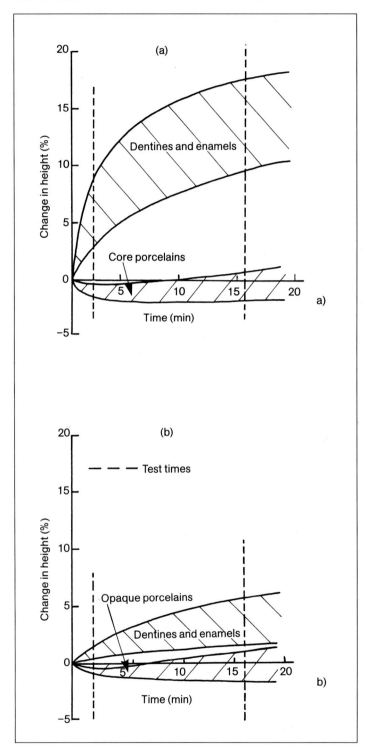

Fig. 7 Pyroplastic flow measurements on (a) jacket-crown porcelains, (b) metal-bonding porcelains.

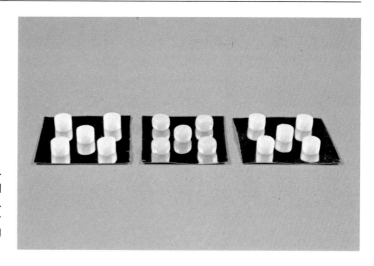

Fig. 8 Pyroplastic flow specimens after heating to the normal
firing temperatures for 16 minutes.
Metal-bonding porcelain – jacket-
crown porcelain – metal-bonding
porcelain.

glasses which constitute dental porcelains, so that appreciable overfiring
may be necessary for bulk deformation. Very accurate firing would be
needed to separate the processes for
glasses containing less Al_2O_3 and
greater proportions of multivalent
glass modifiers.

The effect of overfiring a porcelain restoration, therefore, is a change of contour
due to surface tension, the end-point of
which is the state of minimum surface
energy, termed a sessile drop. This process has been simulated by a test for
pyroplastic flow which is based on measuring the change in height of a porcelain
cylinder on refiring to the normal firing
temperature for an extended period
(Binns, 1977). Figure 6 shows the changes
which take place during the reheating of a
typical specimen of jacket-crown dentine or enamel, and Figures 7a and b show
the deformations found in jacket-crown
and metal-bonding porcelains. Measure-

ments are normally made after firing for
2 min. and 16 min. Jacket-crown core
porcelains are much more resistant to
pyroplastic flow than dentines and enamels, as might be expected from their
content of crystalline alumina. It will be
observed also that metal-bonding dentines and enamels are more resistant
than corresponding jacket-crown porcelains; the appearance of pyroplastic flow
specimens of the two different types of
porcelain can be seen in Figure 8. The
most likely reason for the greater resistance to deformation of the metal-bonding porcelains is the presence in them of
$\sim 40\%$ of small leucite crystals. This
conclusion is confirmed by the work of
Hahn and Teuchert (1980) which showed
that the dilatometric softening point of a
$K_2O–Al_2O_3–SiO_2$ glass increased with
increasing leucite content. As with
jacket-crown core porcelains, metal-
bonding opaques exhibit less pyroplastic
flow than the corresponding dentines
and enamels. This again is probably due

55

to the added crystalline material; although present in proportions less than 10%, the added opacifiers are much finer than the alumina powders added to jacket-crown core porcelains.

Mechanical Properties of Dental Porcelain

As in all systems involving brittle materials, when considering the strength in service of porcelain restorations it is impossible to ignore the effect of design and preparation. A number of photoelastic investigations have been made to illustrate the stress-raising effect of different design factors (*Walton* and *Leven,* 1955), (*Pettrow,* 1961), (*Lehman* and *Hampson,* 1962), (*El-Ebrashi* et al, 1969). Among the more important design considerations are the height of the preparation, the shoulder geometry, sharp line angles, and adequate support. In porcelain-metal restorations stresses due to thermal mismatch between metal and porcelain must also be taken into account.

The thermal matching of metal and porcelain will be considered in some detail later, but it may be said here that *Smyth* (1977) has calculated, on available information, the stresses set up in porcelain layers on metal rods and hollow cylinders for various thermal expansion differences. The results show that stresses comparable with the tensile strength of porcelain can be set up for differences in thermal expansion which might not be considered excessive.

However, to consider the strength of porcelain in isolation, in brittle materials the practical stress level is generally several orders of magnitude less than the theoretical limit provided by the lattice cohesion. Fracture theory, the foundations of which were laid by *Griffith* (1920) and *Inglis* (1913), is based on the concept that stress concentrations are formed around small flaws. In ductile materials sufficient slip systems are present to allow of plastic deformation, and the stress concentrations can be relieved. In most ceramics at low temperature, on the other hand, this is not possible and a relatively small applied stress may be sufficient to initiate crack propagation and cause failure. In crystalline ceramics there are a number of reasons for the formation of flaws within the solid volume. In glasses, on the other hand, which have been melted and fabricated at high temperatures, stress-raising flaws are generally present only on the surface. The chief causes of such flaws are abrasion, corrosion (especially by water vapour) and surface devitrification. Considerable increases in glass strength can be brought about by treatments which produce compressive stresses in the surface layers and neutralize the effects of surface flaws; in crystalline ceramics, on the other hand, the strength increases resulting from such treatments are limited by the internal flaw population to perhaps 50% of the original strength. Dental porcelain is basically glassy in structure, so that the most important flaws are probably in the surface, and due to the causes enumerated earlier. It can therefore be strengthened by the methods applied to glass but to a lesser extent; the application of such techniques will be described in detail elsewhere in this publication. It might be expected that, as with glass, the strength of dental porcelain would be affected by the presence of water, and it has been shown by Southan and Jorgensen (1974) that there is some strength loss by fatigue in the oral environment.

Unlike glass, dental porcelain is fabricated by powder sintering, which can give rise to a volume distribution of flaws such as voids and cracks. Vacuum firing has reduced the effect of voids, and the stress-raising effect of the residual small spherical pores is slight; care must be exercised, however, to avoid causing the expansion of small pores near the surface which can occur during refiring in vacuum. The consolidation of a powder bed against a non-contracting solid surface, particularly a metal surface which may be imperfectly wetted, can give rise to stress-raising voids. Southan and Jorgenson (1972, 1973) observed large irregular voids at the internal surfaces of crowns built up on platinum foil, which they attributed to sporadic, or irregular, condensation and the high contact angle of porcelain on the metal. When a porcelain layer is sintered against a metal surface, the shrinkage of the porcelain next to the metal is restrained but the outer surface is free to contract. This phenomenon is responsible for the cracks frequently observed in core and opaque porcelains, which generally extend only part way through the porcelain layers.

These cracks are filled in and sealed by fusion in subsequent firings, but may leave vestigial cracks or areas of weakness. Another potential source of weakness is the formation of cracks by thermal shock. Although the dimensions of restorations are small, the rates of heating and cooling in dental furnaces are high, and the effects of such temperature changes are accentuated by variations in porcelain cross-section. A test for thermal shock resistance has been devised by Anusavice et al (1981) based on the quenching of porcelain-metal crowns constructed to a standard design. If cracking occurs when the whole restoration is rigid the crack will close up when cold, and be very difficult to see without special crack-detection procedures (Saklad, 1958). Such cracks are likely to propagate in the mouth due to the applied stresses and the effect of corrosion at the crack tip.

The most generally satisfactory method of measuring the strength of a brittle material is by flexure of a rod or bar, which has been the most commonly used method for dental porcelain. Other methods such as the indirect tensile test on a disc specimen (Brown and Sorensen, 1979) or the biaxial flexure measurement, also on a disc specimen (McLean and Hughes, 1965), have been used. Whatever type of specimen is used, it is desirable that the cross-sectional dimensions should be comparable in size with those of porcelain restorations and that the surface textures should be similar. Specimens should, therefore, be subjected to the normal range of firings, finishing with the appropriate glaze firing. During

Table 3   Flexural Strength (MPa) of Dental Porcelains

Jacket-crown Porcelains		Metal-bonding Porcelains	
Aluminous core porcelains	90–120	Opaque porcelains	75–95
Dentine porcelains	60– 90	Dentine porcelains	50–65
Enamel porcelains	60– 80	Enamel porcelains	50–65

this process, however, specimen geometry may become modified by warping, and unwanted stresses set up during testing. As *Wilson* and *Whitehead* (1967) remarked: "Difficulty of fabrication and the complex nature of the fusion process make it extremely difficult, if not impossible, to produce test specimens which are both glazed and consistent in shape and size". A solution to the problem is to surface grind specimens, followed by a glaze firing in air to eliminate flaws and provide surfaces similar to those of restorations. When tested in this way, a number of jacket-crown and metal-bonding porcelains were found to have flexural strengths within the ranges given in Table 3. The mean coefficient of variation for these measurements was 9.2%, a value comparing favourably with the results quoted by *Jones* (1971).

It will be seen that metal-bonding dentines and enamels were found to be slightly weaker than the corresponding jacket-crown materials. As might be expected, the aluminous core porcelains were found to be stronger than jacket-crown dentines and enamels. When fired at the manufacturers' recommended schedules the margin was not as large as had been expected, but as reported by *Jones* (1970) it was found that the strengths of some aluminous core materials could be increased considerably by firing to higher temperatures for longer times. It is perhaps more surprising that metal-bonding opaques were also found to be markedly stronger than the corresponding dentines and enamels, the average increase being ~35%. It might be expected that the addition of fine opacifiers would have some effect on strength, but only a minor one, considering the small proportions added.

Aesthetic Properties of Dental Porcelain – Colour and Translucency

The way in which the visual effect of natural dentition arises is a complex phenomenon, and will only be discussed here as far as is necessary to identify the optical properties of the different types of porcelain needed to produce an acceptable match to the natural tooth. The light incident on the surface of the tooth is partly reflected specularly and partly transmitted into the tooth, where it is again partly absorbed and partly scattered, a proportion being eventually re-emitted from the surface of the tooth. The optical properties of the tooth are not uniform, the outer regions being made up of two main components which vary continuously in thickness over the whole tooth, and have the major effect in producing the complex variation of colour and translucency observed. The two components are the partly translucent dentine which is orange-yellow in colour, and the enamel, which is highly translucent and more neutral in colour. The area providing the dominant colour impression is the middle third of the tooth where the light from a large area and depth of dentine is modified by passing through the outer layer of enamel, which reduce the saturation of the colour. In the incisal third the thickness of dentine decreases as the incisal edge is approached so that the colour becomes rapidly more neutral and the tooth more translucent, particularly close to the incisal edge. In the cervical third the enamel thins progressively to a feather edge so that the tooth colour becomes more orange or even brown, being affected also by pink light from the gum. The envelope of enamel around the tooth increases the translucency in the proximal areas, softening the outline of the tooth. The nature of the tooth surface also contributes to the visual effect, having high gloss on a small scale, but on a large scale an irregular undulating surface traversed by fine grooves, resulting in irregular highlight areas of specular reflection. The individual appearance of teeth is also contributed to by surface defects such as cracks and check lines, areas of staining and calcification faults. To simulate all these visual features of natural teeth a wide range of porcelains is required, comprising perhaps 40–50 different materials. The basic range of colours is found in the dentines, body dentines for building up the bulk of the restoration and more intense, less translucent shades for the gingival area. Enamels have a more restricted range of greyer shades, supplemented by high-translucency clear porcelain for the incisal edge. Since opaque or core porcelains only contribute to the general colour background of the restoration the range of shades is generally less; however dentines and opaques or core porcelains should be approximately colour matched to avoid marked changes in colour with varying dentine thickness. Modifying materials are supplied to alter the colour of the core or opaque base in the incisal and gingival areas. The high concentrations of opacifying oxides needed to hide the metal surface in porcelain-veneer crowns can have a marked effect on the appearance of a restoration because of the high surface reflectivity; an adequate thickness of at least 1.5 mm in the overlaying porcelain is necessary to avoid an overbright appearance and to give a greater depth of translucency. Highly pigmented effect porcelains are also supplied to extend the range of effects possible in the characterization of restorations. Apart from surface application to simulate defects, they can be added to opaques in the cervical area to simulate root dentine and for proximal staining to provide separation between crowns. Surface application of such materials has also been suggested for modifying the general colour when a shade cannot be accurately matched. However, apart from modifying colour these highly pigmented porcelains also increase surface reflection, and it is better to produce modified shades by mixing dentines.

The eye is the final arbiter in such aesthetic considerations as the visual effect of a dental restoration, and is a remarkably sensitive detector of colour difference. However, the nature of a visually observed difference is less readily defined, and the placement of a range of colours in correct relationship to one another is made much easier by the use of instrumental colour measurement. In instrumental methods the intensity of light reflected from a surface, either over the full spectral range, in a spectrophotometer, or within selected wavebands, in a colorimeter, is measured by a photodetector. Both colour perception and colour measurement must be related to a colour-order system in which individual colour samples or colour measurements are placed in colour space. Colour space is 3-dimensional, two dimensions being used to describe the chromaticity of a colour and the third being related to the luminosity or the total light reflected by a surface.

Colour order systems and colour atlases will be described elsewhere, but it may be said that the colour atlas most widely used in dentistry is that of Munsell (*Nickerson,* 1969) the dimensions of which are value (luminosity, related to an achromatic scale from black to white), hue (the nature of the colour, which may be related to a spectral wavelength) and chroma (saturation). Spectrophotometric and colorimetric measurements are most often expressed in terms of the CIE (Commission Internationale d'Eclairage) colorimetric systems. Colour measurements quoted here will be given in terms of the CIELAB system (*McLaren,* 1976), the coordinates of which are L^* (luminance), a^* (redness if positive, greenness if negative) and b^* (yellowness if positive, blueness if negative). The colour space so described is an equal chromaticity one, in that colours equally different in visual perception are represented by points equidistant in colour space.

The process of colour matching for the preparation of a dental restoration starts with the assessment of the basic colour of a tooth by comparison with the elements of a shade guide, which is a series of porcelain standards built up to resemble natural teeth. Since the range of colour variation in natural teeth is, in absolute terms, small, this matching process is a difficult one and to give satisfactory results several conditions must be fulfilled:

1. The observer should have normal colour vision and good visual acuity.
2. Conditions such as lighting and background should be suitable.
3. The shade guide should be well designed.

The nature of the shade guide is of considerable importance. Ideally it should cover evenly the volume of colour space occupied by the majority of natural teeth, the intervals between neighbouring shades being related to the maximum acceptable colour deviation. Finally the arrangement of shades in colour space should be a logical one, which will facilitate a systematic matching procedure. Shade guides should, therefore, be based on the colours of natural teeth. No systematic measurements of tooth colour in vivo have been reported, presumably because of experimental difficulties, but studies of the range of colours in extracted teeth have been made by *Clark* (1933), *Marui* (1963), *Sproull* (1973) and *Lemire* and *Burk* (1975). The investigations of *Clark* and *Marui* were made visually by matching with porcelain specimens and paper tabs, but *Sproull* and *Lemire* and *Burk* used spectrophotometer measurements. It is known that the colours of extracted teeth change on standing in air due to alteration in the fluid balance, which affects particularly the lightness. Measurements could be made as soon after extraction as possible, but the possibility of short-term colour change after extraction remains, to allow for which colour measurement in the mouth would be essential. In Figure 9 the most recent measurements, those of *Lemire* and *Burk,* are plotted in CIELAB co-ordinates. The chromaticity ranges of the three most recent surveys of natural teeth, and the distribution of shades in three shade guides, are shown in Figure 10. It is difficult to get a true idea of the distribution of shade-guide colours from

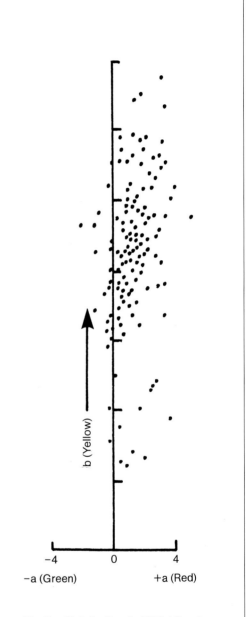

Fig. 9 Distribution in CIELAB colour space of natural tooth colour measurements made by *Lemire* and *Burk*.

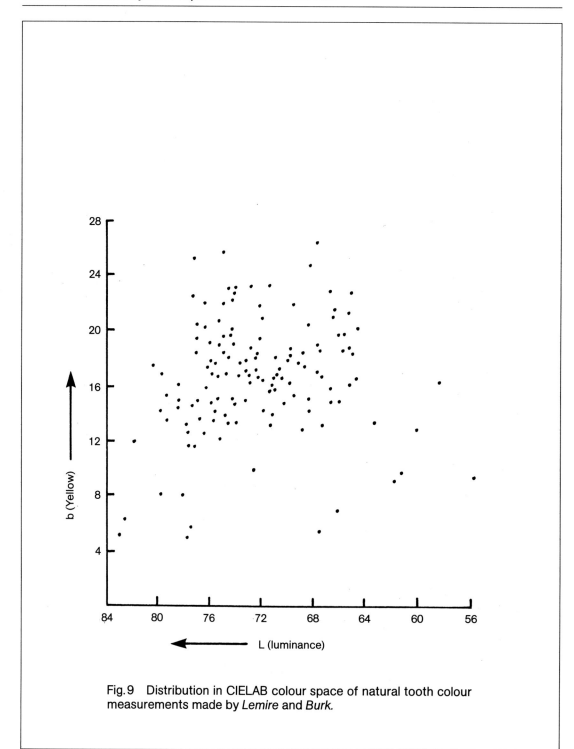

Fig. 9   Distribution in CIELAB colour space of natural tooth colour measurements made by *Lemire* and *Burk*.

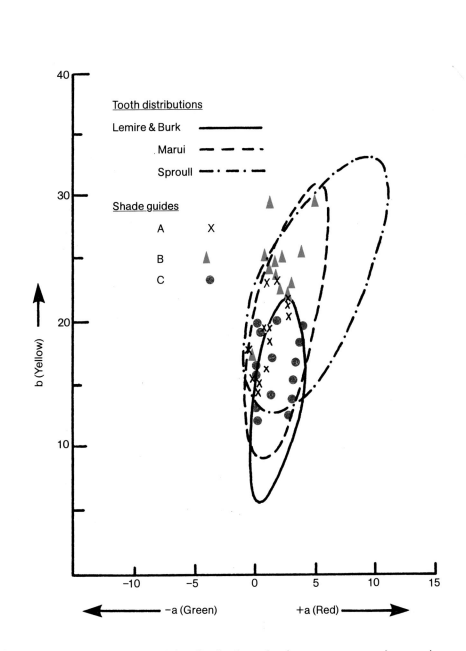

Fig.10 Chromaticity distribution of colour measurements on natural teeth and three porcelain shade guides.

a 2-dimensional representation, but it can be seen that considerable areas of the natural tooth colour distribution are not covered by the shade guides. In addition the distributions in colour space are irregular.

To keep shade-guide numbers within bounds it is probably inevitable that the extremes of the natural tooth distribution will not be included in the shade-guide coverage. However, within the colour space covered it is desirable that the shades should be evenly spread, so that there are no areas that cannot be acceptably matched, and that they should be arranged systematically. If the latter condition is not fulfilled time is wasted in reaching a match and the accuracy of a match cannot be readily checked because the nearest neighbours of the chosen shade are not known. Also, if shades are arranged in a systematic colour array interpolations between neighbouring shades can be made. Suggestions for redesigned shade guides have been made, based on the surveys of natural tooth colour. Both *Clark* and *Hayashi* (using *Marui*'s measurements) advocated the use of grids of shades in the Munsell colour system. The Hayashi system included a large number of shades, impracticable in porcelain samples but reproduced as paper tabs, which do not, however, simulate teeth in texture and translucency. *Clark* developed a porcelain shade guide, reducing the number of shades required by using only one hue, but varying value and chroma. In both systems there would be some very little used shades and the use of a single hue would probably be inade-

quate. *Lemire* and *Burk* produced a shade guide having two sets of nine shades at different value levels, each set having three hue and chroma levels. This shade guide fulfills the requirement of systematic arrangement, but the higher chroma (yellower) teeth evident particularly in Sproull's measurements could not be matched with it. The *Lemire* and *Burk* shade guide is the most practical development, but its coverage would probably need to be increased.

Given a range of shades with which satisfactory colour matches can be made, probably the most important feature of the colour of dental porcelain is its stability during the successive firings involved in the production of a restoration, and the maintainance of translucency in enamels. Changes in colour with refiring can be detected by spectrophotometric measurements, but a sensitive tri-stimulus colorimeter is particularly convenient for measuring small colour differences. Because of the translucency of dentines and enamels such measurements are affected by the nature of the background; in B.S. 5612 (1977) the recommended background for a dentine is the appropriate core porcelain, and for an enamel a black background, representing the oral cavity. Translucency can be assessed by reflectance measurements against dark and light backgrounds. Figure 11 shows the variation in the CIE-LAB colour co-ordinates of several dentines with refiring. It will be seen that the variation observed was mainly in lightness and yellowness; this corresponds to the plane of most variation in natural teeth. The limits shown as dotted lines

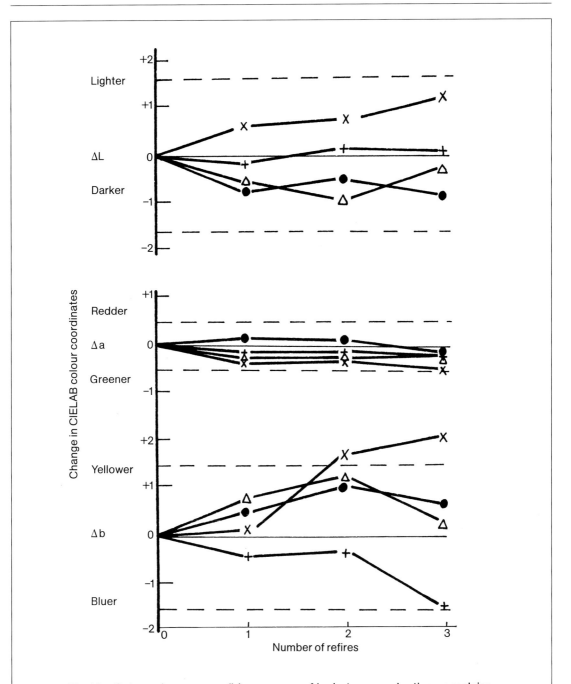

Fig.11 Colour change on refiring a range of jacket-crown dentine porcelains.

Thickness in mm.

MB 1	0.90	0.71	0.62	0.51	0.43
MB 2	0.91	0.76	0.55	0.48	0.44
MB 3	0.92	0.76	0.63	0.53	0.42
MB 4	0.88	0.74	0.58	0.51	0.38
MB 5	0.90	0.75	0.57	0.51	0.41

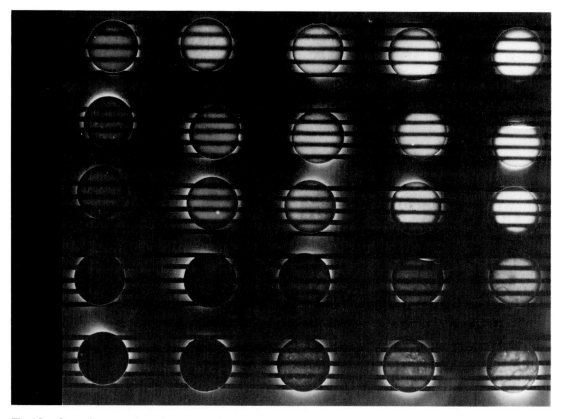

Fig.12   Covering powder of a range of opaque porcelains.

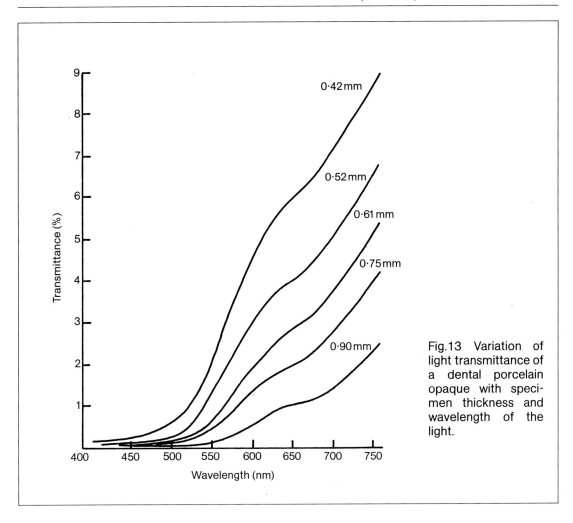

Fig.13 Variation of light transmittance of a dental porcelain opaque with specimen thickness and wavelength of the light.

were arrived at quite independently of the measurements themselves. Colour measurements on a range of shade guides were analysed to derive the mean difference between nearest neighbours, on the principle that the differences between neighbouring shades should be related to the maximum acceptable colour difference.

In the metal-bonding porcelain system it is in theory important that the opaque porcelain should have the maximum possible covering power, on the principal that the thinner the layer needed to mask the metal colour the greater the thickness available for dentine and enamel layers; it should then be easier to match the depth of translucency of a natural tooth. However, current opaques vary considerably in covering power as can be seen from Figure 12, where opaque discs of varying thickness have been placed over masks against a uniformly lit background. Between the discs and the masks a pattern of clear and opaque stripes has been interposed. Gettleman et al (1977) investigated the covering power of opaques by making spectrophotometric measurements on layers of different thicknesses baked-on to a precious metal alloy. As might be expected, covering was most effective for light of shorter wavelengths and less opaque was needed to cover gold-flashed surfaces. Covering power can also be compared by trans-

mission measurements on opaque discs. Figure 13 shows the variation of transmittance with wavelength for different thickness specimens of one opaque, measured by a spectrophotometer. From these curves the reason for the effectiveness of masking at short wavelengths can be seen; the transmission is very low up to 500 nm. but increases rapidly at higher wavelengths.

The transmission of light through a translucent medium is governed by Bouguer's Law:

$$I_x = I_o e^{-ax}$$
(Jenkins and White, 1950)
$$\text{or} \quad \log I_x = \log I_o - bx$$
where
I_o, I_x are the incident and emergent light intensities.
x is the thickness of the specimen.
a and b are constants.

so that if the log of the transmittance at a particular wavelength is plotted against thickness straight-line relationships should be obtained. Figure 14 shows log transmittance-thickness graphs for a range of opaques; similar graphs can be produced for total light transmission using a simple densitometer. Using such measurements, the covering power of opaques can be characterized by transmittance at a standard thickness.

It is widely known that natural tooth structure is fluorescent. This property is obvious under some circumstances, such as in discotheques where effect lights are

used emitting considerable amounts of long-wavelength ultra-violet light, when teeth are seen to emit bluish-white to yellowish-white fluorescence. Fluorescent properties can of course change the appearance of objects in normal daylight, as evidenced by the use of dayglow paints. To find out how far the brightness of natural teeth was affected by their fluorescence, Clarke (1974) carried out spectrophotometric measurements on natural teeth. The results indicated that in normal daylight fluorescence was responsible for $\sim 2\frac{1}{2}\%$ of the total light emitted, a proportion which would not

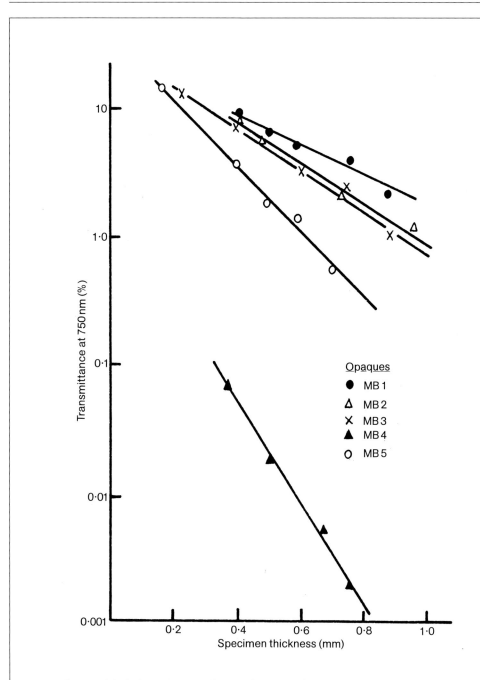

Fig.14   Variation of monochromatic transmittance with specimen thickness for several different opaques.

very noticeably increase the visible brightness. The case for matching in dental porcelain the fluorescence of natural teeth rests, therefore, upon the desire of patients to have restorations which are cosmetically satisfactory under all conditions. The colour of natural fluorescence varies from tooth to tooth and in different parts of the tooth structure, but a typical example can be seen in Figure 15 which shows the fluorescent emission of a molar enamel. Fluorescence was first produced in dental porcelain by the addition to it of small proportions of uranium oxide (UO_2), giving brilliant fluorescence which, however, was green in colour. It was found that the further introduction of cerium oxide (CeO_2) into the glass structure produced a good match for natural tooth fluorescence; suitable proportions of the two oxides might be 1000 ppm of each. A typical emission curve for porcelain containing CeO_2 and UO_2 is also shown in Figure 15; the peaks at 505 and 525 nm are provided by UO_2 and the fluorescence $<490\,\mu m$ is due to CeO_2. When uranium was identified as a possible radiological hazard by *McCullough* and *Moore* (1974) and *O'Riordan* and *Hunt* (1974) attempts were made to develop non-radioactive fluorescence (*Binns* and *Bloor,* 1978; *Smyth,* 1979). Investigation of potential fluorescers showed that when a number of rare-earth oxides were incorporated in the glass structure they produced fluorescent emissions ranging across the whole spectrum, as shown in Figure 16, and it seemed likely that they could be combined to give any desired colour of fluorescence. However there were two

effects which limit the fluorescence obtainable in practice:

1. Self-quenching. In some cases, as the concentration of rare earth is increased the emission increases to a maximum and then falls owing to the resonance between atoms as they approach each other more closely.
2. Interaction. One rare earth may activate another and fail to fluoresce itself; in ternary systems more complicated interactions can take place.

Owing to these limitations the most practical system was found to be provided by cerium oxide–terbium oxide mixtures, which can give fluorescence ranging from bluish-white through neutral-white to greenish yellow. Warmer tones can be produced by the addition of small proportions of dysprosium oxide and samarium oxide. The fluorescence produced by such additions is dependent on the base-porcelain composition, since the emission of ions in glass is affected by the presence of impurities, notably transitional metals such as iron and titanium. Rare-earth ions can also give fluorescence when incorporated in suitable crystalline lattices, and if the host crystals are similar to porcelain in refractive index, or present only in small proportions, such a system can be used to give fluorescence in dental porcelain (*Miyai* et al 1979).

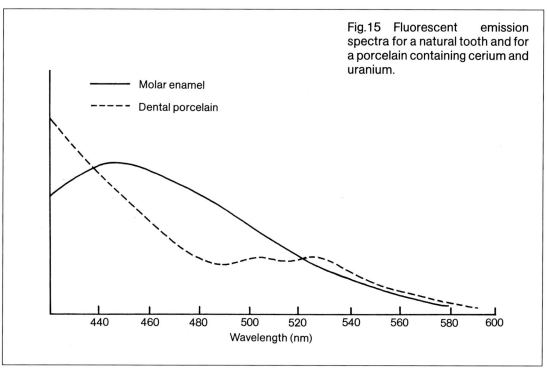

Fig.15 Fluorescent emission spectra for a natural tooth and for a porcelain containing cerium and uranium.

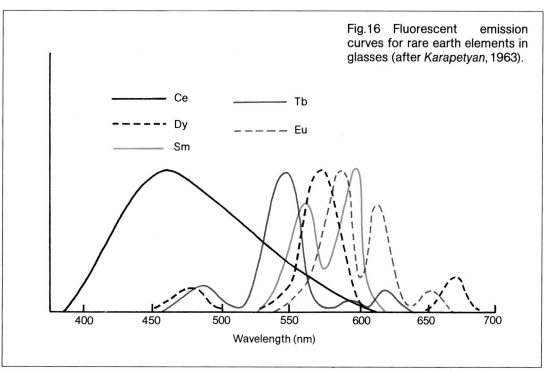

Fig.16 Fluorescent emission curves for rare earth elements in glasses (after *Karapetyan*, 1963).

Compatibility and Bonding in Porcelain Metal Restorations

The first consideration in any composite involving a brittle ceramic phase must be the closeness with which the phases are matched in thermal expansion. The different alloys that can be used to produce copings and frameworks for crowns and bridges have high thermal expansions relative to most glasses and an account has been given of the way in which a suitable high expansion porcelain was produced by the crystallization of a high-expansion crystal phase in a glassy matrix. This process, however, makes the resultant porcelain more liable to variation of thermal expansion than the purely glassy jacket-crown porcelains.

The stress on a metal-porcelain composite system at room temperature is governed by the thermal strain or mismatch M which is given by M = $(\alpha_m - \alpha_p)\Delta T$ where ΔT is the temperature interval between room temperature and the set-point of the glass (the temperature at which it becomes effectively a rigid body); α_m and α_p are the mean thermal expansion coefficients of the metal and porcelain over the interval ΔT.

The normal recommendation is that the porcelain thermal expansion should be less than that of the metal; then M is positive and compressive stress is produced in the porcelain, which can increase its effective strength. However, in the somewhat complicated geometry of a restoration, unwanted stresses may result, for example at margins, which may give rise to flaws if M becomes too large. If, on the other hand, the alloy is completely enclosed by porcelain and M is negative, compressive stress will be produced across the porcelain-metal interface which will increase the effective bond strength; the corollary is, of course, tensile stress in the porcelain. Two further considerations suggest that M should be kept as small as possible:

1. Thermal mismatch will give stresses in the metal which can cause distortion; in particular, thin sections of high-gold alloys will deform under small loads down to relatively low temperatures.
2. Thermal mismatch of any kind will result in shear stresses at the porcelain-metal interface, which will tend to reduce bond strength.

Thermal expansion curves of dental porcelain samples measured after the normal porcelain firing process show, to varying degrees, the characteristics of a rapidly-cooled glass. When a glass is cooled quickly there is not sufficient time for the structural re-arrangement needed to give a more compact configuration, and a 'frozen-in' low-density state results. If such a chilled specimen is reheated slowly to the transformation range the re-arrangement to the higher-density state can take place and the rate of expansion is reduced. Slowly cooled specimens on the other hand exhibit a continuous increase in thermal expansion through the transformation range. The thermal expansion curves resulting from different cooling rates can be seen in Figure 17, which shows the results of two successive measurements on the same porcelain sample; the rate of cooling in the

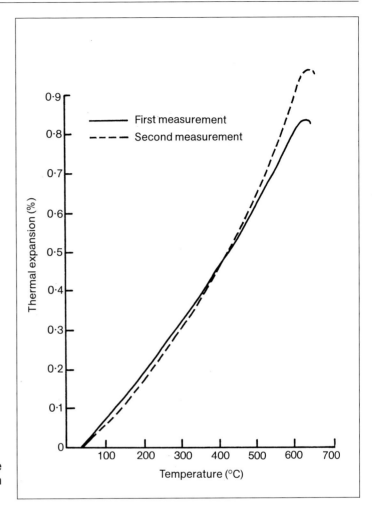

Fig.17 Effect of cooling rate on the thermal expansion of an opaque porcelain.

dilatometer is, of course, relatively slow. Since the state of a porcelain layer in a restoration is that characteristic of the normal rapid cooling it is apparent that samples should not undergo any other thermal treatment before thermal expansion measurement.

The porcelain layers in a restoration are, of course, submitted to a number of heat treatments, during which their thermal expansion properties might change. It has in fact been shown that, with reheating, porcelains may increase or decrease in thermal expansion; measurements on a range of materials reheated up to 3 times have shown changes of $+1.5$ to $-1.7.10^{-6}$ in thermal expansion coefficient from $20-500°C$, the extremes being found in the same porcelain system. Variations in thermal expansion are probably due to changes in leucite content

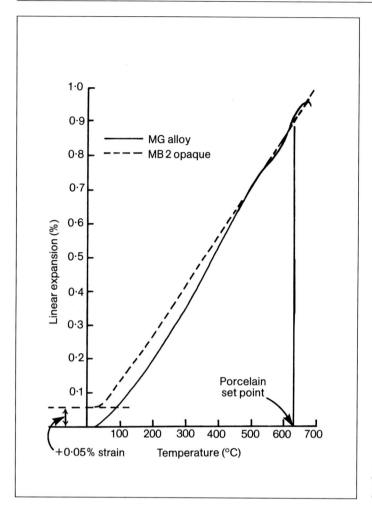

Fig. 18   Use of alloy and porcelain thermal expansion curves to assess residual strain.

because the glass-crystal system is not in equilibrium at the porcelain firing temperature. Although such changes can continue with repeated firing, it has been found that in many cases a steady level of thermal expansion is reached after 5–10 firings. Since such changes in thermal expansion could produce serious thermal mismatch some attention should be given to increasing the thermal stability of metal-bonding porcelains. With certain assumptions, an estimate of thermal mismatch can be made by comparing the thermal expansion curves of metal and porcelain. If one curve is displaced vertically until the two coincide at the set-point of the porcelain, as shown in Figure 18, the mismatch as % strain is given by the vertical distance between the curves at room temperature. The use of this technique is based upon an assumed set-point temperature; for ceramic glazes the set-point is commonly taken to be at the upper end of the transformation range, but it probably depends upon the viscosity-temperature relation for the particular glass and the rate of cooling. It can be determined by the deformation of a composite porcelain-metal specimen, such as in the strip-flexure test used by Dorsch (1979) which gives a measure of the strain and hence the stress developed. Other stresses, such as those introduced by sudden changes of temperature, may be superimposed on those resulting from thermal mismatch so that the resultant stress locally reaches the limiting value for the porcelain. For this reason a thermal shock test has been proposed by *Anusavice* et al (1981) as an indication of porcelain-metal compatibility.

The problems involved in the bonding of porcelains to dental alloys will be considered in detail elsewhere and only a brief outline will be given here of the underlying principles of glass-metal bonding, the application of which to dental systems was reviewed by *Pask* (1977). Clean metal surfaces are normally wetted by molten glasses, but such wetting in itself gives rise only to weak bonding by Van der Waals forces. Reaction with surface oxide facilitates the spreading of molten glass on metals, and can lead to chemical bonding. The strongest bonding occurs when there is chemical equilibrium at the interface relative to the metal oxide, the porcelain at the interface being saturated with the oxide; there should also be a minimum layer of free oxide at the interface. The attainment of this condition depends on the rate of oxide formation and the rates of solution in, and diffusion through, the porcelain. In noble metals the surface oxide is provided by minor base-metal constituents which diffuse to the surface of the alloys when they are heated. In base metal alloys, on the other hand, surface oxide arises from the major constituents. Such metals readily oxidize when heated in air, and the chief danger lies in excessive oxidation, which can be limited by the addition of trace metals to the alloys and close process control.

These principles of glass-metal bonding were established in the main by studies of simple model systems. However, the porcelain-dental alloy system is more complicated in terms of the composition of the two phases and also in the presence at the interface, sometimes, of bonding agents which are themselves complex in composition. In consequence there is still a good deal of uncertainty as to the effects of different materials and treatments on bonding.

Some of the different conclusions on the effects of various factors on porcelain-metal bonding may also be due to the methods used to assess the effectiveness of bonding. If one considers the design of an ideal test for porcelain-metal bonding the following would probably be the chief requirements:

1. The porcelain should be applied to cast metal specimens by a method compatible with those used in building up restorations, and the porcelain component should have dimensions comparable with those of restorations.

2. The porcelain-metal interface should be stressed in a way compatible with the stressing of a restoration in service, and the loading should be such as to encourage fracture propagation along the interface.
3. The test should give an unequivocal answer, preferably quantitative.

Considered in the light of these criteria probably all the tests so far reported would be found wanting.

To provide a rough check on bonding, manufacturers of alloys and porcelains have for a long time used simple tests involving the application of porcelain layers to metal strips, which are then bent, twisted or hammered, and the bonding assessed by the way in which failure occurs. Attempts have been made to define more closely and, if possible, to quantify such simple tests; it is difficult, however, to find a substitute for the inspection of fracture surfaces by a skilled observer. Experience with a simple test, coupled with clinical data, can give a good qualitative assessment of the effectiveness of the bond; it is doubtful whether, in spite of the proliferation of more sophisticated tests, there is at present any greater certainty of assessment. Although a quantitative test would be desirable, some authorities doubt whether any numerical values are meaningful. A common approach to bonding is to consider it on the weakest link basis–to say, for example, that if fracture occurs in the porcelain the bond strength is adequate (the alternative conclusion might, of course, be that the porcelain strength is inadequate!). Failures are classified as cohe-

sive or adhesive, and identified by the interfaces exposed (O'Brien, 1977). However, unless there is a very definite failure in adhesion it is commonly observed that fracture propagates through the porcelain close to the interface, leaving a discontinuous, sometimes thin, coating of porcelain on the metal. It seems likely that a plane of weakness exists in the porcelain close to the interface due to intermittent failure of wetting or a higher concentration of voids than in the bulk of the porcelain. On such a surface visual inspection will often suggest that there are areas of bare metal over which bonding has failed, which on further optical or scanning electron microscopy examination are found to be at least partly covered by a thin layer of porcelain.

In this review, shortage of space precludes detailed description of the very various bond test methods that have been devised, and the author must assume that the reader has some general acquaintance with bond testing. An attempt has been made in Table 4 to summarize and classify the published tests. The most widely used method of assessing bonding has been the pull-through shear test of *Shell* and *Nielsen* (1962); examples of its use can be seen in papers by *Leone* and *Fairhurst* (1967), *Anthony* et al (1970), *Goeller* et al (1972), *Moffa* et al (1973) and *Lubovich* et al (1977). Such a test, however, is likely to be subject to the "pinch effect", in which the measured adhesion is affected by the residual radial stresses resulting from thermal mismatch. It may be noted that high bond strength values would result from the condition normally regarded as

Table 4   Range of Tests for Porcelain-Metal Bonding

Authors	Type	Details
Nally (1969)	Direct tension	Porcelain fused between two metal rods.
Kelly et al (1969)	Direct tension	"Mushroom" of porcelain fused to the end of a metal rod.
McLean and *Sced* (1973)	Tension – shear	Porcelain fused to metal cone, stressed along axis of cone.
Silver et al (1960)	Tension – shear	Porcelain fused between two metal rods. Cantilever bend test.
Wight et al (1977)	Tension – shear	Porcelain fused between two overlapping strips. Tested in shear with off-axis loading.
Shell and *Neilson* (1962)	Shear	Ring of porcelain fused round metal rod. Pull-through test.
Chong and *Beech* (1980)	Shear	Porcelain cylinder fused to flat metal surface. Sideways loading at interface.
Schmitz and *Schulmeyer* (1975)	Shear	Rectangular porcelain specimen fused to flat metal surface. Sideways loading.
Knap and *Ryge* (1966)	Shear	Porcelain layer fused to cylindrical surface of metal rod, which is stressed axially in tension.
Lavine and *Custer* (1966)	Flat strip test	Strip flexed with porcelain in tension.
Fairhurst (1977)	Circular strip test	Strip flexed with porcelain in compression.
Carter et al (1979)	Flat strip test	Porcelain applied to both sides. Strip deformed in torsion.
Claus (1981)	Flat strip test	Porcelain surface impacted with spherical-ended striker.

harmful, in which the porcelain expansion is higher than that of the metal. *Shell* and *Nielsen* oberved, in their original paper, that measurements were only made on porcelain-metal pairs of matched thermal expansion; however, in view of the lack of information on the set-points of porcelains, and the large variations in thermal expansion on firing, it would be difficult to guarantee freedom from residual stress, even if it were desirable to limit testing to such pairs.

Tests have also been devised (*Chong* and *Beech*, 1980) (*Schmitz* and *Schulmeyer*, 1975) in which shear is applied to a plane interface. The resulting test configuration, however, in which a block of porcelain is fused on to a flat metal surface, is rather far from the geometry of a restoration. There is also the possibility in such a test of the application of a bending moment to the porcelain component; this is avoided in the *Chong* and *Beech* test by loading at the interface, which may, however, give rise to localized stresses. In the test developed by *McLean* and *Sced* (1973) the specimen configuration, in which a porcelain layer is built up on a conical metal surface, is similar to that of a porcelain crown. The loading is such that the stress system acting at the interface will combine tension and shear and the cone angle encourages the fracture path to follow the interface. However, it has been found that the measured failure stresses do not always match the type of failure observed, probably owing to varying degrees of stiction between the metal components used, so that inspection of the fracture surfaces is a more reliable indication of the effectiveness of bonding.

Several of the methods developed are strip tests in which layers of porcelain are applied to metal strips or tabs, which are then deformed by flexure or torsion until failure of the porcelain layer occurs. In the most common type of test the strips are flexed so that the porcelain is in tension, and the failure of the bond assessed at a standard deflection. In such a system fracture is initiated first at the free surface of the porcelain, and cracks propagate towards the porcelain-metal interface. Further failure then depends on the strength of the bond and the shear stress at the interface. The latter, however, depends on the dimensions of the components and their elasticities; stress analysis would be needed to determine the interfacial shear stress. A more promising configuration for a flexural strip test would seem to be with the porcelain in compression when failure would not be due to tension in the porcelain but by shear, either at the interface or in the porcelain. Stress analysis for composite beams may be used to determine the distribution of shear stresses, and the stress level at the interface, for any deflection. A test of this kind has been developed by *Fairhurst* (1977).

It will be seen from the examples discussed that objections can be raised to most of the methods devised. The need, however, is to decide which gives the best indication of clinical performance. Each of the wide variety of methods has been used independently to determine the effect of changes in the factors capable of affecting bonding, such as the metal and porcelain components used, the metal pre-treatment and its surface roughness, the use of bonding agents, and so on. Many significant differences in bonding have been found, but as observed by *Fairhurst* (1977) "None of these tests have been able to predict clinical failure or success". Very little work has been done, however, in which different methods have been compared. More systematic investigation is required, in which a range of tests would be applied to systems known to give differences in clinical performance so that the relative effectiveness of the different tests can be compared.

References

Anthony, D. H., Burnett, A. P., Smith, D. L. and *Brook, M. S.* (1970): Shear Test for Measuring Bonding in Cast Gold Alloy–Porcelain Composites. J. Dent. Res. 49: 27.

Anusavice, K. J., Ringle, R. D., Morse, P. K., Fairhurst, C. W. and *King, G. E.* (1981): A Thermal Shock Test for Porcelain–Metal Systems. J. Dent. Res. 60: 1686.

Binns, D. B. (1962): Some Properties of Crystal–Glass Composites. Science of Ceramics 1: 315.

Binns, D. B. (1977): The Chemical and Physical Properties of Dental Porcelain. "Dental Porcelain: The State of the Art – 1977", Ed. H. N. Yamada, Univ. S. Calif. School of Dentistry, Los Angeles 1977: p. 25.

Binns, D. B. and *Bloor, I. K.* (1978): Fluorescing Agents for Dental Porcelain. Brit. Pat. 1, 529, 984.

Brown, M. H. and *Sorensen, S. E.* (1979) Aluminous Porcelain and its Role in Fixed Prosthodontics: J. Prosthet. Dent. 42: 507.

Budworth, D. W. (1969): A Minimum Value for the Density of Random Close Packing of Equal Spheres. J. Mater. Sci. 4: 374.

Carter, J. M., Al-Mudaffar, J. and *Sorensen, S. E.* (1979): Adherence of a Nickel-Chromium Alloy and Porcelain. J. Prosth. Dent. 41: 167.

Chong, M. P. and *Beech, D. R.* (1980): A Simple Shear Test to Evaluate the Bond Strength of Ceramic Fused to Metal. Austral. Dent. J. 25: 357.

Clark, E. B. (1931): An Analysis of Tooth Colour. J. Amer. Dent. Assoc. 18: 2093.

Clarke, F. J. J. (1974): Spectrophotometric and Fluorimetric Properties of Dental Porcelain and Teeth. National Physical Laboratory, Rept. MOM 0583/C(0891/C).

Claus, H. (1981): Investigatory Tests into the Bonding Strength between Dental Porcelain and Metal Alloys. Dental Labor (5).

Cutler, I. B. (1969): Sintering of Glass Powders During Constant Rates of Heating. J. Amer. Ceram. Soc. 52: 14.

Cutler, I. B. and *Henrichsen, R. E.* (1968): Effect of Particle Shape on the Kinetics of Sintering of Glass. J. Amer. Ceram. Soc. 51: 604.

Dorsch, P. (1979): A Method of Calculating Stresses in Metal-Porcelain Composites. Ber. Dt. Keram. Ges. 56: 328.

El-Abrashi, M. K., Craig, R. G. and *Peyton, F. A.* (1969): Experimental Stress Analysis of Dental Restorations, Part III The Concept of the Geometry of Proximal Margins, Part IV The Concept of Parallelism of Axial Walls. J. Prosth. Dent. 22: 333, 346.

Fairhurst, C. W. (1977): Metal Surface Preparation and Bonding Agents in Porcelain–Metal Systems. "Alternatives to Gold Alloys in Dentistry", Ed. T. M. Vallega, DHEW Publication No. (N14) 77–1227.

Frenkel, J. (1945): Viscous Flow of Crystalline Bodies under the Action of Surface Tension. J. Phys. (USSR): 385.

Gettleman, L., Herzberg, T. W., Webber, R. L. and *Moffa, J. P.* (1977): Effect of Metal Surface Treatment on the Masking Power of Opaque Porcelain. "Dental Porcelain: The State of the Art – 1977", Ed. H. N. Yamada, Univ. S. Calif. School of Dentistry, Los Angeles 1977: p. 161.

Goeller, I., Meyer, J. M. and *Nally, J. N.* (1972): Comparative Study of Three Coating Agents and their Influence on Bond Strength of Porcelain Fused to Gold Alloys. J. Prosth. Dent. 28: 504.

Griffith, A. A. (1920): The Phenomenon of Rupture and Flow in Solids. Phil. Trans. Roy. Soc. Lond. A 221: 163.

Hahn, C. and *Teuchert, K.* (1980): Importance of the Glass Ceramic System $K_2O–Al_2O_3–SiO_2$ in Dental Porcelain. Ber. Dt. Keram. Ges. 57: 208.

Hermansson, L. and Carlssen, R. (1978): On the Crystallization of the Glassy Phase in Whitewares. Trans. Brit. Ceram. Soc. 77: 32.

Hoshikawa, T. and Akagi, S. (1972): Formation of Leucite and Thermal Expansion in $SiO_2-Al_2O_3-K_2O-Na_2O$ Glasses. Yogyo-Kyokai-Shi. 80: 42.

Inglis, C. E. (1913): Stresses in a Plate due to the Presence of Cracks and Sharp Corners. Trans. Inst. Nav. Archit. 55: 219.

Jones, D. W. (1970): Dental Refractories and Ceramics. Ph. D. Thesis, University of Birmingham.

Jones, D. W. (1971): Statistical Parameters for the Strength of Dental Porcelain. Dent. Pract. 22: 55.

Jenkins, F. A. and White, H. E. (1950): Fundamentals of Optics, New York: McGraw Hill, p. 197.

Karapetyan. G. O. (1963): Luminescence of Glass with Rare Earth Activators. Bull. Acad. Sci. USSR, Phys. Ser. 27: 791.

Kujczynski, G. C. and Zaplatynskyj, I. (1956): Sintering of Glass. J. Amer. Ceram. Soc. 39: 349.

Kulp, P. R., Lee, P. W. and Fox, J. E. (1961): An Impact Test for Dental Porcelain. J. Dent. Res. 40: 1136.

Lehmann, M. L. and Hampson, E. L. (1962): A Study of Strain Patterns in Jacket Crowns on Anterior Teeth Resulting from Different Tooth Preparations. Brit. Dent. J. 113: 337.

Lemire, P. A. and Burk, B. (1975): Color in Dentistry, J. M. Ney Co., Hartford Conn. USA.

Leone, E. F. and Fairhurst, C. W. (1967): Bond Strength and Mechanical Properties of Dental Porcelain Enamels. J. Prosthet. Dent. 18: 155.

Lubovich, R. P. and Goodkind, R. J. (1977): Bond Strength Studies of Precious, Semiprecious and Nonprecious Ceramic-Metal Alloys with Two Porcelains. J. Prosthet. Dent. 37: 288.

McCleary, R. K. (1961): Mechanical Packing of Spherical Particles. J. Amer. Ceram. Soc. 44: 513.

McLean, J. W. and Hughes, T. H. (1965): The Reinforcement of Dental Porcelain with Ceramic Oxides. Brit. Dent. J. 119: 251.

McLean, J. W. and Sced, I. R. (1973): Bonding of Dental Porcelain to Metal I, The Gold Alloy-Porcelain Bond. Trans. Brit. Ceram. Soc. 72: 229.

Marui, M. (1963): Colour of the Tooth Crown. J. Japanese Stomatological Soc. 35: 412.

Miyai, K., Suzuki, N. and Kuzi, I. (1979): Fluorescent Dental Porcelain. U.S. Pat. 4, 158, 641.

Moffa, J. P., Lugassy, A. K., Guckes, A. D. and Gettleman, L. (1973): An Evaluation of Nonprecious Alloys for Use with Porcelain Veneers I. Physical Properties. J. Prosthet. Dent. 30: 424.

Moore and McCullough (1974): The Inclusion of Radioactive Compounds in Dental Porcelain. Brit. Dent. J. 136: 101.

Nally, J. N. (1969): Chemico-Physical Analysis and Mechnical Tests of the Ceramo-Metallic Complex. Int. Dent. J. 18: 309.

Nickerson, D. (1969): Color Eng. 7 (5).

O'Brian, W. J. and Ryge, G. (1965): Contact Angles of Drops of Enamels on Metals. J. Prosthet. Dent. 15: 1094.

O'Riordan, M. C. and Hunt, G. J. (1974): Radioactive fluorescers in dental porcelain. National Radiological Protection Board NRPB R 25.

Pask, J. A. (1977): Fundamentals of Wetting and Bonding between Ceramics and Metals. Alternatives to gold alloys in dentistry. Ed. T. M. Valluga. DHEW Publ. No (NIH) 77–1227, p. 235.

Pettrow, J. N. (1961): Practical Factors in Building and Firing Characteristics of Dental Porcelain. J. Prosthet. Dent. 11: 335.

Saklad, M. J. (1958): The Disclosure of Cleavage and Fracture Lines in Porcelain Restarations. J. Prosthet. Dent. 8: 115.

Schmitz, Kh. and Schulmeyer, H. (1975): Determining the Adhesive Strength of Metal-Ceramic Composite Systems. Dental-Labor (12).

Shell, J. S. and Nielsen, J. P. (1962): Study of the Bond between Gold Alloys and Porcelain. J. Dent. Res. 41: 1424.

Smyth, M. B. and Lee-You, J. (1979): Fluorescent Artificial Teeth. U.S. Pat. 4, 170, 823.

Southan, D. E. and Jørgensen, K. D. (1972): Faulty Porcelain Jacket Crowns. Austral. Dent. J. 17: 436.

Southan, D. E. and Jørgensen, K. D. (1973): An Explanation for the Occurrence of Internal Faults in Porcelain Jacket Crowns. Austral. Dent. J. 18: 152.

Southan, D. E. and Jørgensen, K. D. (1974): The Endurance Limit of Dental Porcelain. Austral. Dent. J. 19: 7.

Sproull, R. C. (1973): Colour Matching in Dentistry II. Practical Application of the Organization of Colour. J. Prosthet. Dent. 29: 556.

Vines, R. F., Semmelman, J. O., Lee, P. W. and Fonvielle, F. P. (1958): Mechanism involved in Securing Dense, Vitrified Ceramics from Preshaped, Partly Crystalline Bodies. J. Amer. Ceram. Soc. 41: 304.

Walton, C. B. and Leven, M. M. (1955): A Preliminary Report of Photoelastic Tests of Strain Patterns within Jacket Crowns. J. Amer. Dent. Ass. 50: 44.

Weinstein, M., Katz, S. and Weinstein, A. B. (1962): Fused Porcelain-to-Metal Teeth. U.S. Pat. 3, 052, 982.

Wight, T. A., Baumann, J. C. and *Pellen, G. B.* (1977): An Evaluation of Four Variables Affecting the Bond Strength of Porcelain to Nonprecious Alloy. J. Prosth. Dent. 37: 570.

Wilson, H. J. and *Whitehead, F. I. H.* (1967): Comparison of Some Physical Properties of Dental Porcelain. Dent. Pract. 17: 350.

The Strength and Strengthening Mechanisms of Dental Ceramics

Derek W. Jones

Strength

Critical Strain of Ceramics

Any discussion of the strength of dental porcelain material and the methods by which it can be strengthened must also have as a prerequisite a definition of dental porcelain. Dental porcelain is essentially a borosilicate and/or feldspathic glass which may or may not contain dispersed crystalline metallic oxide components. The exacting aesthetic requirements of dental porcelain have largely dictated its development and compositional limitations (*Jones,* 1971). Crystalline structures are generally stronger than non-crystalline structures since the atoms are in a state of maximum packing density. Thus a glass structure is generally weaker than a metallic oxide crystalline or polycrystalline ceramic since the interatomic distances will be greater. It has been pointed out previously by *Jones* (1971) that although the properties of dental porcelain are intrinsically a function of composition, other factors have an overriding effect upon observed mechanical properties.

Although we can regard traditional dental porcelain as a glass, our dental prosthesis are produced by a process of fusion of frit particles, rather than from a glass melt as in the fabrication of most industrial glass articles. The imperfections present in a fused dental ceramic which arise due to incomplete fusion give rise to faults which limit strength. Incomplete fusion at the interface also results in a prismatic effect which may influence the translucency. Crystallised glasses (devitrification produced by heat treatment) are also generally found to be tougher as well as stronger than uncrystallised glasses. It has been shown (*Hing,* 1975) that the strength increases as the inverse of the square root of the mean free path in the intercrystalline glass whereas the fracture surface energy increases with the inverse of the mean free path. Glass-ceramics with fine-grained structure obtained from complex compositions may form thermally and mechanically incompatible phases which may cause some reduction in strength particularly after prolonged crystallization at higher temperatures. *Hing* (1975) also found that the fracture toughness of glasses in the Li_2O–SiO_2 system did not vary significantly with glass ceramics of fine grained as opposed to those with medium grain size, although the mode of fracture was said to be quite different.

Although crystallised glasses are stronger, such a system is not generally applicable to dentistry since crystallization will adversely affect the translucency. Some of the dental porcelains used for fusing to metal have a composition with sufficient Na_2O to increase the thermal coefficient of expansion in order to be compatible with the metal. The use of a higher proportion of Na_2O which opens up the network structure in order to increase the thermal expansion coefficient may also run the risk of devitrification as a result of disruption of the Si–O bridging.

A glass by definition when cooled from the liquid state to form a solid possesses a viscosity greater than $10^{14.5}$ poises, if no crystallization occurs it becomes a glass in which no long-range order or three-dimensional periodicity occurs. However, the theory that glass structure is based upon a continuous random network (*Zachariasen*, 1932; *Warren*, *Biscoe*, 1938) may be an over simplification, other models have been postulated which include some degree of order within the structural units of the glass which are then dispersed at random within a low order matrix network (*Sugarman*, 1967). In the various types of glass and ceramic materials we are perhaps dealing with a graduation from strictly short range order to one of long range order of the atomic structure. It is further known that

the specific location of ions within a glass structure may dramatically effect the physical properties and strength. The term glass may embrace various types of materials but generally refers to a material which is both transparent and brittle at room temperature. The largely covalent and/or ionic bonded structure of ceramics and glass result in the following characteristic properties.

1. Brittleness (even when strong), hard wear resistance.
2. Good resistance to chemical degridation.

Such properties are ideally suited for the use of glass-like materials as a restorative to replace natural tooth enamel.

Various attempts have been made to derive a theoretical strength for glass-like materials, such calculations are of necessity only approximate since many of the essential data for material properties are lacking in accuracy. However, various workers, *Griffith* (1920), *Condon* (1954), and many others (*Sugarman*, 1967; *Astbury*, 1968; *Eagan* and *Swearengen*, 1978; *Kingary*, 1960), have suggested theoretical strength values of the order of 1 to 7 GPa. More recent theoretical estimates (*Eagan* and *Swearengen*, 1978) of the intrinsic strength of glass are based upon the premise that fracture is controlled by the strength of the silicon-oxygen bond. Calculation of the force required to rupture this bond in fused silica suggests a theoretical strength of 18 GPa for glasses. According to *Eagan* and *Swearengen* (1978) some values as high as 14.7 GPa have been measured on specially prepared specimens. The practical

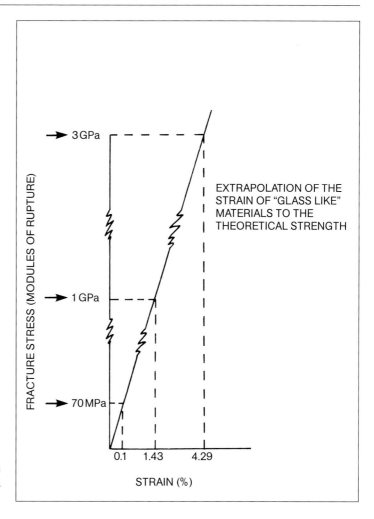

FRACTURE STRESS (MODULES OF RUPTURE)

3 GPa

1 GPa

70 MPa

EXTRAPOLATION OF THE
STRAIN OF "GLASS LIKE"
MATERIALS TO THE
THEORETICAL STRENGTH

0.1   1.43   4.29

STRAIN (%)

Fig. 1   The extrapolation of strain
in a brittle glass like material for a
theoretical stress of 3 GPa.

strength of bulk glasses are generally considered to be 100 to 1000 times smaller than the theoretical values. As a rough guide, the ceramic materials in everyday use have a strength value about one tenth the strength of similar materials prepared in a controlled laboratory process, and about one hundredth of the strength of fine near perfect crystals or whiskers. Most glasses have moduli of elasticity of the order of 30–50 GPa. It would seem that if we assume that the factors limiting the attainment of theoretical strength do not affect modulus of elasticity and assuming that Hooke's law operates to the breaking stress, strains of the order of 4 % should theoretically be possible with a fracture stress of 3 GPa as illustrated in Figure 1. The extrapolation of the strain for a theoretical fracture stress of 18 GPa would lead to a staggering 26% strain value. However, in practice it is noted that for a wide range of ceramic and glass-like materials ranging from pure oxide structures such as carbides, nitrides to glasses and heterophase cements and refractory materials, the critical strain at fracture will only range between 0.05 up to 0.2%. "Ceramic" materials thus have a very characteristic critical strain of the order of 0.1%. *Astbury* (1968) has suggested that this may perhaps be as much as two orders of magnitude below the theoretical value for an ionic crystal. If we take the values shown in Figure 1 for theoretical strain at 1 or 3 GPa we can see that we have some 14 to 43 times less strain at fracture in practice (0.1%) than the theoretical values would seem to predict (i.e. 1.43 and 4.29%). The limitations of the critical strain are dependent upon atomic spacing, microcrack length, or in the case of crystalline ceramics the crystal size, which will limit the degree of dislocation movement. In the case of dental porcelain materials the critical strain is mainly limited by the fabricational defects.

Several researchers have measured the modulus of elasticity of ceramic materials by means of resonant-bar techniques (*Spinner* and *Tefft*, 1961; *Rosinger* et al, 1974; *Richie*, 1973; *Richie* et al, 1974). *Richie* (1973) advocated an improved dynamic system using a four point loading bend test in which a continuous measurement of dynamic modulus of elasticity was made as a function of the applied stress. It was suggested that the technique would make it possible to study the mechanisms which might cause observed departure from linearity such as cracks or flaws. It was found by *Ritchie* et al (1974) that the dynamic modulus of notched bars of Al_2O_3 dropped rapidly just prior to failure.

Frey and *Mackenzie* (1967) determined the dynamic elastic properties of glass/Al_2O_3 and glass/ZrO_2 composite systems by means of an ultrasonic-pulse reflection technique in which a quartz-crystal transducer was bonded to the end face of cylindrical samples. The theoretical values for the modulus of elasticity for two levels of volume inclusions (20% and 40%) of the dispersed phase were calculated and compared to the experimental data. The experimental and theoretical values for the four types of samples reported by *Frey* and *MacKenzie* (1967) are shown in Table 1.

Table 1

	Glass/crystalline composite	
	20% Al_2O_3	40% Al_2O_3
Experimental Elastic Modulus GPa	118.0	157.0
Theoretical Elastic Modulus GPa	121.0	156.0
	20% ZrO_2	40% ZrO_2
Experimental Elastic Modulus GPa	106.0	131.0
Theoretical Elastic Modulus GPa	110.0	128.0

(after *Frey* and *Mackenzie* 1967)

It was concluded by *Frey* and *Mackenzie* (1967) that the theoretical values for modulus of elasticity could be calculated (by means of *Haskin*'s analysis) and that the experimental data presented indicated a close relationship to the theoretical values. It was further stated that the flexural strength of glass/crystalline composite systems are influenced by the elastic properties of the dispersed phase. As can be seen from the data Table 1 the glass Al_2O_3 composites exhibited a higher moduli of elasticity than the glass/ ZrO_2 materials and it is further indicated that the larger volume fraction of dispersed phase produced a higher mean value for moduli of elasticity. However, as shown from data by *Jones* (1970) in Figure 2 low volume inclusion may not significantly influence the modulus of elasticity of glass/crystalline composites. Samples D, F and G have 5–15% by weight of dispersed alumina, whilst samples H and I have 40–50% by weight of alumina.

Yu. M. Rodichev et al (1977) have made a comparison between the modulus of elasticity data for glassy materials using strain gauge tests in both tension and compression and compared this with data from a dynamic resonance method. It was found that the dynamic elastic modulus of glass materials was on average some 7% higher than the static modulus obtained by means of strain gauge tests. The difference was said to be due to the relaxation processes involved. Although the data recorded for static moduli of elasticity for both compressive and tension tests were found to be not significantly different, a greater variation in the data obtained for the tensile tests was noted. The values obtained for a glass ceramic material were:

Static strain Gauge Method

	GPa	Variation Coefficient
Tension	103	± 4.87
Compression	106	± 2.92

Dynamic Sonic Method

	110	± 0.83

A strain gauge technique was used (*Jones* et al 1972) to obtain values of elastic modulus and critical strain for failure for a range of nine dental ceramic materials at two rates of loading. Using a three point loading slow bend test (0.01 cm/min.) it was found that all materials failed at about 0.10% strain. In contrast a slow impact test (800 cm/min.) gave a higher value of 0.14% strain at failure. The mean elastic modulus values for the different types of porcelains (using a slow bend test 0.1 cm/min.) ranged from 99.5 GPa for an aluminous core material to 56.8 GPa for a low fusing feldspathic material as shown in Figure 2. In addition, samples of fused alumina rod used in construction of all ceramic bridges were also tested for comparison, these samples gave a mean value of 418 GPa. Each specimen was loaded up to approximately two-thirds of its anticipated breaking strength (based upon previously determined strength evaluations) the force was then removed. This procedure was repeated three times and the specimens finally taken to fracture. In each

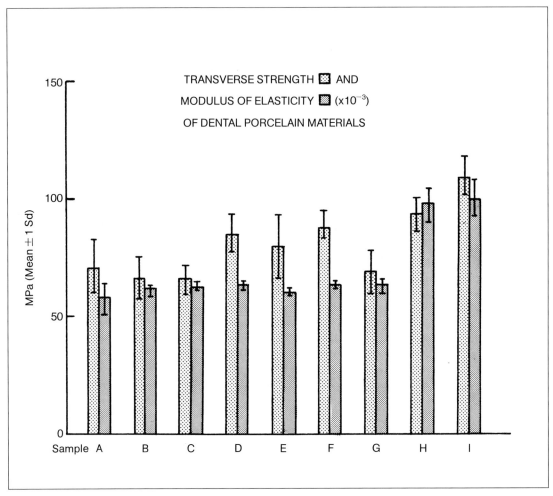

Fig. 2   Transverse strength and modulus of elasticity for dental porcelain materials. Samples D, F, and G have 5–15% by weight of dispersed alumina, whilst samples H and I have 40–50% by weight of alumina.

case the loading, unloading and reloading cycles produced identical results. Dynamic tests were also carried out for five different porcelain materials at slow impact speed of 800 cm/min., this being the estimated maximum speed of chewing (*Jones* et al, 1970). With the dynamic method it was not possible to apply and remove the force as in the case of the slow speed test and only one result could be obtained for each of the fifteen specimens tested. The results for both slow bend and dynamic tests are shown in Table 2 for comparison. The values for the

Table 2   Modulus of Elasticity of Dental Porcelains

(by the strain gauge method)

Samples	Mean Modulus (GPa ± 1 sd)	
	*Slow bend	**Impact
A	57 ± 15	66.5 ± 19
B	61 ± 3.3	75 ± 2.6
C	63 ± 6.3	76 ± 4
G	63 ± 6.3	78 ± 7
I	99.5 ± 8	125 ± 3.1

(After *Jones* et al, 1972)

impact modulus of elasticity ranged from 66.5 GPa for a low fusing feldspathic porcelain up to 125.4 GPa for an aluminous core porcelain with 40–50% alumina present.

Since in practice all dental ceramic materials tend to fail at the same "critical strain" of the order of 0.1%, any increase in strength and also toughness can only be achieved by an increase in the elastic modulus. This concept is illustrated in Figure 3 in which three ceramic materials, all failing at the same "critical strain" have different failure stress and consequently variations in the slope of the elastic modulus.

As can be seen from Figure 3, an increase in strength and toughness can be achieved by increasing the elastic modulus, provided that the strain at fracture remains constant. This was found to be the case with the inclusion of particles of polycrystalline alumina into a feldspathic glassy matrix (*Spinner* and *Tefft* 1961). It was also shown by *Jones* et al (1972) that the inclusion of up to 15% (by weight) of alumina particles in the veneer and body porcelain samples D, F and G illustrated in Figure 2, indicated no significant difference in the elastic modulus as compared to the unmodified glass frit sample E. However, when 40–50% (by weight) of alumina particles are included as in samples H and I of aluminous core porcelain material, it was found that the elastic modulus was significantly increased by approximately 50%. This value is, however, still far below that recorded for samples of sintered polycrystalline alumina rod, which were found to be some six times stiffer than conventional dental porcelain (*Jones* et al, 1972). The theoretical strength values for brittle materials is estimated to be of the order of 1/10 that of the modulus of elasticity. The practical strength of many engineering ceramic materials is in general variable but is of the order of 10 to 150 times smaller than the theoretical value predicted from their elastic moduli. In the case of dental porcelain materials it has been found (*Jones*, 1970) that the practical strength values

* Slow bend tests, three point loading 10:1 span to depth ratio, strain rate 0.01 cm/min.
** Impact, three point loading 10:1 span to depth ratio, strain rate 800 cm/min.
The specimen size used was 25x4x2 mm. Samples A, B and C are feldspathic glassy porcelain. Samples G and I have 15 and 45% by weight of dispersed alumina particles respectively.

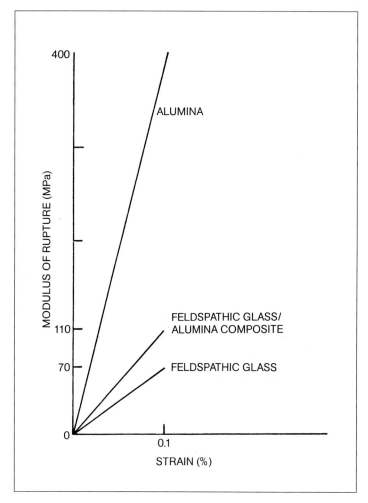

◄

Fig. 3 Three ceramic materials, all failing at the same 'critical strain', but with different failure stresses and consequently variations in the elastic modulus, and toughness.

Fig. 4 A regression analysis plot of modulus of rupture versus modulus of elasticity X10⁻³ for dental porcelain materials. ►

are as much as 100 times smaller than the theoretical values extrapolated from the modulus of elasticity data. Only very fine fibres of such materials as glass, silica or alumina have been produced which have tensile strength values at all close to the theoretical predicted limits.

The bar diagram (Fig. 2) illustrates the relative modulus of elasticity values for a range of dental porcelains, together with the modulus of rupture values. It can be

seen that there is a reasonably close relationship between the fracture strength and the modulus of elasticity which has a value larger by a factor of 1000. Samples H and I in Figure 2 are aluminous (core) porcelains. Samples D, E and F indicated a significant difference between the modulus of rupture and the modulus of elasticity X10⁻³. Samples D and F are feldspathic glass porcelains containing a small percentage of alumina (10–15% by

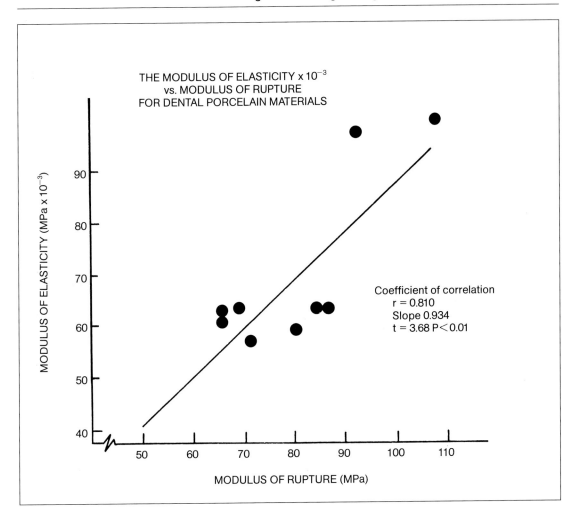

THE MODULUS OF ELASTICITY x 10⁻³
vs. MODULUS OF RUPTURE
FOR DENTAL PORCELAIN MATERIALS

Coefficient of correlation
r = 0.810
Slope 0.934
t = 3.68 P<0.01

weight 10–50 mμ size) as a reinforcing phase within the glassy matrix. Sample E is an experimental synthetic glass of feldspathic composition. It can be assumed in general that the modulus of elasticity of a dental porcelain arises from the bulk texture of the sample. In contrast the maximum stress and critical strain at fracture are limited by the presence of fabricational faults and defects. The effect of small percentages of so called reinforcing phase will be dependent upon the interaction between the matrix glass and the dispersed phase (as discussed on page 117). A regression analysis plot of modulus of rupture versus modulus of elasticity X10⁻³ (Fig. 4) gave a significant correlation (r = 0.810; t = 3.68; P< 0.01). In general we can thus assume that we can extrapolate the modulus of elasticity from the modulus of rupture data with a reasonable degree of accuracy.

Mechanical Properties of Feldspathic Dental Porcelain

In the heterogeneous structure of dental ceramics which may include glass, crystal and fabricated defects, it is inevitable that the mechanical properties will be dominated largely by "texture" than by structure. This will no doubt explain why the strength values of dental porcelain are approximately some $X10^{-2}$ compared to the extrapolated theoretical values. According to *Kingery* (1960), we must have a healthy scepticism for "average" strength values of ceramics, since these values can be affected by temperature, atmosphere, loading rate, microstructure, porosity surface treatment and loading geometry.

The author (*Jones,* 1971) has previously listed twelve factors which may affect the mean and distribution of measured transverse strength values of dental porcelain. These were said to be:

Test Variables

1. number of test specimens,
2. bulk of material under stress,
3. span to depth ratio,
4. ambient test conditions,
5. type, duration (rate) of loading,

Specimen Variables

6. chemical composition of the frit,
7. fabrication, temperature/time of firing or heat treatment,
8. viscosity,
9. crystalline inclusions or precipitations,
10. surface condition,
11. porosity (quantity size-shape), micro-cracks and other fabricational defects,
12. micro-structure, texture, frit mean particle size and distribution, shape of frit particles.

These twelve factors contribute in varying degrees to both the critical stress to cause fracture and to the statistical scatter obtained. Fabricational defects arising from the relatively rapid sintering technique used in conjunction with the fusion of dental frit materials tend to dominate the measured strength values obtained. An accurate and reliable measure of the mean fracture strength of dental ceramic materials under uniaxial stress whilst valuable as a comparison amongst different porcelain materials and fabricational techniques is not, however, a prerequisite for the design of the dental restorative structure, since the bulk and shape of such structures are dictated by desirable clinical criteria and the limitations of space.

The techniques which have been used for the measurement of mechanical strength determinations on dental porcelain materials are varied and diverse. The mode of failure of ceramics and glassy materials will be related to the inherent low tensile strength. Tensile tests although desirable for glassy ceramic materials are very difficult to perform since great care has to be taken to ensure that the gripping of the specimen ends does not damage or pre-stress the test area. Perhaps the most difficult problem, however, is the need to ensure that only tensile stresses are applied to the test sample. The direct tensile testing of industrial glasses in the form of fibres and rods is well established, *Thomas* (1960) and *Symmers* et al (1962) have described tensile testing apparatus. However, such test systems are not suitable for dental ceramic specimens fabricated by realistic and conventional dental procedures.

Jones (1971) has discussed the possible use of a diametral compression or perhaps even a brittle ring test. Such a test would enable specimens having a realistic bulk and shape to be tested. However, the fabrication of specimens for such tests would present considerable problems. The specimens during the firing-sintering process would need to be contained within a platinum foil matrix or some form of mould. The major problem would be the difficulty in controlling the specimen dimensions, shape and surface integrity. However, some workers (*McPhee*, 1977; *Meyer* et al, 1976) have undertaken "diametral" (indirect tensile) compression tests on cylindrical porcelain specimens. Conventional compression tests have also been used (*McLean* and *Hughes*, 1965) to test dental porcelain, although the test presents problems associated with complex frictional and shear stresses across the loaded surfaces.

Considerable research has been carried out recently at the Institute of Strength Problems–Academy of Science U.S.S.R. involving the biaxial compressive strength testing of glassy porcelain materials (*Pisarenko* et al, 1978; *Okhrimenko*, 1976 and 1980; *Poleshko*, 1975; *Kvitka*

and *Dyachkov*, 1980). The materials investigated were mainly electrical porcelains, pyroceramic glasses and various technical glasses. In some cases the specimen cylinders were secured into the recess of a ring on the loading plates by cold setting resin adhesives (*Kvitka* and *Dyachkov*, 1980). A preliminary study of the shear strength of dental porcelain using a direct shear test was undertaken by *Johnston* and *O'Brian* (1978). The data produced is important since an estimate of shear strength based upon other strength values for dental porcelain is not yet established. In spite of the difficulty in obtaining reliable data, it is generally accepted that there is an approximate relationship between tensile, compressive and flexural strength for brittle materials. Generally the values suggest that the compressive strength is some ten times that of the tensile strength whilst the flexural strength (modulus of rupture) is approximately double the tensile value. *Karpilovskii* and *Letskaya* (1979) have evaluated electrical porcelain by means of tensile, compressive and static bending tests and found a linear relationship between the data. It was concluded, however, that the most sensitive test method was the bending test and the least sensitive the compressive test. The data reported indicated that the bending strength was approximately twice that of the tensile strength and some three times less than the compressive strength.

Modulus of Rupture

Because of the difficulties encountered in performing reliable direct tensile tests on materials which exhibit no appreciable plastic deformation, three or four point bending tests are the most commonly used method of testing the strength of glass and ceramic materials. The simple bend test is readily adaptable to various test conditions. Elementary theory predicts that the sample will fail as a result of maximum tensile stresses in the lower curved surface of the loaded beam. The value recorded for this maximum tensile "fibre-stress" at the instant of fracture is therefore in effect a measure of the uniaxial strength of the specimen.

Newnham (1975) has discussed the limitations of the simple theory involved in performing bend tests and has made recommendations and suggested guidelines for the design of the test to minimise deviations from elementary theory. *Newnham* (1975) further detailed the possible deviations of stresses from predicted values due to the effects of shear stresses, local high stresses at loading points and friction at the loading and support points. It was pointed out that friction may cause serious overestimation of the uniaxial strength unless suitable precautions are taken.

Five assumptions which are made in using the simple bending theory were listed by *Newnham* (1975):

1. The elastic deformation will be linear for both tension and compressive stresses up to the point of fracture.
2. Shear stresses in the loaded beam are negligibly small.
3. The test sample is not constrained in the thickness direction in order to prevent through-thickness stresses developing.
4. The support members and load-points are frictionless (the use of glazed test samples will help to minimize friction).
5. There are no local stress concentrations due to contact at the load and support points which may impose couples which tend to constrain the specimen.

It is generally agreed that the four-point bend test is superior to the three-point test since in the former no shear stresses should be present in the central position of the beam, since this is subject to a constant bending moment. In contrast the three-point bending tests may experience shear stresses throughout their length. Constraint due to excessive thickness of the beam may also occur although specimens of practical dimensions will deform in a 'plain stress' mode so that no through-thickness stresses develop (*Newnham,* 1975). Friction at the supports was said by *Newnham* (1975) to develop bending couples opposing the bending movement of samples of silicon nitride, this resulted in bend strength values being some 13 % higher for supports which were fixed as opposed to supports which were set in bearings and free to rotate.

Although much work has been carried out over the years to assess the strength of various dental porcelain materials, a comparison of results reported by different researchers is difficult. There has been considerable variation in the size of specimens, specimen preparation, degree of firing, rate of loading and span to depth ratio. However, modulus of rupture values would seem to range between 28–70 MPa for the different types of feldspathic dental porcelain materials. This rather large range in values may be explained by the test methods and conditions used. Several workers (*Jones,* 1970; *Jones,* 1971; *Milligan,* 1953; *Shevlin,* 1959; *Puluboyarinov,* 1956; *Jones* et al, 1972; *Schonborn,* 1953; *Binns,* 1965) have found that the test conditions affect the determination of mechanical strength of glassy structures.

According to *Milligan* (1953), consistent cross breaking strength values are obtained only when the ratio of span to depth of the test specimen is greater than ten to one. *Shevlin* and *Lindenthal* (1959) also found that breaking strength of ceramics was dependent upon the ratio of span to cross sectional area and the rate of loading. *Puluboyarinov* (1956) discussing the bend strength of ceramics has said that the modulus of rupture values increase with decreasing distance between the specimen supports. This was explained by the fact that the test involves not only pure bending but also involves some partial shearing stresses as emphasized by other workers (*Jones* et al, 1972; *Binns,* 1965). *Schonborn* (1953) also found that tensile and bending strength values of ceramic materials decreased in specimens with increasing cross section and increasing length. However, in spite of these problems *Binns* (1965) and *Newnham* (1975) have concluded that there is considerable agreement that for brittle materials such as ceramics the most satisfactory strength test is a cross breaking strength or modulus of rupture measurement of some sort.

Jones et al (1972) using a modulus of rupture (three-point loading) transverse test investigated some six variables which might have an influence upon the measured strength values. It was concluded that the differences observed in reported strength values by different research workers was likely to be associated with the specimen size, the ratio of span to depth or cross sectional area. A regression analysis plot of mean values for five different feldspathic materials in which the specimens were tested with span to depth ratios of 5:1 and 10:1 is shown in Figure 5. A strong correlation was found (r = 0.921; t = 4.09; P < 0.05) between the data obtained at the two span to depth ratios. It can be seen from the slope of the line that the values for the 10:1 ratio are in general lower. It can also be seen that two different span to depth ratio tests gave the same order of ranking for the five different materials.

This data is in general agreement with the work of *Binns* (1965), who reported that a significant increase in modulus of rupture occurred with span to depth ratios of 4:1 or less. The 5:1 span to depth ratio would seem to be on the border line for the above trend. The maximum shear stress would tend to increase as the distance between the supports decreases.

In view of the difficulty encountered in producing long thin specimens of dental porcelain for transverse testing, it would seem reasonable, based upon the work of *Jones* et al (1972), to recommend a span to depth ratio of 10:1 for a standard test procedure. The use of bulky speci-

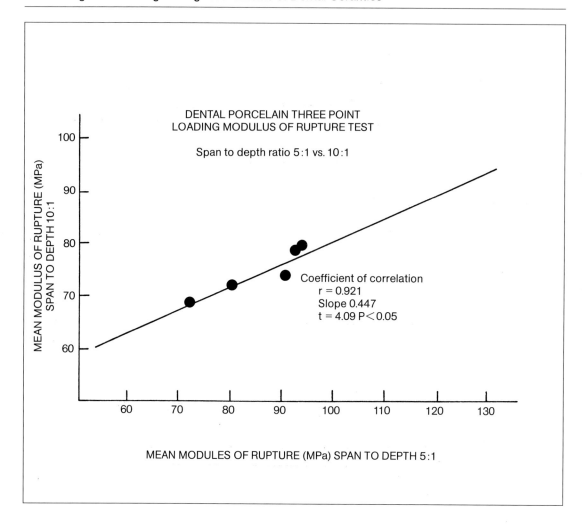

mens with smaller span to depth ratios will tend to give preferentially higher values for modulus of rupture due to the effects of complex shearing and compressive stresses. This is especially true for materials dependent upon bulk texture for strength as compared to those materials which are more dependent upon surface phenomenon. The materials depicted in the regression analysis (Fig. 5) being of the feldspathic glass type would be less dependent upon bulk texture for strength than alumina reinforced materials.

The Effect of Strain Rate upon Stress at Fracture

The fracture strength of dental ceramic materials determined by a modulus of rupture test has been found to be significantly influenced by strain rate (*Jones* et

Fig. 5 A regression analysis plot of mean values of five different feldspathic materials tested for modulus of rupture with a span to depth ratio of 5:1 plotted versus strength values for a 10:1 span to depth ratio.

◀

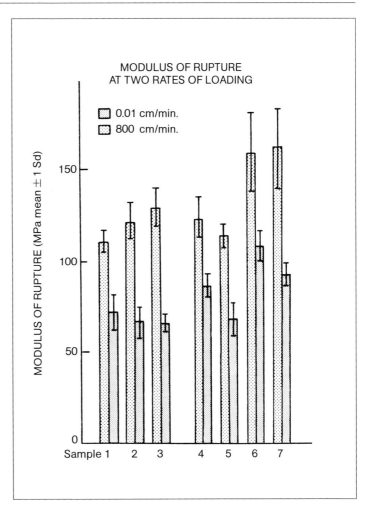

Fig. 6 Modulus of rupture for dental porcelain materials at two rates of loading (0.1 cm/min and 800 cm/min). Samples 1, 2 and 3 are feldspathic glass materials, whilst 4 and 5 are feldspathic glass plus 5–15 % alumina. Samples 6 and 7 contain 40–50 % alumina dispersed phase. ▶

al, 1972). The mean values for modulus of rupture were between 40 and 90 percent higher when the strain rate was increased from 0.1 cm/min. up to 800 cm/min. The mean values ± 1 sd for seven different dental porcelain materials are shown in the bar diagram, Figure 6. It may be seen that a significant difference was obtained for the slow bend test between samples 4 and 5 and between samples 6 and 7; however, such differences were not ob-

tained at the higher strain rate. Samples 1, 2 and 3 are feldspathic glass materials, whilst samples 4 and 5 are feldspathic glass plus 5–15 % dispersed phase of alumina. Samples 6 and 7 contain 40–50 % alumina dispersed phase. A regression analysis plot of the modulus of rupture at two rates of loading is shown in Figure 7. This would suggest that in general we can reasonably predict the impact strength from a slow bend test since

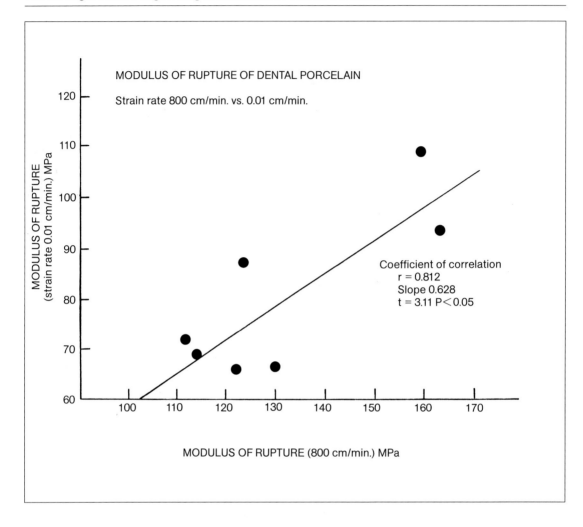

a significant correlation was found (coefficient of correlation 0.812; t = 3.11 P < 0.05). *Vardar* and *Finnie* (1977) have discussed the failure mechanism of brittle solids under very short duration tensile loading tests. The failure mechanism was said to be basically different from prolonged or static loads in which the initiation and propagation of a single inherent flaw may lead to failure. In contrast under short duration loading or impact, many cracks have to initiate and propagate in order to link up and create a fracture surface. The initiation of a large number of cracks no doubt explains the higher force generated for impact fracture.

Fig. 7 A regression analysis plot of the modulus of rupture at two rates of loading for dental porcelain materials. This data would suggest that in general we can reasonably predict the impact strength from the slow bend test.
◄

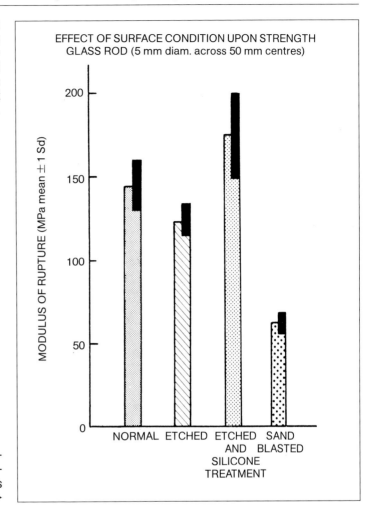

Fig. 8 The effect of surface condition upon the strength of laboratory grade soda-lime-silica glass rod. ▶

Surface and Bulk Texture, the Limiting Factors for Strength

The Surface

The surface of glass-like materials has a predominant effect upon the strength. It is well known that near perfect surfaces on glass materials will produce strength values which are considerably higher. Littleton was quoted by Preston (1933) as saying that "we measure not the strength of glass, but the weakness of its surface". The well known work of Griffith (1920) established that glass contained numerous microscopic flaws and cracks. It was also established that for most glass materials the surface faults would have a greater influence than the internal ones. Later work (Thomas, 1960; Otto and Preston, 1950; Ernsberger, 1962) has considerably improved our understanding of the dependence of the strength of glass upon surface condition. According to *Sugarman* (1967), flaws in the surface of glass of the order of 10A wide would produce substantial stress raisers with consequent lowering of strength. *Ernsberger* (1962) has used an ion exchange technique which he claims identifies the presence of Griffith flaws on the surface of glass. Various workers (*Sugarman,* 1967) have used silicone coating treatments combined with H. F. etching to improve the strength of glass. Some have claimed strength increases of the order of two and a half times that obtained by other toughening methods.

The effect of surface condition upon the strength of laboratory grade soda-lime-silica glass rod is illustrated by the bar diagram in Figure 8. The mean values ±1 sd illustrate that etching followed by a treatment with a silicone surface coating produced a significant recovery in strength. The surface was etched with H.F. solution for 1 second. The catastrophic 50 % reduction in strength for samples which had been sand blasted is also illustrated. The lowering of strength of the glass rod by H. F. etching was considered to be due to the removal of a stressed (compressive layer) produced during fabrication and the sharpening and enlargement of surface faults.

An evaluation of the effect of removal of the surface glaze from two dental feldspathic porcelain materials is illustrated by the bar diagram in Figure 9. It can be seen that etching with H. F. produced a significant reduction (40%) in strength for material A but not for material B. It was found that the silicone treatment significantly improved the strength of material A but not material B. The scatter in strength was lower in the case of the etched material A. This is considered to be due to the increase in the number of likely initiation sites for fracture.

The silicone (chlorosiloxane) treatment of the dental porcelain did not produce the increase in strength which occurred in the case of the glass rod. A possible reason for this could be that the glass rod strength is predominantly dictated by surface condition, whilst in the case of the sintered dental porcelain, strength appears to be limited by other factors, this seems to be particularly so in the case of porcelain sample B in which etching or silicone treatment had little or no effect. In the case of sample A, however, which exhibited a 40% reduction in strength as a result of etching, a significant recovery of some half of this strength loss was achieved by silicone treatment, when the mean strength values came to within 22% of that measured for the normal untreated condition.

One can conclude that dental porcelain frit material A is much more dependent upon surface condition for its strength than material B which relies more upon the bulk texture. A further factor which would influence the relative behaviour of dental porcelain samples A and B would be the relative etch rate which could be influenced by the higher percent of alumina in the frit B. In general it would be true to say that dental porcelain materials because of the method of fabrication would tend to be as much if not more dependent upon bulk texture imperfections rather than surface defects. However,

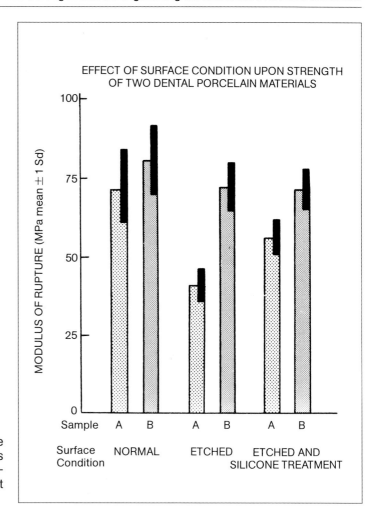

Fig. 9 The effect upon the strength of two dental porcelains i) removing surface glaze by etching with H. F. acid, and ii) treatment with a chlorosiloxaine solution.

one cannot generalize as illustrated by the data shown in Figure 9.

It is well-known that plate glass which has been ground and polished will not withstand such a high stress as sheet glass which has been drawn from the melt and then flame or fire-finished. According to Sugarman (1967), flame or fire-polishing is an established method for restrengthening glass weakened by grinding and it may increase the strength by as much as 400 %.

The mean surface roughness of glazed dental feldspathic porcelain has been measured by Sherrill and O'Brien (1974) as being 0.24 μm, whilst the surface of aluminous porcelain core material was reported as being 0.54 μm. Barghi et al (1975) reported that the as glazed porcelain has a significantly smoother surface than any mechanical polishing agent or technique.

Most dental porcelains are reliant upon a self glazing process to produce the final

101

surface. However, some so called over-glaze frit materials have been available from time to time. The use of such materials in theory should enable the surface defects to be minimized. A study of four different over-glaze frit materials (*Turner et al, 1977*) concluded that their use resulted in a smoother and less pitted surface when compared to the self glazing process. A slight mismatch in the thermal coefficient of expansion of the glaze and the underlying porcelain which will result in a compressive stress at room temperature is necessary. If the glaze has a lower coefficient of thermal expansion than the body porcelain, it will be put under compressive stress on cooling, conversely if the glaze has a higher coefficient of thermal expansion it will be placed into tension. If tensile stresses develop the glaze will tend to craze, only in the case of very substantial stresses will problems occur with failure due to excessive compression or as it is known 'shivering'. *Kingery* (1960) has calculated that acceptable compressive stresses in typical glazes on ceramic ware are of the order of 70 MPa. *McLean* (1977) has pointed out the danger of using an over glaze technique which may result in crazing or shivering, this danger was said to be increased due to the placing of the over-glaze onto an already glazed surface. The thickness of the glaze will also have an influence as well as small changes in composition (which may effect coefficient of thermal expansion) of the surface layers of the glaze which may occur due to diffusion or contamination phenomenon. Crazing has often been observed on ceramic crowns (which have been over-glazed) some years after being in the mouth. The glaze used in such cases may well have made use of sodium in its composition to lower the fusion temperature and viscosity. This would have a marked effect upon increasing the thermal expansion coefficient, thus making it more likely that the glaze would contract more than the underlying porcelain and would thus be placed into tension. The presence of sub-micro-cracks and faults on the surface would in the presence of moisture lead to the possibility of stress corrosion cracking of the glaze which may lead to the observed crazed appearance after a period of several years. *Taylor* (1947) has pointed out that solids under tension are at a higher potential energy and therefore are more susceptible to chemical attack than when stress free. He also predicted that the conditions of the ambient atmosphere would affect the activation energy of the fracture process.

Surface Hardness

It is well known that chemisorbed surface active species can have a significant affect upon the microhardness of certain minerals. The effects of chemical environments on some mechanical behaviours have been generically termed Rebinder effects after the Russian academician who first demonstrated the phenomenon in 1928. A study was made by *Westbrook* and *Jorgensen* (1968) of the effects of absorbed water on the microhardness of different crystal faces of a range of minerals, including oxides, silicates, fluorides, carbides, sulphides and carbonates. It was found that in almost every case the absorbed water caused softening. The theory put forward to explain the so called Rebinder effect is that surface-active environments cause reductions in microhardness as a direct consequence of chemisorption-induced reductions in the surface free energy of the solid. It is suggested that the indentation process involves, in part, the creation of a new surface area at the tip of the indenter, and since the chemisorption results in a reduction in surface energy the indenter can penetrate further for a given load.

Ceramic materials are the hardest and most inert restorative materials used in dentistry. Hardness determinations of natural tooth enamel and dentine have been determined by means of a diamond indentation test by several workers (*Avery* et al, 1961; *Craig* and *Peyton,* 1958; *Jones,* 1970). A comparison of the microhardness of various porcelain frit materials, porcelain teeth, fused silica, quartz and natural tooth are shown in Figure 10. The mean values for the frit samples were based upon 50 indentations per sample whilst the values obtained for the glassy phase of denture teeth were based upon 20 indentations per sample. Little variation in mean hardness values are seen for the porcelain frit materials, the quartz and fused silica by comparison are significantly harder. All of the dental ceramics are significantly harder than natural tooth enamel. No correlation has been found between hardness and other mechanical properties of dental porcelain materials (*Jones,* 1970).

Georoff and *Babcock* (1973) have indicated that they found a linear relationship between the microindentation hardness and the composition of various SiO_2–CaO–Na_2O and SiO_2–Na_2O–Al_2O_3 glasses. Other workers (*EL-Batal* and *Ghoneim,* 1977; *Ainsworth,* 1954; *Roberts,* 1965) have related chemical composition to the microhardness of glass, one such study, (*EL-Batal* and *Ghoneim,* 1977) found that the substitution of monovalent alkali oxides in place of CaO decreased the micro hardness. The effect was greatest in glasses containing Lithia, and least in glasses containing potash, with glasses containing sodium having intermediate values. *Roberts* (1965) found that variations of Al_2O_3, B_2O_3 or SiO_2 within practical limits gave only small changes in hardness for ceramic glaze materials in the system Na_2O–CaO–PbO–Al_2O_3–B_2O_3–SiO_2. The total range of hardness found by *Roberts* was 520–640. This compares with the mean values for dental frit porcelains shown in Figure 10 which ranged from 566 ± 74 up to 612 ± 67. The hardness value for fused silica (silica glass) in Figure 10 is given as 808 ± 145. This in a sense represents the upper limit in hardness for a glass since any substitution of silica by Na_2O or K_2O will disrupt the si–o–si– bonds. Whilst there is no direct relationship between hardness and other mechanical properties it is generally believed that some loose correlation exists between abrasion-scratching and hardness. Since the surface integrity of ceramics and glass play such a significant role in dictating strength a good resistance to abrasion is a necessary ideal. In the case of dental ceramic restorations the presence of the

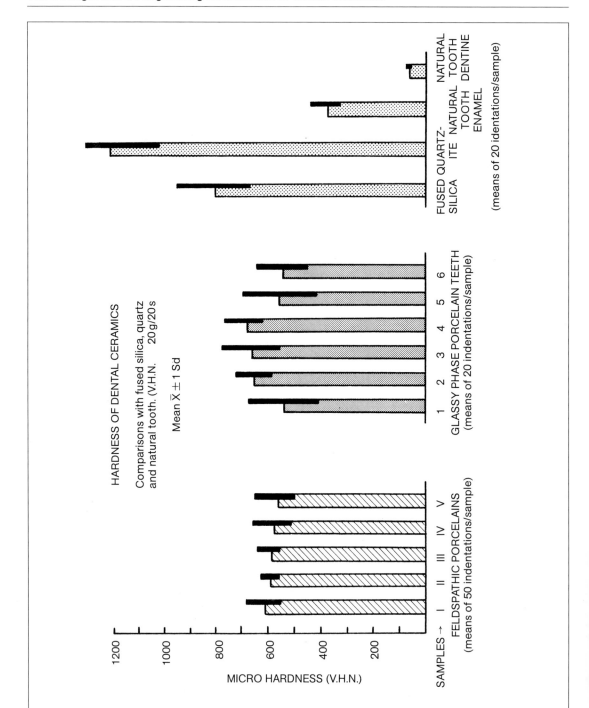

Fig. 10   A comparison of micro-hardness of various porcelain frit materials, porcelain teeth, fused silica, quartz and natural tooth.

original surface glaze will aid in resisting staining or plaque retention.

Bulk Texture

The bulk texture of dental ceramic materials is dominated by the presence of imperfections between the fused interfaces of the original frit particles. It is the presence of these fabricational and textural imperfections, which arise due to incomplete fusion, that limit the strength of dental porcelain materials. The size of these defects are dictated by the size and distribution of the original frit particles. A comparison of strength values for a feldspathic glass frit having large and small particle size has been made by *Jones* and *Wilson* (1975). Although it was found that the sample with the smaller particle size had a mean strength value some 30% higher, this was not significantly different due to the high coefficient of variation.

It would seem reasonable to postulate that any incomplete sintering between particles, or separation of the fused interface due to thermal stresses on cooling, will tend to result in faults or flaws which will limit the strength. It has been postulated by *Jones* and *Wilson* (1975) that the use of smaller frit particles will lead to smaller average flaw size throughout the specimen. However, there may not be a significant increase in the number of such flaws since the smaller sized frit particles will undergo more rapid and efficient sintering. It was suggested that this will not only lead to a reduction in faults due to incomplete fusion between particles, but will also give an improved surface glaze.

Table 3

Material	Modulus of Rupture MPa	Coefficient of Variation
Feldspathic frit 'Small' (S) (mean particle size ~ 5–10 µm)	78	16.3
Feldspathic frit 'Large' (L) (mean particle size ~ 10–50 µm)	55	11.6

The Effect of Porosity upon Strength

Porosity is regarded as a most undesirable feature for any restorative dental material, dental ceramics are no exception in this regard. It is well known that the presence of porosity will affect both the translucency and strength (*Semmelman,* 1957). A further problem is that subsurface porosity may be uncovered by grinding, thus exposing a surface which will accumulate debris and result in plaque accumulation and retention. The modern method of so called vacuum firing has largely overcome the problem of porosity for the sintering of frit materials for producing crowns and fixed units.

It is generally accepted that the major effect of texture upon strength in industrial ceramic and glass materials is due to porosity (*Kingery,* 1960). The presence of

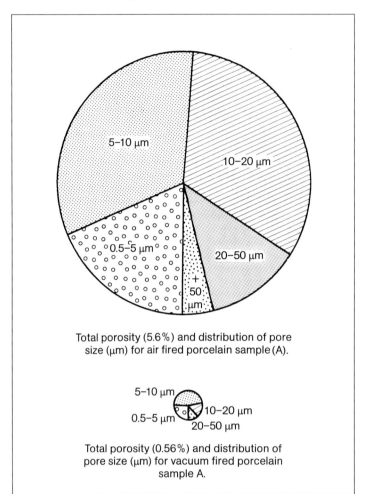

Total porosity (5.6%) and distribution of pore size (μm) for air fired porcelain sample (A).

Total porosity (0.56%) and distribution of pore size (μm) for vacuum fired porcelain sample A.

Fig. 11 Porosity in a dental feldspathic porcelain sample (A). The total porosity is indicated by the relative size of the circle for both air fired and vacuum fired materials. The segments of the circles represent the relative distribution of porosity size. The porosity data was obtained by means of an image analyzing instrument.

pores obviously reduce the total cross sectional area over which the force is applied, and in addition the pores (faults) may act as stress concentrators. Various analytical relationships have been suggested for relating strength to the degree of porosity (*Coble* and *Kingery,* 1956; *Duckworth,* 1953; *Murray* et al, 1960; *Creyke,* 1968). In general it has been claimed and the extrapolated data suggests that strength may increase by as much as 50% when porosity is reduced from 10% down to zero. Such relationships are, however, based upon experiments involving sintered alumina and other pure oxide systems (*Coble* and *Kingery,* 1956). According to *Creyke* (1968), commercial electrical high voltage porcelains have about 4% closed pores in the body, and about 5 to 7% in the glaze. The effect of this porosity was considered to reduce the theoretical strength

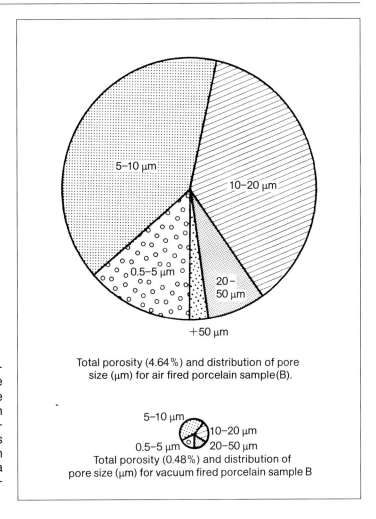

Total porosity (4.64%) and distribution of pore
size (μm) for air fired porcelain sample (B).

5–10 μm
10–20 μm
0.5–5 μm   20–50 μm
Total porosity (0.48%) and distribution of
pore size (μm) for vacuum fired porcelain sample B

Fig.12 Porosity in a dental feld-spathic porcelain sample (B). The total porosity is indicated by the relative size of the circle for both air fired and vacuum fired materials. The segments of the circles represent the relative distribution of porosity size. The porosity data was obtained by means of an image analyzing instrument.

by 25%. *Murray* et al (1958) discussing the effect of low porosity values have suggested that a larger scatter in the strength data for measurements in samples with low porosities, indicates that strength is becoming less dependent upon total porosity and more upon surface defects. It should be noted that the porosity generally found in pure oxide systems is of an irregular shape in contrast to the rather spherical type of poros-

glassy feldspathic dental frit porcelain materials.

An evaluation of porosity in dental porcelain materials was undertaken by *Jones* and *Wilson* (1975) using an image analyzing instrument (Quantiment 'B'). The total porosity measured as a function of cross sectional area of sample is shown for two materials in Figures 11 and 12. The total porosity is indicated by the relative size of the circle, whilst the segments of the

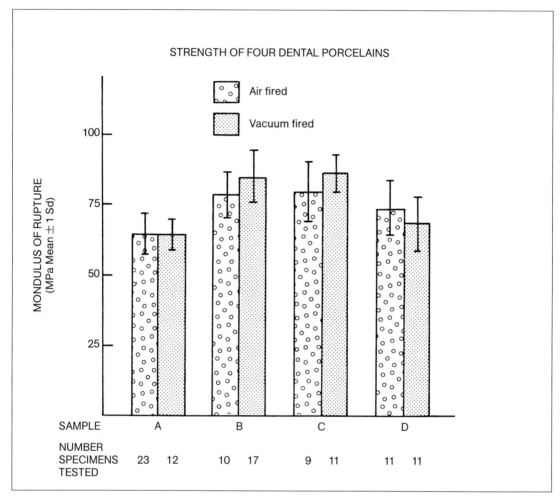

Fig. 13   A comparison of the strength of four samples of dental porcelain. No significant difference is observed for the air fired and vacuum fired materials.

circles represent the relative distribution of porosity size. The two materials shown were fired both in air as well as in reduced pressure (so called vacuum fired). The porosity measurements were made on fractured transverse strength test specimens which had been sectioned to give a representative random view of porosity, and then mounted in resin, ground and polished for optical examination by reflected light. Each value of porosity was based upon five specimens, some thirty fields of view were examined optically for each material involving an area of the order of 400 mm^2 per material. The total number of blow holes counted and measured for each sample ranged from as high as 3000 down to 300.

The dramatic reduction in porosity resulting from the use of 'vacuum' firing can be seen in both cases. Sample A having a total air fired porosity of 5.6% which was reduced to as low as 0.56% for the vacuum fired samples. A similar reduction was observed for sample B which was reduced from 4.6% down to 0.48%. A similar reduction in porosity was also observed for other samples in addition to the two shown in Figures 11 and 12, in all cases the porosity was reduced approximately by a factor of ten.

A comparison of the effects of porosity upon strength of four samples of dental porcelain can be seen in the bar diagram Figure 13. The mean value ± 1 sd are shown for two of the same air fired and vacuum fired samples (A and B) whose porosity is indicated in Figures 11 and 12. The number of specimens tested for each material is also indicated at the base of the bar ranging from 11 up to 23. Samples A and C are veneer porcelains, whilst B and D are so called body porcelains all four materials being used in conjunction with aluminous porcelain systems.

It can clearly be seen that the ten fold reduction in total porosity does not significantly affect the transverse strength of these four materials. This result lends strength to the suggestion that the predominantly spherical porosity found in glassy feldspathic dental porcelains may only act as stress raisers of low power, and thus such porosity will not have such

a catastrophic effect upon strength as in the case of irregular porosity which tends to occur with many pure oxide ceramic systems. *Meyer* et al (1976) have also reported that they found no significant difference in strength for air or vacuum fired dental glassy veneer porcelain materials.

It is possible that irregular shaped porosity may occur more frequently in the alumina/feldspathic (composite) core porcelain materials used for the all ceramic crowns. This is borne out by the data of *McLean* and *Hughes* (1965) who found an inverse relationship between porosity and strength for aluminous core porcelain materials. An analysis by *Jones* (1970) of over 1000 specimens of various types both air and vacuum fired dental porcelain frit materials indicated that there was no significant difference between the coefficient of variation for the air versus the vacuum fired materials. The persistent scatter in data which is related to the imperfections in the samples did not appear to be affected by vacuum firing with its related reduction in total volume of porosity. Other studies have also indicated that there may be a relationship between porosity and strength for alumina reinforced glass composite systems in which the limited amount of glassy phase may result in irregular shaped porosity between alumina particles (*Jones*, 1970; *Jones* et al, 1972; *Harman* and *Wiener*, 1969).

The Action of Moisture on the Fracture of Ceramics

The strength of glass and ceramic materials is strongly influenced by the presence of surface flaws as discussed earlier in this chapter. However, it has also been mentioned that in the case of most dental porcelain materials other fabricational defects within the bulk texture of the material will tend to play a very significant role in controlling the strength of dental porcelain.

It is now well established that the chemical environment may have a greater effect on the strength than the size of the flaws which are on the surface of the glass or ceramic. The time-dependent strength of glass and ceramics often referred to as "static fatigue" is now accepted as being due to the influence of water in moist ambient conditions. It is generally believed that static fatigue results from a stress dependent chemical reaction between water vapour and the surface faults in the glass or ceramic which cause the flaw to grow to critical dimensions which then allows spontaneous crack propagation (*Hasselman* 1968; *Hillig* and *Charles*, 1965; *Gurney* and *Pearson*, 1949; *Southan*, 1975; *Douglas*, 1967; *Fox*, 1979; *Wiederhorn*, 1972; *Ritter*, 1968; *Southan* and *Jorgensen*, 1974; *Wiederhorn*, 1966). According to *Hasselman* (1968), the role of absorbed moisture in static fatigue is that it lowers the energy required at the crack surface to create vacancies at the crack tip, thereby decreasing the apparent activation energy for crack growth. Much of the work on static fatigue is based upon the theoretical model for stress corrosion put forward by *Hillig* and *Charles* (1965) in which the stress accelerated reaction of the glass with water was related to the time to failure at low stress. Various workers (*Gurney* and *Pearson*, 1949; *Southan*, 1975; *Douglas*, 1967; *Fox*, 1979; *Wiederhorn*, 1972; *Ritter*, 1968; *Southan* and *Jorgensen*, 1974; *Wiederhorn*, 1966; *Smothers*, 1958; *Shoemaker*, 1973) have demonstrated that delayed fracture in glass occurs as a result of chemical reaction between the surface of the glass and water vapour. Comparisons of samples tested in moist air and those tested in vacuum dry air have shown in some cases a 33% difference (*Gurney* and *Pearson*, 1949). The reduction in strength due to the presence of water acting within the small surface faults or cracks which causes a stress enhanced chemical reaction is known as static fatigue. The phenomenon is somewhat analogous to stress corrosion cracking in metals in which the conjoint action of a tensile stress and the presence of a corroding medium may work together in crack nucleation and propagation.

Shoemaker (1973) has illustrated how static fatigue may limit the loadbearing capacity of glass. Similar diagramatic representations to those used by *Shoemaker* are applied to the static fatigue of glassy dental porcelain materials and are illustrated in Figures 14–17. It has been shown by *Jones* et al (1972) that various dental porcelain materials are susceptible to rate of loading (Figures 6 and 7). In general, glass materials loaded at a rapid rate require a higher force to fracture. Long-term loading of glass with stresses

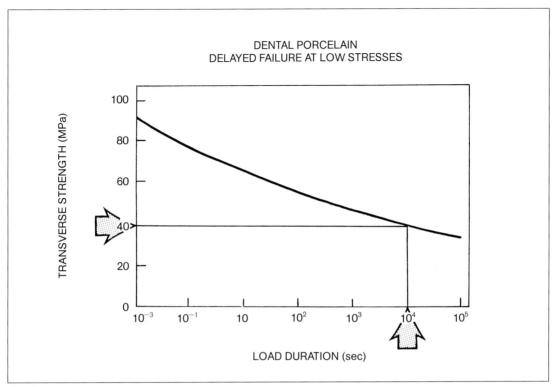

Fig. 14 The time to failure versus stress plot illustrates that the delayed failure of dental porcelain may occur at 40 MPa when loaded for 10^4 seconds, whilst a higher stress would result in failure in a much shorter time.

well below those considered necessary to cause fracture will, however, result in fracture after several hours. An example of this phenomenon is illustrated in Figure 14 in which a dental porcelain may fail at a stress of 40 MPa when loaded for 10^4 seconds whilst the application of higher stresses would result in failure in a much shorter time. In other words, dental porcelain subjected to rapid or short-term loading is stronger than porcelain under slow or long-term loading conditions. In the clinical situation a porcelain crown may fail for no apparent reason after several months or years due to stresses induced during fabrication or at the time of cementation.

The presence of faults or flaws in the surface of the glassy dental porcelain and the presence of either a dry or wet environment together with the effects of dynamic and staticly applied stresses are shown in Figure 15. For a given hypothetical flaw severity X, the dynamic stress Y_1 of 145 MPa might be necessary in order to cause fracture in a dry atmosphere with no chemical action by moisture as indicated at point A, whilst in a wet environ-

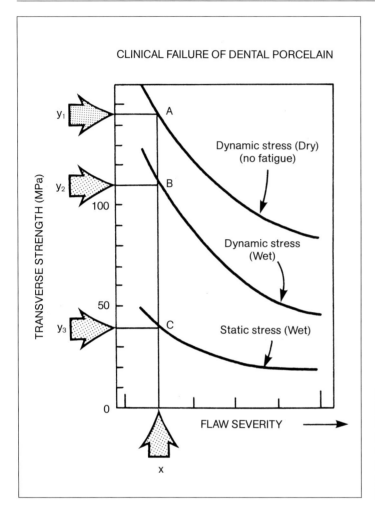

CLINICAL FAILURE OF DENTAL PORCELAIN

TRANSVERSE STRENGTH (MPa)

y_1 A

Dynamic stress (Dry)
(no fatigue)

y_2 B

100

Dynamic stress
(Wet)

50

y_3 C   Static stress (Wet)

0

FLAW SEVERITY ⟶

X

Fig. 15   Failure of dental porcelain may occur for a given hypothetical flaw severity X at a dynamic stress Y, at point A, in dry air, whilst in a moist environment a stress Y 2 would cause fracture at point B, static fatigue failure may occur at a low stress Y 3 at point C.

ment a lower dynamic stress Y_2 such as 110 MPa would be sufficient to cause fracture at B, in contrast the static failure of a similar sample at a stress of Y_3 may cause failure at C to be as low as 40 MPa. Strength values for a given test condition cannot be used for failure predictions for other environmental conditions unless possible differences in slow crack growth behaviour are taken into account. Since in the case of dental ceramics we cannot avoid the moist environment, the values for dry strength may be regarded as being of academic interest only. Figure 16 perhaps illustrates more realistically the dental situation in which dynamic or static stresses operate in a wet environment and the ceramic surfaces will contain variations in the severity of fabricational defects. With a flaw severity of X, failure will occur at Y stress for long-term loading. The never fail zone is suggested by

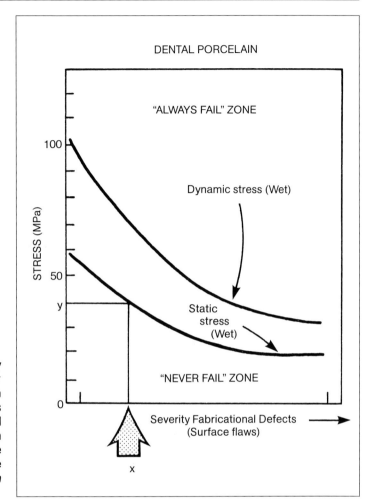

DENTAL PORCELAIN

"ALWAYS FAIL" ZONE

Dynamic stress (Wet)

Static stress (Wet)

STRESS (MPa)

100

50

y

0

"NEVER FAIL" ZONE

Severity Fabricational Defects (Surface flaws)

x

Fig. 16 This diagram realistically illustrates the clinical situation for the failure of dental porcelain, in which dynamic and static stresses operate in a wet environment, and the ceramic surface will contain various fabricational defects. The never fail zone is suggested by the work of *Southan* and *Jorgensen* (1974).

the work of *Southan* and *Jorgensen* (1974) from which it would appear that an endurance 'limit' could exist for dental porcelain. The 'never fail' endurance limit zone would be dependent upon the blunting of faults by chemical action at a stress level which would not cause crack sharpening.

The three-dimensional failure criteria for dental porcelain is illustrated in Figure 17. It can be seen that the stress to cause

failure will be lower as flaw severity increases together with increased times of loading. The susceptibility of dental porcelain to strain rate having been clearly demonstrated by the work of *Jones* et al (1972) and the effect of moisture has been confirmed by the work of *Southan* (1975) and *Sherrill* and *O'Brien* (1974). *Douglas* (1967) has produced data from a study of simple binary glasses which illustrates that reactions between the

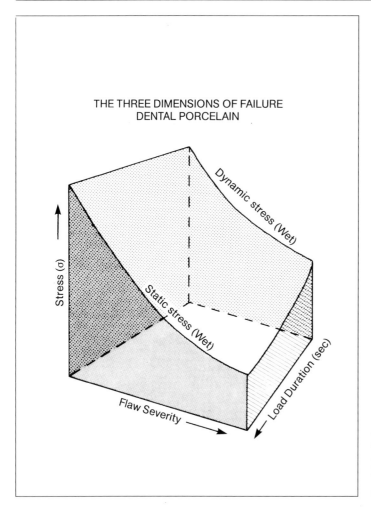

THE THREE DIMENSIONS OF FAILURE
DENTAL PORCELAIN

Fig. 17 The three dimensional failure criteria for dental porcelain. The stress to cause failure will be lower as flaw severity increases together with increased times of loading.

glass and aqueous solutions can occur over a wide range of pH. It was also shown that the reaction products from low pH interaction may result in an even more hostile environment which will lead to even greater decomposition of the glass network structure. It is clear from the work of *Douglas* that reactions occurring within a crack or crevice at the surface of glass could easily provide conditions for a rapid change of pH resulting in a de-composition of the glass within the crevice. *Fox* (1979) has studied the thermodynamic equilibria between water and several glass forming oxides. The results suggest that solution equilibria set up at the surface region of a glass by the dissolution of oxide constituents control the stability of the silica matrix. This was said to be directly related to the static fatigue susceptibility of the glass. *Fox* (1979) pointed out that stannic and titanium oxides are commonly used in industry to coat glass surfaces to increase strength and improve the resistance to static fatigue. It was stated that tin may be present in more complex association with the constituents of glass. SnO_2 and TiO_2 which behave amphoterically in aqueous solutions are said to be considerably less soluble than others. By producing chemical equilibria between the oxide constituents of a glass and water it was concluded that static fatigue could be controlled.

The pH and hence the stability of silica at the crack tip was said to be dependent upon the type of oxides present. It was claimed that resistance to static fatigue can be improved by adjusting the pH at the crack tip to a value which stabilises the silica matrix and considerably reduces the dissociation in aqueous environments. The use of SnO_2 and TiO_2 should be capable of moving the pH at the crack tip into a range in which the silica matrix has a greater chemical stability.

The work of *Douglas* (1967) indicated that alkali ions would be preferentially extracted from glass below pH 9 whilst above pH 9 there would be a dramatic fall in the rate of alkali extraction. It was further indicated by the work of *Douglas* (1967) that preferential removal of the network SiO_2 progressively occurs above pH 9. *Wiederhorn* (1972) has shown that chemical interaction between components of the glass and the reaction products in solution at the crack tip can influence the fracture process. Specimens of glass were fractured whilst immersed in slurries of ground glass to provide a variable hydroxyl ion concentration at the crack tip. The hydroxyl ion concentration of the slurries was found to correlate with crack motion. This finding supported the suggestion that static fatigue is in fact a stress-corrosion process in which the hydroxyl ions play an important role. Crack motion was assumed to result from a stress-corrosion enhanced reaction controlled by the OH^- ion concentration at the crack tip.

Work by *Smothers* (1958) demonstrated that the strength of unglazed industrial feldspathic porcelain test bars in air decreased with increased relative humidity at the time of breaking. It has also been shown (*Shoemaker*, 1973; *Richter* et al, 1980) that delayed fracture of commercial sintered alumina is significantly influenced by normal atmospheric moisture. Other work (*Pearson*, 1956) has shown that both delayed fracture (static fatigue) and dynamic fatigue of sintered alumina were functions of atmospheric attack.

It has been shown that environmental moisture does have an influence upon the fracture strength of dental ceramic materials (*Sherrill* and *O'Brien*, 1974). Specimens of dental porcelain tested by transverse three point loading in the dry condition, were approximately 27% stronger than those tested in water. A similar reduction in strength was said to occur for glassy feldspathic type porcelains as well as aluminous porcelain materials.

Ritter (1968) has discussed the phenomenon of crack sharpening by the synergistic co-acting stress and chemical solution at the crack-tip, and the possible alternative in which the crack could become blunted by chemical action and become balanced at some intermediate stress, less than that required to cause spontaneous crack propagation. *Southan* (1975) has postulated that this phenomenon could account for the existence of a so called endurance limit for dental porcelain.

Southan and *Jorgensen* (1974) subjected disc specimens of dental porcelain to stresses which were well below that which would initially cause fracture. The samples were subjected to short incremental loading tests in the presence of moisture for up to one week. The study was said to confirm the concept of an endurance limit for dental porcelain. The authors expressed concern that this endurance limit could be low enough to be less than the functional loading which might be experienced by a ceramic crown. It was pointed out that any stress above the endurance limit could be harmful; and it was conceivable that subsequent loading which may be nominally below the endurance limit may lead to failure.

Methods of Improving Strength

As discussed previously on page 85 there is a very large differential between the theoretical strength of ceramics and glass and the strength obtained in practice. There are several approaches to the possible strengthening of glass like dental porcelain materials which will allow utilization of a greater proportion of the materials inherent strength. We can produce a relatively flaw free surface and protect it against subsequent damage or defects by fusing it onto a ductile metal substrate. Strengthening can also be achieved by dispersing within the glassy structure a high modulus of elasticity second phase which will reduce flexibility and increase toughness. Other systems could be devised which will aid in the healing of surface defects by incorporation of elements which will blunt cracks during moisture contamination. The creation of a compressive stress at the surface will tend to inhibit crack opening. Some techniques developed to generate compressive stress at the glass surface are temporing, surface crystallization and ion exchange. In dentistry we are limited to those strengthening techniques which do not unduly affect the degree of translucency of the ceramic.

Dispersion Strengthening

The method of dispersion strengthening by incorporating crystalline reinforcing components within a borosilicate feldspathic glass matrix was developed and applied as a dental ceramic technique by *McLean* and *Hughes* (1965). The system made use of a high proportion of polycrystalline alumina particles 45–50% by weight embedded in a feldspathic glass matrix as an inner core for the ceramic crown, surrounded by a semi-translucent outer veneer. This type of dental ceramic has in recent years almost completely replaced the use of traditional feldspathic porcelain as the all porcelain crown material. The outer veneer materials having a lower thermal coefficient of expansion than the aluminous core are therefore placed under compressive stresses on cooling.

The properties of multiphase brittle solids have been studied by several investigators (Frey and Mackenzie, 1967; Jones, 1970 and 1971; McLean and Hughes, 1965; Sherrill and O'Brian, 1974; Jones and Wilson, 1975; Hasselman and Fulrath, 1966; Binns, 1962; Batchelor and Dinsdale, 1961; Harman and Wiener, 1969; Brown and Sorensen, 1979; Selsing, 1961; Dinsdale et al, 1967). The concept of the addition of a second phase to a glass in order to produce a glass-crystal composite in which the relatively high strength and elastic modulus of the crystalline oxide are used to increase toughness and reduce flexibility is well established. Frey and MacKenzie (1967) evaluated the strength and elastic properties of glass with the addition of Al_2O_3 and ZrO_2 as a second phase. Consideration was given to the elastic properties of the components, the relative thermal expansion coefficients, the degree of interfacial bonding between the component phases and the volume fraction of the crystalline phase. The glass-Al_2O_3 composite was found to be stronger than the ZrO_2 formulation. The difference in strength was attributed to the higher elastic modulus of the Al_2O_3 composite.

Jones (1971) has discussed the statistical parameters for the strength of dental porcelain. Transverse tests on over 1000 specimens from different batches and types of dental materials were found to give a 'mean' coefficient of variation value for the differential groups of 12.37, with a standard deviation for this mean of 4.5. On this basis 68% of transverse strength tests on sintered dental porcelain beam specimens should have a coefficient of variation of this order, ranging from 8–16. The various groups of aluminous core dispersion strengthened materials tested were found to generally have a coefficient of variation at the lower end of this range with a mean value of the order of 8.6.

Hasselman and Fulrath (1966) observed the effect of Al_2O_3 inclusions on the modulus of elasticity of a composite, a fracture theory was postulated based upon restricted flaw size as a function of the volume fraction of the dispersed phase. The hypothesis put forward suggested that crystalline dispersions within the glass matrix limit the size of Griffith flaws and thus strengthen the composite. The flaws in glass were said to be considerably larger than those in high strength crystalline ceramics. It was calculated using the Griffith theory that the flaw size in the glass was of the order of 50 µm, whereas in the case of crystalline alumina the flaw size would be only a few microns.

The strength of the glass/alumina composite was said to be a function of the volume fraction of the dispersed phase at low volume fractions, whilst dependent upon both the volume fraction and particle size of the dispersed phase at high volume fractions. Frey and MacKenzie (1967) however, said that a hypothesis which postulates strengthening as a

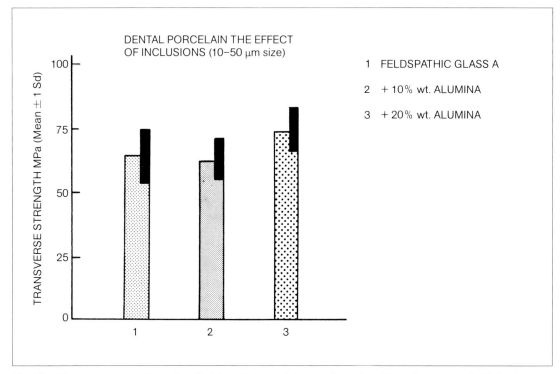

Fig. 18   The transverse strength of feldspathic dental porcelain glass 'A' on its own and with inclusions of 10% and 20% by weight of alumina of 10–50 μm particle size.

result of restricted flaw size was not applicable to the materials in their study.

A feldspathic (electrical) porcelain composition with a second dispersed phase of solid alumina was evaluated by *Batchelor* and *Dinsdale* (1961). The strength of the composite was said to be 50% above that of the matrix porcelain on its own when 25% by weight of alumina phase was present. It was found that both strength and modulus of elasticity progressively increased with the proportion of crystalline phase present. Maximum strength was obtained when alumina was used that had a particle size distribution in which 75% were smaller than 5μm. *Dinsdale* et al (1967) proposed that the system was behaving as a constant strain model, the strain in both glass matrix and in the higher modulus of elasticity filler being of the same order. In such a situation the high modulus elasticity phase will take a higher proportion of the applied stress. This is illustrated in the stress strain diagram figure 3, for alumina, feldspathic glass and alumina/feldspathic glass composite. From the work of *Binns* (1962) using hot pressed discs of glass matrix and alumina, and *Jones* (1970) and

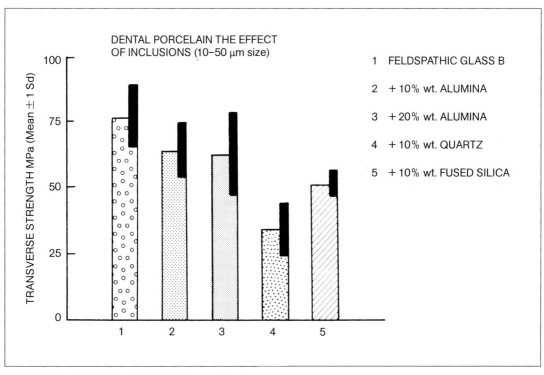

Fig. 19   The transverse strength of a feldspathic dental porcelain glass 'B' on its own and with inclusions of 10% and 20% of alumina, and 10% of quartz and fused silica by weight (10–50 μm particle size).

Jones et al (1972, 1975) using conventional dental systems it would seem that alumina/glass composites behave partly as a constant strain system. The energy to promote crack propagation in such composite systems has been found to be higher than that necessary to cause fracture of the glass matrix material on its own (Jones, 1970).

The effect upon transverse strength of inclusions of small fractions (10 to 20% by weight) of alumina of between 10 and 50 μm particle size dispersed in two different feldspathic glass systems has been studied by Jones (1970) and Jones

et al (1975). Evaluations were made of the effect of inclusions of phases with obvious gross mismatch of coefficients of thermal expansion with the glass matrix, such as quartz and fused silica. The results for inclusions of alumina 10 and 20% by weight within a feldspathic porcelain 'A' matrix are shown in Figure 18. The feldspathic glass 'A' on its own is not significantly different from the composites containing 10 and 20% of alumina as a dispersed phase. It can be seen from the bar diagram, Figure 19, that feldspathic glass 'B' gave values for the alumina/ glass composites which were again not

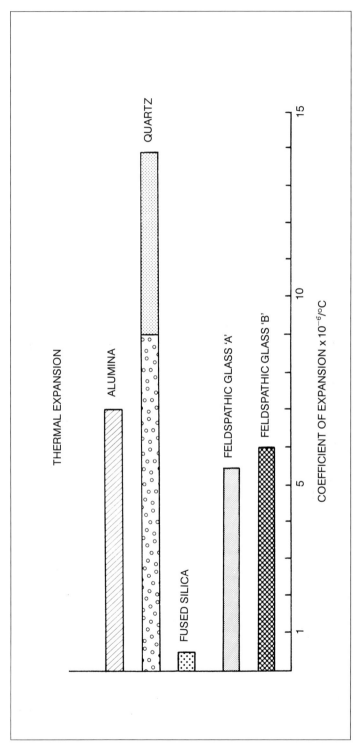

Fig. 20 The bar diagram shows the relative coefficients of thermal expansion for the feldspathic glass and the inclusions shown in Figures 18 and 19.

significantly different from the matrix glass on its own. The feldspathic glass 'B' had a higher viscosity than glass 'A' and would not be expected to provide as good a wetting of the alumina as glass 'A'. It can be seen from the bar diagram, Figure 19, that the inclusion of 10% quartz with its high coefficient of thermal expansion or the fused silica with its low coefficient of thermal expansion both cause a significant reduction in strength compared to the feldspathic glass 'B' on its own. This clearly illustrates the effect of gross mismatch of expansion coefficients upon the strength of glass/solid phase composites.

These findings would seem to support the results of *Hasselman* and *Fulrath* (1966) and the work of *Binns* (1962) in that no increase and even the suggestion of a reduction in strength is possible with low concentrations of solid phase inclusions in a glass matrix. This will be especially true in the case of mismatch of coefficients of thermal expansion and lack of interfacial bonding. The values for the coefficients of expansion of the various phases used are illustrated in the bar diagram, Figure 20. The variation between the values for the feldspathic glass, crystalline quartz and the amorphous silica, largely explains the observed reduction in strength for these composites as shown in Figure 19. In contrast it can be observed that the coefficient of expansion of the alumina phase is only slightly higher than the feldspathic glass 'B' matrix material. This small mismatch in coefficients would result in the matrix glass being placed into compression on cooling, which might be expected to increase

the strength of the glass/alumina composite. However, it would appear that this will only be the case when alumina is present in proportions greater than 20% by weight.

Binns (1962) reported that a glass-Al_2O_3 composite with angular Al_2O_3 particles produced cracking of the matrix glass on cooling in those cases in which the thermal expansion coefficient of the glass was higher than that of the alumina. *Frey* and *MacKenzie* (1967) also found similar cracking occurring for spherical inclusions with the use of a glass matrix having a significantly higher coefficient of thermal expansion than the inclusions. Further work by *Frey* and *MacKenzie* (1967) indicated that two glasses with coefficients one just slightly higher, the other just slightly lower than the alumina did not result in cracking.

The inclusion of alumina with 40–50% by weight into a feldspathic glass has clearly indicated significantly increased strength and modulus of elasticity as illustrated in the bar diagram in Figure 2, samples H and I, and in Figure 6, samples 6 and 7.

The bar diagram in Figure 21 indicates that the relative differences in strength between a feldspathic porcelain and an aluminous core material remain of the same order independent of strain rate. The slow bend test values indicate that the aluminous porcelain is some 20% cent stronger whilst the impact transverse test show it to be 18.4% stronger. The inclusion of alumina into a feldspathic glass in sufficient quantities produces a significant increase in strength and modulus of elasticity. The

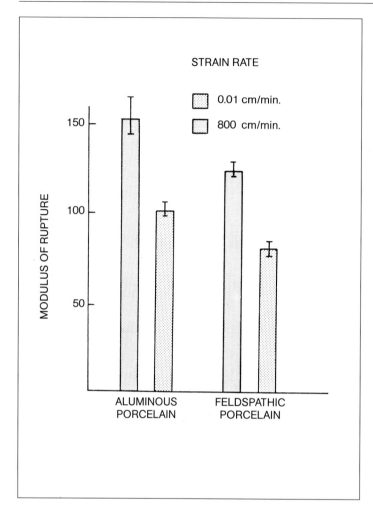

Fig. 21 The relative difference in strength for a feldspathic porcelain, and an aluminous core porcelain at two rates of loading. ◀

Fig. 22 The expression $Y = 4 PL^3/bd^3E$ indicates that the deflection of a beam Y is inversely proportional to the modulus of elasticity E. Where P = load or force, L the length of the beam, b the breadth and d the depth of the beam. As illustrated if the depth of the beam is reduced by 50%, the deflection Y is increased by 8 times. ▼

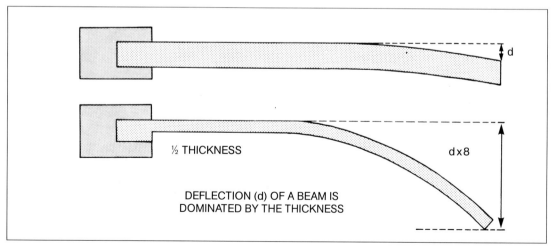

composite of glass and alumina is not only stronger but is also stiffer and therefore tougher than the original glass as illustrated in Figure 3. The aluminous core material should always be used in sufficient thickness when aesthetics permit in order to reduce the flexibility in areas of high stress. As illustrated in Figure 22, the flexibility of a section will be dictated more by thickness than by the modulus of elasticity of the structure. Thus the advantage of the higher modulus of the aluminous core material can only be beneficial if present in sufficient thickness.

Fusion of Ceramics to Metals

The art of sealing metals to glass is very old, and has been part of manufacturing processes for centuries. However, in spite of this, our understanding of the fundamental reasons as to why a glass to metal seal can exist is only partly understood. This is despite the fact that experience of the exact conditions required to optimize the metal to glass bond have been known and practiced for some time. In the fifties and sixties *Pask* and Coworkers (1953–1962) undertook fundamental studies of simple glass-metal systems. By means of sessile contact angle measurements and electron microprobe analysis, much progress was made in the understanding of metal-glass bonding, however, many questions still remain unanswered. *Hull* and *Berger* (1934) wrote almost 50 years ago that the requirements necessary in order to obtain a good glass to metal seal are easily defined:

1. The glass must wet the metal.
2. The stresses resulting from thermal expansion and contraction must not exceed the tensile strength of the glass.

It was further stated that the necessary conditions for fulfilling these requirements could be stated in advance of any evidence.

a) Any glass ('dental porcelain') will wet and adhere to any clean, gas-free metal, provided that the metal is covered with an adherent layer of oxide, and the temperature is raised to the point where this oxide partially dissolves into the glass.

b) Properly annealed seals will be strain-free at all temperatures if, and only if, the coefficients of expansion of glass and metal are the same over the whole temperature range from room temperature up to the annealing point (*Hull* and *Berger,* 1934).

These requirements laid down by *Hull* and *Berger* (1934) almost 50 years ago have stood the test of time very well, our problem, if we have one, is that of attempting to comply with these requirements.

Brecker (1956) reported a significant development with the use of dental ceramics in 1956 when porcelain (glass) was fused to certain gold alloys to form crowns and bridges. *Mathe* (1933) is given credit as one of the earliest to report such systems, although *Fenn*

(1932) actually described a method for casting porcelain onto metal to form a post crown the previous year in 1932. The motivation for fusing porcelain to gold alloys was due to the desire for combining the aesthetics of porcelain and the tensile strength and ductility of the gold alloy. Previous metal to ceramic bonding had been used with iridio platinum and palladium alloys which were difficult to cast (*Brecker, 1956*). Many problems had to be overcome in the development of the gold alloy/ceramic bonding techniques. Some of the early alloys had shortcomings, they were said to be difficult to cast, produced a poor fit and some even caused discolouration of the porcelain. These problems are largely a thing of the past and the technique is now a well established part of dental practice. Many of the original ceramic fused to gold materials soon became obsolete as a result of changes and improvements. In 1964 it was reported that some 35% of all crowns and bridges constructed in the U.S.A. were fabricated from porcelain fused to metal (*Mumford, 1965*). Some seventeen years later the percentage is regarded as being of the order of 95% or above (*Jones, 1982*). The striving to find less expensive substitutes for the gold, palladium, platinum and silver alloys has, however, put further complications in the way of achieving an acceptable bond between a well fitting metal casting and an aesthetic ceramic veneer. A significant proportion of the fixed ceramic fused to metal restorations produced in dentistry are now using base metal alloys.

The Nature of Attachment Forces at the Metal Porcelain Interface

A considerable number of theories have been put forward to explain the mechanism of attachment forces for glass or porcelain-to-metal seals. (*Zackay* et al, 1953; *Mitoff,* 1957; *Fulrath* and *Mitoff,* 1957; *Volpe* et al, 1959; *Cline* et al, 1961; *Hegan* and *Ravitz,* 1961; *Adams* and *Pask,* 1961; *Pask* and *Fulrath,* 1962; *Hull* and *Burger,* 1934; *Aksay* et al, 1974; *Jach* et al, 1980; *Borom* and *Pask,* 1965 and 1966; *Vickery* and *Badinelli,* 1968; *O'Brien* and *Ryge,* 1964 and 1965; *Lavine* and *Custer,* 1966; *Fowkes,* 1962; *Good,* 1966.) One of the main problems is that even in simple glass compositions bonding to simple alloys or even to single metals there is still considerable doubt as to the precise mechanism (*Jach* et al, 1980). It is clear that when we move to more complex glass compositions such as dental porcelain and complex multiphase alloys with between 5 and 8 constituents, a clear understanding of the reactions at the interface may be impossible to achieve.

It is generally accepted that some sort of oxide layer of an unspecified nature must be present for a strong 'bond' to occur. However, some important questions have been raised by *Jach* et al (1980):

1. How thick does the interface layer have to be?

2. Is the layer an oxide of the metal or does it contain modifying cations and only resemble an oxide?

3. Do concentrations change gradually over this interface layer or alternatively are there sharp changes in composition on either side of the interface?

In an attempt to answer some of these questions, *Jach* et al (1980) used Auger Electron Spectroscopy to evaluate a simple sodium disilicate glass and its reaction with iron. It was said that in the system being studied fracture may occur as a result of gross elemental concentration changes occurring. It was found that the 'reaction zone' while decreasing with time and temperature of heating did not vary widely. The thinning down of the reaction zone was said to be due to dissolution of the oxide into the glass. A 'very thin reaction zone' was n e v e r o b - s e r v e d, it was concluded that the iron and glass n e v e r c a m e i n t o c o n t a c t without some sort of intermediate oxide layer.

The break line at which adhesive failure was said to occur was found to coincide with a rapid drop in the Na^+ concentration profile which may affect the apparent strength of the reaction zone. It was speculated that the role of Na^+ may be crucial to our understanding of the strength of the glass/metal bond.

An important series of seven papers was published by *Pask* and Co-workers between 1953 and 1961 in which they studied in depth the fundamental properties of glass to metal bonding and the wetting of metals by molten glass. A reasonable interpretation of the nature of adhesion of glass to metal was made possible by this extensive work. It was said by *Pask* and *Fulrath* (1962) in sum- marizing their eight years work that inter- facial energies, contact angles and the nature of the interface in glass metal seals became much more meaningful when the factors responsible for the interface are interpreted as driving forces, as well as equilibrium forces.

It was pointed out (*Pask* and *Fulrath*, 1962) that the surface of molten glass can easily arrange itself in such a way that it consists essentially of a layer of oxygens whose electrovalence is balanced normally and they are effectively screening (internal) adjoining silicon cations whose co-ordi- nation number remains at 4, this struc- tural arrangement results in a compara- tively low surface energy for the molten glass. In contrast, metals which have a high co-ordination number have much less effective screening of atoms exposed at the surface and as a result exhibit a high surface energy. A low sur- face energy of the liquid glass and a high surface energy of the metal substrate present the ideal situation for wetting and adherence to take place. A liquid and a solid will produce a good interfacial bond if the resultant energy of the system is lower than the sum of the surface energies of the two principal phases involved.

It was found that contact angle measure- ments for glass on metals were often not consistent with the anticipated values based upon theoretical reasoning and calculations (*Volpe* et al, 1959; *Cline* et al, 1961). In such cases the inconsistency was found to be due to changes in the surface energy of the metal as a result of chemisorption. Absorbed carbon as well as water vapour were found to significantly affect the wetting of a metal by a molten glass. It was theorized by *Pask* and *Fulrath* (1962) that a molten glass in contact with an oxidised metal surface attempts to increase its O/Si ratio by dissolving the oxide. A dynamic condition will thus exist with the dissolved oxide diffusing from the molten glass interface into the bulk of the liquid until the liquid glass is saturated with oxide. Because the bonding in the glass and in the oxide are similar in nature, a balance of bonds may exist and chemical bonds across the phase boundary may be maintained (*Pask* and *Fulrath*, 1962). If the liquid is frozen to a glass (super cooled liquid) it is expected that the strong chemical bonds will persist.

Pask and *Fulrath* (1962) further theorised that if all of the available oxide was completely dissolved from the surface of the metal, b e f o r e the glass was saturated with oxide (for its particular composition), the mobility of the molten glass will allow its surface to be rearranged at the interface to produce a minimum energy state consisting essentially of charge satisfied oxygens and well screened silicon atoms. A liquid glass surface which has a large number of charge satisfied oxygens in contact with a metal surface would result in a weak interface bond when cooled to form a solid glass.

The ideal adherence situation has been described by *Pask* and *Fulrath* (1962) as requiring strong chemical bonds at the interface which are characterized by a 'transition layer' of metal atoms exhibiting both metallic and ionic-covalent bonds and adjoining chemically bonded oxygen atoms which are also part of the glass structure. However, the more recent work by *Jach* et al (1980) seems to suggest that this ideal 'very thin transition layer' may not be produced in practice.

Hull and *Burger* (1934) also wrote that if the oxide on a metal surface is thin or the heating prolonged to such an extent that all of the oxide is absorbed, adherence may become weak. It was further stated that if on the other hand the oxide layer is too thick, the adherence of metal oxide to metal will be weak. These authors (*Hull* and *Burger,* 1934) concluded in simple terms that it is evident that the problem of adherence of glass to metal is a problem of oxidation. It was further stated that since the metal oxide represents a phase which is soluble in both metal and glass, it is qualified to act as a 'cement'.

In summary it can be said that the chemical bond theory (*Pask* et al, 1953–1962) at the interface between glass-metal systems requires a balance of bond energies and a continuous electronic structure across the interface which will be attained when equilibrium compositions are present and maintained at the glass-metal interface. The thermodynamic equilibrium occurs when both phases of glass and metal become saturated at the interface with the metal oxide of the lowest valence cation of the substrate metal. It was pointed out that a driving force for a reaction will exist in a glass-metal system if thermodynamic equilibrium is not present (*Boron* and *Pask,* 1965 and 1966).

Predictability of Clinical Failures

Warpeha and *Goodkind* (1976) have stated that unexpected clinical failures still occur with the metal ceramic system used in dentistry. Three of the most common types of failure were said to be cleavage through the porcelain-metal interface, fracture through the opaque or body porcelain, and crazing of the surface of the restoration. In attempting a laboratory evaluation of bond strength between metal and ceramic, we may argue that if a cohesive fracture occurs within the ceramic the bond is of adequate strength, since it exceeds the strength of the porcelain. This may only be true, however, if the test configuration causes the maximum stress to occur at the interface between ceramic and metal.

Research on the metal-ceramic restoration has tended to be overwhelmingly concerned with evaluating the bond strength, however, most bond strength studies have not related to clinical failure. A large number of different test systems have been employed to evaluate the mechanical bond strength of dental porcelain to various alloys. Whilst there is no complete agreement as to the type of test to be used, there is a general agreement that the type of test specimen configuration will significantly affect the data produced. A report from the Council on Dental Materials, Instruments and Equipment of the ADA (1981) has suggested four types of test data for evaluating porcelain-metal compatibility. These comprised:

1. Relative thermal coefficient of expansion measurements of alloy and ceramic.
2. Thermal shock tests to evaluate the maximum temperature differential that a metal/ceramic system can endure.
3. A three point loading bend test for evaluating bond failure.
4. Multiple firing of a long-span bridge to determine if and when a porcelain will crack.

Riley (1977) has summarized bonding of dental porcelain to metals as follows: "A great deal of research will be required to achieve predictability with respect to bond strength. There are many treatment variables, numerous alloys, and little standardization with respect to testing. Even the relative importance of the different bonding forces may vary from one alloy to another. Despite the problems, research efforts must continue so that eventually techniques will become predictable by having a scientific rather than an empirical base."

Thickness and Flexibility

Weiss (1977) has suggested that it is possible to use much thinner copings for base metal alloys for ceramic fused to metal restorations than when using gold alloys. The suggestion was made that the coping section could be reduced from 0.3 mm for a single gold alloy unit down to 0.1 to 0.2 mm for a base metal alloy unit, a reduction in thickness of between 66 and 33%.

It was further suggested that multiple

units could be reduced in thickness by 50 to 60%. However, as discussed on page 86, the limiting factor for dental ceramics is the critical strain of the order of 0.1%. This is equally true whether the ceramic is bonded to a metal or is in the form of an all ceramic restoration. The ease of flexing of the metal substrate (coping framework) will dictate the level of stress necessary to cause fracture of the ceramic veneer.

We can use a simple cantilever beam loaded at its free end to very much over simplify and represent the complex stress-strain behaviour of cast metal copings having different thicknesses. The expression $Y = 4PL^3/bd^3E$ illustrates that the deflection of a beam Y is inversely proportional to the modulus of elasticity E where P = the load or force, L the length of the beam, b the breadth and d the depth of the beam. Thus by doubling the modulus E we can reduce the deflection (Y) of the beam by 50%.

However, as illustrated in Figure 22, if the depth of the beam is reduced by 50%, the deflection Y is increased by eight times. Thus it is clear that the thickness of a section has a much greater effect upon deflection than the materials modulus of elasticity. Assuming the oversimplification of the beam theory applied to a metal coping, the relative thickness of base metal and gold alloy frameworks can be estimated. Using this beam theory it can be calculated that in order to maintain the same deflection when using a material which has double the modulus of elasticity it is only possible to reduce the thickness by some 16%. This means that if a gold alloy coping has a thickness

of 0.3 mm, the thickness can only be reduced by 48 μm when using a base metal alloy having double the modulus of elasticity, without increasing the flexibility of the coping above that of the gold alloy. It must be remembered that thin sections of crowns at the margins may be too flexible and thus unable to prevent the strain exceeding the critical level of 0.1%. Thickness and flexibility in situations of limited space, combined with brittle fracture at 0.1% strain are the dominant features which complicate the use of ceramic materials as substitutes for natural tooth tissue.

Bonding of Ceramics to Tin Plated Platinum Foil

A new ceramic bonded to metal system was developed by *McLean* and *Sced* (1976). Porcelain was fused to a platinum foil matrix by means of an oxidised layer of tin plating. The foil matrix remaining as a permanent part of the finished crown and thus provided a ductile metal at the fitting surface which would prevent crack propagation from faults at the surface of the porcelain. The system developed also made use of aluminous core porcelain which has a fracture strength and modulus of elasticity and therefore toughness greater than conventional porcelain (as discussed on page 116).

The new system of bonded platinum foil has been developed commercially with new aluminous porcelains compatible with the technique (Vita-Pt* Vita-Zahnfabrik, Bad Säckingen, West Germany).

One advantage of this technique is that the tin oxide on the fitting surface of the finished crown can be chemically bonded to the tooth structure by means of polyacrylate type cements.

Holmquist and Pask (1976) made the very important observation that absorbed carbon significantly interferes with the wetting of platinum by glass. The carbon on platinum will greatly decrease the surface energy and will result in a much increased contact angle with molten glass. It was further noted that absorbed carbon was only removed from platinum by oxidation at ambient pressures of $\approx 5 \times 10^{-3}$ to 10^{-1} torr in the range 700–1000°C. It was noted that ordinary vacuum pressures of $\approx 10^{-5}$ torr will not affect any absorbed carbon. The normal use of platinum foil in the traditional build-up of the all ceramic dental crown relies on the easy removal of the porcelain after the final firing schedule. The non adherence of dental porcelain to platinum foil when constructing the traditional all ceramic crown can be largely explained by the fact that platinum will tenaciously retain absorbed carbon. The fact that a good bond can be achieved between platinum and porcelain by means of using a flash coating of tin and then oxidizing the tin, fits in well with the findings of Holmquist and Pask (1976). The platinum surface is unable to become contaminated by carbon due to the oxide film which is subsequently taken into solution by the molten glass.

It has been pointed out by both Parikh (1958) and by Holmquist and Pask (1976) that water vapour will also have an effect upon the wetting of a metal surface by a glass. The surface tension of a soda-lime-silica glass was lowered significantly as a result of the presence of moisture (Parikh, 1958). Holmquist and Pask (1976) found that a humid atmosphere resulted in the glass absorbing water, subsequently the spreading and wetting of the platinum substrate by the glass when molten was greatly increased. Moisture is thus thought to play a significant role in the spreading and wetting by molten glass on the surface of metals. In the dental situation considerable moisture will be present as a result of aqueous solutions used to produce a slurry to build up the frit prior to firing.

The chemisorption of various gasses onto platinum has been studied by Lang et al (1972). The major contaminants on the platinum surfaces were found to be carbon monoxide from the ambient atmosphere and carbon which diffuses from the bulk of the crystal at high temperatures above 700°C. Whilst the chemisorption of hydrocarbons onto a platinum surface requires little or no activation energy, in contrast it has been shown that chemisorption onto a gold surface requires a very much larger activation energy.

It seems that the wettability of platinum by dental porcelain will be very high if we can prevent the platinum surface acting as a contact catalyst for carbon compounds. The tin plating and oxidation technique developed by McLean and Sced (1976) seems to be an excellent method by which to achieve this. It is conceivable that the bond achieved between oxidised platinum foil and dental porcelain could be in large part due to

129

Van der Waals forces and mechanical locking resulting from the close proximity (good wetting) of the platinum foil and the porcelain once the tin oxide has been taken into solution. The good wetting of the platinum foil has been confirmed by the work of Sarkar and Jeansonne (1981), who also suggest that some chemical interaction takes place between the tin oxide and the porcelain phase.

Southan (1977) has discussed the problem of achieving a good adaptation of aluminous core porcelain to the platinum foil. Defects were found at the metal ceramic interface in the adaptation of core porcelain to tin coated platinum foil in aluminous bonded crowns. Southan (1977) suggested that better wetting of the foil might be achieved by covering the tin coated foil with a feldspathic glass identical in composition to the matrix of the core porcelain prior to the build-up of the core material. It has previously been demonstrated by Jones et al (1975) that the densification of aluminous porcelain requires longer firing schedules than are often used in practice.

Poor areas of bonding between the porcelain and surface of the foil could possibly occur due to two factors: 1. contamination by carbonacious products or 2. poor plating of the flash coating of tin.

The fusing of porcelain onto platinum foil rather than using a cast substrate of gold or base alloy may well result in less residual strain within the ceramic veneer on cooling, since the thin foil will be able to adjust itself more readily to locked-in stresses to relieve the strain.

The thickness of the platinum foil will not be sufficient to strengthen by reducing the flexibility to any extent. The main strengthening process will be due to the elimination of microcracks at the surface of the porcelain and protection from moisture contamination of the fitting surface of the cemented porcelain crown which could otherwise cause static fatigue.

Ion Exchange Strengthening

Surface Crowding

A method which has been used to improve the strength of glass-like materials is that which involves the substitution of alkali ions at the surface. The increased strength occurs as a result of compressive stresses. Commercial glass products can be strengthened by as much as ten fold or more when compared to products in the annealed state (Capps et al, 1980). The reported strengthening obtained for dental porcelain materials is however much more modest than this, although still very impressive.

Several researchers have reported strength increases for dental porcelain due to ion exchange techniques. These range from impressive 140% increases reported by Von Breustedt et al (1975) and 47 to 122% by Southan (1970) whilst Pendry and Bradshaw (1971) obtained strength increases of the order of 30 to 90% for a variety of dental porcelain formulations and Jones (1977) reported increases of up to 45% for a feldspathic porcelain.

The chemical strengthening techniques involve placing the fired crown or porcelain specimen into a molten salt, which contains the necessary alkali ions for substitution into the glass matrix structure.

The vast majority of ion exchange strengthening studies of dental porcelain have involved substitution of large potassium ions at temperatures below the strain point for the glassy porcelain. The strengthening process in such cases is understood to be due to the compressive stresses produced by substituting large for small ions which distort or crowd the surface of the silicate network.

However, the main problem with these techniques has been the unrealistic length of time specified for salt bath treatments in order to achieve the increased strength. The work reported by *Von Breustedt* et al (1975) which resulted in 140% strength increases required a 48 hour immersion in a molten potassium nitrate bath. *Dunn* et al (1977) used the same salt bath with times of between one and four hours at a temperature of 400° C. *Southan* (1970) reported treatment times of 19 and 24 hours.

Modified Thermal Expansion of Surface

A different method for obtaining compressive stress at the surface has been reported by *Jones* (1977). This involves much shorter treatment times of only a few minutes, at temperatures above the strain point of the glass. Samples were immersed in a potassium bromide salt which was found to provide successful treatments above the strain point. The aim was to substitute potassium for

sodium ions in the surface of the porcelain. This would result in a lowering of the thermal coefficient of expansion of the outer layers of the sample, and on cooling the surface would be placed into compression.

Glazed specimens of air fired feldspathic porcelain 25 x 4 x 2 mm were immersed into the salt bath at a temperature of 830°C for periods of 5, 12, 20 and 30 minutes. The depth of penetration of potassium ions was determined by micro probe analysis. Control tests were carried out in which samples were given the same thermal treatment as samples in the salt bath. These samples showed no significant variation in strength from the untreated samples. Some samples were also given the salt bath treatment after being etched with 40% hydrofluoric acid for ten seconds.

The modulus of rupture results for the ion exchange treated samples and controls are shown in Table 5. Surface profile measurements of samples taken before and after salt bath treatments gave similar values, suggesting that there was no significant alteration to the surface due to chemical polishing, thus any observed increase in strength could be attributed to the compressive stresses resulting from the ion exchange treatment.

It can be seen from Table 5 that a significant increase in strength was obtained for sample A with treatments in the KBr bath at 830° C for 12, 20 and 30 minutes. The highest mean value being obtained for the 12 minute treatment, this was significantly higher than the strength for the samples treated for 30 minutes.

Table 5   The effect upon strength of ion exchange treatment. (2 x 4 mm specimens across 20 mm centres, rate of strain 0.01 mm/minute)

Material	No. of Specimens	Condition	KBr salt treatment Time at 830°C	Modulus of rupture MPa mean	s.d.	*Depth of penetration of K+ ions
	10	normal	none	57.11	5.44	„
A	7	etched	none	53.3	11.09	„
	7	**etched	none	54.65	9.24	„
	8	normal	5 min.	69.26	13.37	100–200 μm
	7	etched	12 min.	75.04	10.96	N.D.
	7	normal	12 min.	80.40	7.64	250–300 μm
	7	normal	20 min.	75.67	9.38	N.D.
	7	normal	30 min.	68.3	1.98	400–500 μm
	10	normal	none	65.6	10.43	–
B	5	normal	12 min.	72.2	3.61	N.D.
	11	normal	none	80.41	11.66	–
C	6	normal	12 min.	72.7	11.85	N.D.

* determined by a micro probe analysis test.   ** etched plus 12 minutes in air at 830°C.

After *Jones, D. W.* (1977)

Fig. 23   Electron micro probe analysis results, showing the effect of immersion of Type A sintered feldspathic porcelain samples in potassium bromide bath at 830° for different times. The E.M.P.A. results for potassium are given as: – i) electron image (left) and ii) potassium and background scan (right), the length of scan being in each case 540 μm.
(a) Untreated sample.   (c) 12 minute immersion.
(b) 5 minute immersion.   (d) 30 minute immersion.   ▶

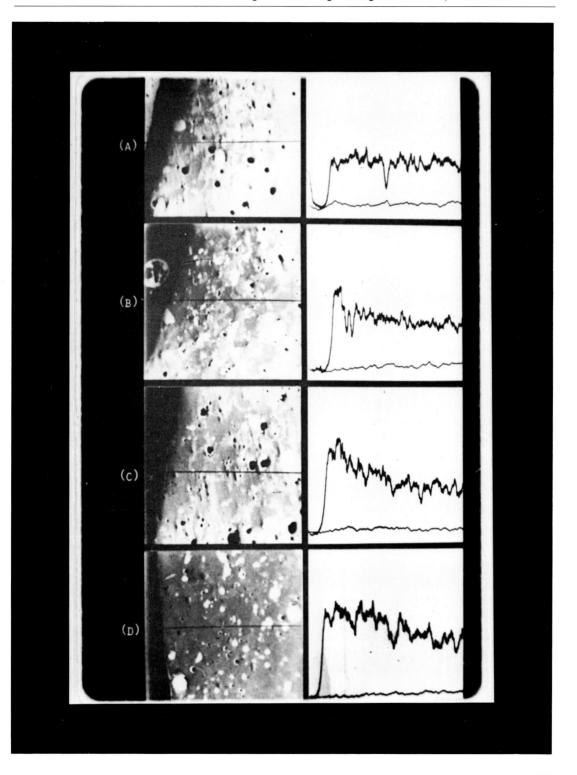

Samples B and C did not show a significant difference in strength following the salt bath treatment.

The modulus of rupture values shown in Table 5 can be contrasted with the electron micro probe analysis data which indicates the distribution of potassium in the glass frit samples. This is shown together with the electron images of the regions concerned and the lines scanned in Figure 24. The electron images indicated the inhomogeneity of the specimens, the white regions and some of the larger circular black regions are porosity; other black regions and different shades of grey indicate variations in composition. The irregularity of potassium scans is attributed to inhomogeneity, the small scale fluctuations being statistical. The background (off peak) x-ray levels are superimposed, these scans being made at a faster speed and have a correspondingly higher relative statistical error.

Electron images and scans for an area of a sample which had received a 30 minute salt bath treatment are shown in Figure 24d. This indicates that the potassium content near to the surface of the specimen had almost doubled, compared with the untreated sample 24a. The penetration of the potassium for the 30 minute treatment had extended to between 400–500 μm. The images and scans for samples which had received 5 and 12 minute salt bath treatments are shown in Figures 24b and 24c respectively. A comparison with the untreated sample 24a indicates that the shorter 5 and 12 minute treatments gave correspondingly smaller penetrations of the order of 100–200 μm and 250–300 μm respectively. It can be seen from this data that the maximum strengthening effect does not necessarily correspond to the maximum depth of penetration of the potassium ions. Indeed it would seem that the optimum penetration to provide the most effective compressive stress is of the order of 250 μm. The highest mean value of 80 MPa occurred following a 12 minute salt bath treatment. This represented a 45% increase in strength over values for the untreated material.

The use of short treatment times for dental porcelains has obvious advantages from a practical standpoint. The treatment temperature used was above the strain point of the porcelain. The strengthening phenomenon occurring with this technique is attributed to a reduction in the coefficient of thermal expansion of the surface layer by replacement of sodium by potassium ions. This change in coefficient of thermal expansion will produce a compressive stress on cooling, since the interior of the sample will undergo a greater contraction thus placing the outer surface skin into compression. Samples B and C which were not as susceptible to the strengthening treatments although they had similar amounts of sodium present. The major differences in composition were due to the amounts of alumina which the three materials contained. Material A had 8.4% alumina, whilst B and C had 14 and 17% respectively. Sample C was in fact significantly stronger than sample A. It is perhaps a sad thought that we can only use ion exchange to strengthen the surface of glassy materials which are already weak in both the chemical and physical sense.

As previously discussed (see page 115) the solubility of glasses in water has been shown to be a function of stress in many cases. The possible leachability of glass which has been subjected to an ion exchange treatment has been studied by *Rothermel* (1967). The solubility of alkali aluminosilicate glasses in water and acids has been shown to be a function of surface stress. Alkali aluminosilicate glasses treated by ion exchange to produce a surface which was in compression were found to be less prone to solubility than glasses which had similar chemical composition at the surface and were in a relatively unstressed state. Samples produced under conditions which resulted in less ion exchange had lower compressive stresses at the surface and were also more soluble.

According to *Rothermel* (1967) when potassium from a salt bath was exchanged for sodium in the glass, leachability was said to be inversely proportional to the percentage of ions exchanged at the surface. The use of an ion exchange strengthening treatment would seem to reduce the possibility of ions leaching from the surface rather than increasing the risk. *Jones* (1977) has suggested that additional work is needed on the development of dental porcelain frit compositions specifically designed to undergo ion exchange treatment.

Olsen (1978) studied the static fatigue behaviour of a glass which had been strengthened by ion exchange. *Ritter* (1970) and *Phillips* (1973) had both concluded that static fatigue should not occur in chemically strengthened glass until residual compressive stresses are overcome by imposed tensile stresses which exceed the static fatigue threshold stress. The time dependent tests conducted by *Olsen* (1978) on chemically strengthened glass were said to suggest a flaw growth mechanism which could be static fatigue.

Summary

Limitations to the Strength of Dental Ceramics

1. The strength of dental ceramics is largely limited by fabricational defects. The major structural features limiting the strength of dental sintered frit materials are the size of the internal and surface flaws which arise due to incomplete fusion. The size of the flaws or defects is dictated by the size and distribution of the original frit particles and the firing time and temperature used. Porosity (up to 5%) of the spherical type in glassy porcelain does not have a major influence upon strength. However, porosity at the interface with a metal substrate could be quite critical, as could porosity of an irregular shape in aluminous porcelains.

2. Dental ceramics have to function in a moist environment which may allow static fatigue to operate and cause the propagation of fractures at relatively low stress levels, due to the stress-enhanced chemical reactions between water and the ceramic at the crack tip.

3. The clinical constraints on the permitted bulk of ceramic material which may be used, are a major limitation for the strength of dental ceramic restorations. A thinner section of ceramic will be much more flexible and thus more easily reach the critical strain of 0.1 %. Thus limited bulk in situations in which only small strains are permitted presents a major problem.

4. One of the major requirements of dental ceramics is the need to produce a translucent aesthetic restoration. This requirement limits the use of stronger crystalline ceramic materials.

Improvements in the Strength of Dental Ceramics

The strength of dental ceramic restorations can be improved by three methods:

1. Limiting the tensile stresses at the surface by fusing the porcelain onto an oxide coated "ductile metal" substrate, which will prevent the tensile stresses propagating cracks from small faults at the fitting surface. This is achieved by fusion to a cast alloy structure or by fusion to tin plated platinum foil.

2. Increasing the modulus of elasticity, strength and toughness by incorporating a high proportion of "crystalline ceramic phase" into the glassy matrix. The dispersed phase will also act to impede the propagation of cracks.

3. Development of compressive stresses at the surface of the ceramic, such that any applied force must first overcome the locked in compressive stress before the surface can be placed into tension. Chemical strengthening ion exchange techniques can produce this effect by either a distortion or crowding effect at the surface, or by a lowering of the coefficient of thermal expansion of the surface layer. In either case the surface layer would be placed into compression on cooling.

As pointed out by *Southan* (1977) "any strengthening process must either remove flaws, stiffen the material or protect its surface from moisture contamination".

References

Adams, R. B. and *Pask, J. A.* (1961): Fundamentals of glass-to-metal bonding; VII. Wettability of iron by molten sodium silicate containing ion oxide. J. Am. Ceram. Soc. 9:44, pp. 430–433.

Ainsworth, L. (1954): The diamond pyramid hardness of glass in relation to the strength and structure of glass. Part I 'An investigation of the D.P.H. test applied to glass'. J. Soc. Glass Technol. 38:479.

Aksay, I. A., Hoge, C. E. and *Pask, J. A.* (1974): Wetting under chemical equilibrium and nonequilibrium conditions. J. Phys. Chem. 12:78, pp. 1178–1183.

Astbury, N. F. (1968): Metals, plastics, ceramics – competition or complementation – The role of ceramics. Met. Mat. and Metallurg. Rev. 2:299.

Avery, J. K., Visser, R. L. and *Knapp, D. E.* (1961): The pattern of mineralization of enamel. J. Dent. Res. 40:1004.

Barghi, N., King, C. J. and *Draughn, R. A. A.* (1975): Study of porcelain surfaces as utilized in fixed prosthodontics. J. Prosthet. Dent. 34:315.

Batchelor, R. W. and *Dinsdale, A.* (1961): Some physical properties of porcelain bodies containing corundum. Trans 7th Int. Ceram. Cong., London, 31.

Binns, D. B. (1962): Some physical properties of two phase crystal-glass solids. Science of Ceramics, Ed. G. Stewart. New York: Academic Press, pp. 315–334.

Binns, D. B. (1965): The testing of alumina ceramics for engineering applications. J. Brit. Ceram. Soc. 2:294.

Borom, M. P. and *Pask, J. A.* (1965): Physical chemistry of glass-metal-interfaces. Paper 81, pp. 11, Proc. VII Int. Glass Cong., Vol. I, Brussels Inst. Nat. du Verre, Charleroi, Belgium.

Borom, M. P. and *Pask, J. A.* (1966): Role of adherence oxides in the development of chemical bonding at glass-metal-interfaces. J. Am. Ceram. Soc. 1:49, pp. 1–6.

Brecker, C. S. (1956): Porcelain baked to gold, a new medium in prosthodontics. J. Prosthet. Dent. 6:801.

Brown, M. H. and *Sorensen, S. E.* (1979): Aluminous porcelain and its role in fixed prosthodontics. J. Prosthet. Dent. 5:42, pp. 507–514.

Capps, W., Schaeffer, H. A., Cronin, D. J. (1980): The effect of striae on the strength of glass. J. Am. Ceram. Soc. 9–10:63, pp. 570–573.

Cline, R. W., Fulrath, R. M. and *Pask, J. A.* (1961): Fundamentals of glass-to-metal bonding; V. Wettability of iron by molten sodium disilicate. J. Am. Ceram. Soc. 9:44, pp. 423–428.

Coble, R. L. and *Kingery, W. D.* (1956): Effect of porosity on physical properties of sintered alumina. J. Amer. Ceram. Soc. 39:377.

Condon, E. V. (1954): Physics of the glassy state, I constitution and structure. Amer. J. Phys. 22:43.

Craig, R. G. and *Peyton, F. A.* (1958): Microhardness of enamel and dentine. J. Dent. Res. 37:661.

Creyke, W. E. C. 1968): Delayed facture of glazed porcelain. Trans. Br. Ceram. Soc. 67:339–365.

Dinsdale, A., Camm, J. and *Wilkinson, W. J.* (1967): Mechanical strength of ceramic tableware. Trans. Br. Ceram. Soc. 66:367.

Douglas, R. W. (1967): Glass technology. J. Brit. Ceram. Soc. 4:75.

Duckworth, W. (1953): Discussions of Ryshkewitch paper by Winston Duckworth. J. Amer. Ceram. Soc. 35:65.

Dunn, B., Levy, M. N. and Reisbick, M. H. (1977): Improving the fracture resistance of dental ceramics. J. Dent. Res. 56:1209.

Eagan, R. J. and Swearengen, J. C. (1978): Effect of composition on the mechanical properties of aluminosilicate and borosilicate glasses. J. Amer. Ceram. Soc. 61:28.

El-Batal, H. A. and Ghoneim, N. A. (1977): Microindentation of glasses: Part I Cabal Glasses. Glass & Ceramic Bulletin 24, 48–59.

Ernsberger, F. M. (1967): Detection of strength-impairing surface flaws in glass. Advances in Glass Technology. New York: Plenum Press. Proc. Roy Soc. A257.

Fenn, B. (1932): Porcelain cast onto metal. Brit. Dent. J. 53:11, 100.

Fowkes, F. K. (1962): Determination of interfacial tension, contact angles and dispersion forces. J. Phys. Chem. 66:382.

Fox, P. G. (1979): The thermodynamic stability of oxides in aqueous solutions and its relevance to static fatigue in silicate glasses. Phys.&Chem. of Glasses 21:161–166.

Frey, W. J. and Mackenzie, J. D. (1961): Mechanical Properties of Selected Glass Crystal Composites. J. Mat. Sci. 2:124–130.

Fulrath, R. M., Mitoff, S. P. and Pask, J. A. (1957): Fundamentals of glass-to-metal bonding; III. Temperature and pressure dependence of wettability of metals by glass. J. Am. Ceram. Soc. 40:8, 269–274.

Georoff, A. N. and Babcock, C. L. (1973): Relation of microindentation hardness to glass composition. J. Amer. Ceram. Soc. 56:97–99.

Good, R. J. (1966): Estimation of surface energies from contact angles. Nature 212:276.

Griffith, A. A. (1920): The phenomenon of rupture and flow in solids. Phil. Trans. Roy. Soc. (London), A 221:163.

Gurney, C. and Pearson, S. (1949): The effect of the surrounding atmosphere on the delayed fracture of glass. Proc. Phys. Soc. B 62:469–476.

Hagan, L. G. and Ravitz, S. F. (1961): Fundamentals of glass-to-metal bonding; VI. Reaction between metallic iron and molten sodium disilicate. J. Am. Ceram. Soc. 44:9, 428–429.

Harman, C. G. and Wiener, I. (1969): Sintered glass, basis composites for porcelain prostheses. IADR Abst., Washington.

Hasselman, D. P. H. (1968): Proposed theory for the static fatigue behaviour of brittle ceramics. Ultra fine grain ceramics, p. 297. New York: Syracuse Univ. Press, Ed. Burke, Reed and Weiss, Proc. 15th Sagamore Army Materials Research Conf.

Hasselman, D. P. H. and Fulrath, R. M. (1966): Proposed fracture theory of a dispersion strengthened glass matrix. J. Am. Ceram. Soc. 49:68–72.

Hillig, W. B. and Charles, R. J. (1965): High Strength Materials. Ed. V. F. Zackey, p. 682. New York: John Wiley.

Hing, P. (1975): Mechanical properties of ceramics (2). Proc. Brit. Ceram. Soc. 25:13–25.

Holmquist, G. A. and Pask, J. A. (1976): Effect of carbon and water on wetting and reactions of B_2O_3 containing glasses on platinum. J. Am. Ceram. Soc. 59:384–386.

Hull, A. W. and Berger, E. E. (1934): Glass to metal seals. Physics 5:12, 384–405.

Jach, J., Joshi, A. and Sengupta, D. (1980): The use of auger spectroscopy in the study of the interface in glass metal seals. Semiconductors and Insulators, 5:111–122.

Johnston, W. M. and O'Brien, W. J. (1978): Shear strength of dental porcelain. J. Dent. Res. 57 Special Issue A 291, Abst. 868.

Jones, D. W. (1970): Dental Refractories and Ceramics. Ph. D. Thesis. University of Birmingham, England.

Jones, D. W. (1971): Ceramics in Dentistry. Dent. Techn. 24:55–60.

Jones, D. W. (1971): Factors influencing test methods and strength of dental porcelain. Trans. and J. Brit. Ceram. Soc. 70, 124.

Jones, D. W. (1971): Statistical Parameters for the strength of dental porcelain. The Dent. Pract. 22:2, 55–57.

Jones, D. W. (1977): Chemical strengthening of three dental porcelain materials. Dental Porcelain, the State of the Art. Ed. H. Ymado. Los Angeles: University of California, p. 342.

Jones, D. W., Jones, P. A. and Wilson, H. J. (1972): The Modulus of Elasticity of Dental Ceramics. Dent. Pract. 22, 170.

Jones, D. W., Jones, P. A. and Wilson, H. J. (1972): The relationship between transverse strength and testing methods for dental ceramics. J. Dent. 1, 85.

Jones, D. W. and Wilson, H. J. (1975): Some Properties of Dental Ceramics. J. Oral Rehab. 2:379–396.

Jones, D. W. (1982): Glass and porcelain as dental restorative materials.Biocompatibility of Dental Restorative Materials, CRC Press.

Jones, D. W. and Wilson, H. J. (1975): Porosity in Dental Ceramics. Brit. Dent. J. 138, 16.

Jones, P. A., Wilson, H. J. and Osborne, J. (1970): Impact properties of dental materials. Brit. Dent. J. 129, 565.

Karpilovskii, L. P. and Letskaya, N. V. (1979): Comparative assessment of methods of determining the strength of electrical porcelain. Glass and Ceramics 35 : 553–555.

Kingery, W. D. (1960): Introduction to Ceramics. London: John Wiley + Sons.

Kvitka, A. L. and Dyachkov, I. I. (1980): Choice of the optimum sample shape for compression testing of brittle materials. Communication 3. Trans. in Strength of Mat. (USA) 11 : 518–520.

Lang, B., Joyner, R. W. and Somorjai, G. A. (1972): Low energy electron diffusion studies of chemisorbed gasses on stepped surfaces of platinum. Surface Sci. 30 : 454–474.

Lavine, M. H. and Custer, F. (1966): Variables affecting the strength of bond between porcelain and gold. J. Dent. Res. 45 : 32–36.

Mathe, Von. D. (1933): Über die Hejemannsche Emailkrone. Dt. Zahnärztl. W. 36 : 1093–1098.

McLean, J. W. and Hughes, H. (1965): The reinforcement of dental porcelain with ceramic oxides. Brit. Dent. J. 119, 251.

McLean, J. W. and Sced, I. R. (1976): The bonded alumina crown I. The bonding of platinum to aluminous dental porcelain using tin oxide coatings. Aust. Dent. J. 21 : 2, 119–127.

McLean, W. J. (1977): Dental Porcelain – the State of the Art 1977. Ed. Yamada. Discussion, Pub. U.C.L.A., p. 66.

McPhee, R. E. (1977): Hot compressed porcelain process of ceramo metal restorations in dental porcelain. Ed. H. Yamada. Dental Porcelain the State of the Art 1977. Pub. U.C.L.A.

Meyer, J. M., O'Brian, W. J. and Yu, C. U. (1976): Sintering of dental porcelain enamels. J. Dent. Res. 55, 696

Milligan, L. H. (1953): Note on modulus of rupture of cylindrical ceramic rods when tested on a short span. J. Am. Ceram. Soc. 36, 159.

Mitoff, S. P. (1957): Fundamentals of glass-to-metal bonding; II. Reactions of tantalum and sodium silicate glass. J. Am. Ceram. Soc. 40 : 4, 118–120.

Mumford, G. (1965): The porcelain fused to metal restoration. Dent. Clin. North Am. 241, 9th (March).

Murray, P., Williams, J. and Livey, D. T. (1958): Mechanical Properties of Non-metallic Brittle Materials. Ed. Walton. Butterworth, London: Butterworth, p. 269.

Newnham, R. C. (1975): Strength tests for brittle materials. Proc. Brit. Ceram. Soc. 25. Mechanical Properties of Ceramics. 2 : 281–293.

O'Brien, W. J. and Ryge, G. (1964): Relation between molecular force calculations and observed strength of enamel-metal-interfaces. J. Am. Ceram. Soc. 47 : 5–8.

O'Brien, W. J. and Ryge, G. (1965): Contact angles of drops of enamel on metal. J. Prosthet. Dent. 15 : 1094–1100.

Okhrimenko, G. M. (1980): Compressive strength of electrical porcelain. Trans. in Strength of Mat. (USA) 11 : 1128–1132.

Okhrimenko, G. M. et al (1976): Stress in the working zone of glass and pyroceramic samples under biaxial compression by the Moire-Band Method. Trans. in Strength of Mat. (USA) 8 : 915–921.

Olsen, C. E. (1978): Static fatigue behaviour in chemically strengthened glass. Symp. on Fract. Mech. of Ceram. Proc. P.A. State Univ., July 27th–29th, 1977, pub. Plenum.

Otto, W. H. and Preston, F. W. (1950): Evidence against oriented structure in glass fibres. J. Soc. Glass Tech. 34, 63.

Parikh, N. M. (1958): Effect of atmosphere on surface tension of glass. J. Amer. Ceram. Soc. 41 : 18–22.

Pask, J. A. and Fulrath, R. M. (1962): Fundamentals of glass-to-metal bonding; VIII. Nature of wetting and adherence. J. Am. Ceram. Soc. 45 : 12, 592–596.

Pearson, S. (1956): Delayed fracture of sintered alumina. Proc. Phys. Soc. (London) 69 : 444B, 1293–1296.

Pendry, N. R. and Bradshaw, W. (1971): Chemical strengthening of dental porcelain. Trans. J. Br. Ceram. Soc. 70, 124.

Phillips, C. J. (1972): Fracture, an advanced treatise. 7, Chapt. 1, Academic Press.

Pisarenko, S., Okhrimenko, G. M. and Rodichev, Yu. M. (1978): Deformation resistance and breaking strength of glass and glass-ceramics under biaxial compression. Trans. Strength of Mater. 9, 993–999.

Poleshko, A. P. (1975): The problem of testing glass in compression. Trans. Strength of Mat. (USA) 7, 1537–1539.

Preston, F. W. (1933): The surface strength of glass and other materials. J. Soc. Glass Tech. 17 : 5–8.

Puluboyarinov, D. N. and Volosevich, G. W. (1956): Trudy Mosk. Khim-tekhnl. Inst. 21, 85.

Report. Council on Dental Materials, Instruments and Equipment of ADA. J. Am. Dent. Ass. 102 : 1, 71–72.

Richie, I. G.(1973): Improved resonant bar techniques for measurement of dynamic elastic moduli and a test of the Timoshenko Beam Theory. J. Sound Vib. 31, 453–468.

Richie, I. G., Rosinger, H. E. and Shillinglaw, A. J. (1974): Measurement of dynamic Young's Modulus during four point bend tests. J. Amer. Ceram. Soc. 57:10, 453–454.

Richter, H., Seidelmann, U. and Soltesz, U. (1980): Slow crack growth and failure prediction for alumina in simulated physiological media. Evaluation of Biomaterials. Ed. G. D. Winter, J. L. Leray, and K. de-Groot, John Wiley & Sons Ltd., Chapter 18, p. 227.

Riley, E. J. (1977): Ceramo-metal restoration – state of the science – symposium on ceramics. Dent. Clin. North Am. 21:4, 669–682.

Ritter, J. E. (1968): Deep submersible vehicles. Glass Indust. Official Publication, Soc. Glass (Dec.), p. 603.

Ritter, J. E. (1970): Static fatigue acid-etched, soda-lime-silica glass rods. Physics and Chem. of glasses, 11:1, 16.

Roberts, W. (1970): The Micro-indentation hardness of glazes. Trans. and J. Brit. Ceram. Soc. 64:33–58 .

Rodichev, Y. M., Okhrimenko, G. M. and Kashtalyan, Yu. A. (1977): Determining Young's Modulus in technical glasses and sitals. Problemy. Prochnosti 6:74–79 .

Rosinger, H. E., Richie, I. G. and Shillinglaw, A. J. (1974): Systemic study of room temperature elastic moduli of silicon carbide. Mater. Sci. Eng. 16, 143.

Rothermel, D. L. (1967): Effects of stress on durability of ion exchange. J. Am. Ceram. Soc. 50, 574.

Sarkar, N. K. and Jeansonne, E. E. (1981): Strengthening mechanism of bonded alumina crowns. J. Prosthet. Dent. 45, 95–102.

Schonborn, H. (1953): Der Einfluß der Versuchsbedingungen auf die Bestimmung der mechanischen Festigkeit des Glases. Silikattechnik, 4, 531.

Selsing, J. (1961): Internal stresses in ceramics. J. Am. Ceram. Soc. 44, 419.

Semmelman, J. O. (1957): A method of measuring porosity of porcelain teeth. J. Dent. Res. 36:945–949.

Sherrill, C. A. and O'Brien, W. J. (1974): Transverse strength of aluminous and feldspathic porcelain. J. Dent. Res. 53, 683.

Shevlin, T. S. and Lindenthal, J. W. (1959): Modulus of rupture versus rate of loading. Am. Ceram. Soc. Bull. 38, 491.

Shoemaker, A. F. (1973): When glass parts fail – look for static fatigue. Mach. Desig. 45:30, 154–158.

Smothers, W. J. (1958): Effect of water on mechanical strength of selected ceramic compositions. J. Amer. Ceram. Soc. 41:11, 440–444.

Southan, D. E. (1970): Strengthening modern dental porcelains by ion exchange. Aust. Dent. J. 15, 507.

Southan, D. E. (1975): Dental Porcelain. Scientific Aspects of Dental Materials. Ed. Von Fraunhofer. Butterworths, p. 277.

Southan, D. E. and Jørgensen, K. D. (1974): The endurance limit of dental porcelain. Aust. Dent. J. 19, 7.

Southan, D. E. (1977): Defects in Porcelain at the Porcelain-to-Metal Interface. Dental Porcelain, the State of the Art, 1977. Ed. H. Yamada. Los Angeles: University of California, p. 143.

Spinner, S. and Tefft, W. E. (1961): Method for Determining Mechanical Resonance Frequencies and for Calculating Elastic Moduli from these Frequencies. Amer. Soc. Test Mater. Proc. 61, 1221–1238.

Sugarman, B. (1967): Strength of Glass. J. Mat. Sci. 2: 275–283.

Symmers, C., Ward, J. B. and Sugarman, B. (1962): Studies of the mechanical strength of glass. Phys. and Chem. of Glasses 3, 76.

Taylor, N. W. (1947): Mechanism of fracture of glass and similar brittle solids. J. Appl. Phys. 18:11, 943–955.

Thomas, W. F. (1960): An Investigation of the factors likely to affect the strength and properties of glass fibres. Phys. and Chem. of Glasses 1, 4.

Turner, K. A., Weinstein, A. B., Eames, W. B. and Price, W. R. (1977): Natural glaze versus overglaze in ceramo-metal restorations. J. Ga. Dent. Ass. 50, 22.

Vardar, O. and Finnie, I. (1977): The prediction of fracture in brittle solids subjected to very short duration tensile stresses. Intern. J. Fract. 13:115–131.

Vickery, R. C. and Badinelli, L. A. (1968): Nature of attachment forces in porcelain-gold systems. J. Dent. Res. 47:5, 683–689.

Volpe, M. L., Fulrath, R. M. and Pask, J. A. (1959): Fundamentals of glass-to-metal bonding; IV. Wettability of gold and platinum by molten sodium disilicate. J. Am. Ceram. Soc. 42:2, 102–106.

Von Breustedt, A., Pahlke, M. and Retmeyers, K. (1975): A new possibility of improving the breaking strength of mineral facets by ion exchange. Stomatol, D.D.R. 25, 235.

Warphea, W. S., Goodkind, R. J. (1976): Design and technique variables affecting fracture resistance of metal-ceramic restorations. J. Prosthet. Dent. 35:3, 291–298.

Warren, B. E. and Biscoe, J. (1938): Fourier analysis of x-ray patterns of soda-silica glass. J. Amer. Ceram. Soc. 21, 259.

Weiss, P. A. (1977): New design parameters, utilizing the properties of nickel chromium superalloys. Dent. Clin. North Am. 21, 769–785.

Westbrook, J. H. and *Jorgensen, P. J.* (1968): "Effects of Water Desorption on Indentation Microhardness Anisotropy in Minerals". American Minerologist, Vol. 53, 1899.

Wiederhorn, S. M. (1966): Effects of environment on the fracture of glass. Environment Sensitive Mechanical Behaviour. Eds. Westwood and Stoloff. Gordon Beach, N.Y.

Wiederhorn, S. M. (1972): A chemical interpretation of static fatigue. J. Amer. Ceram. Soc. 55, 81.

Zachariasen, W. M. (1932): The atomic arrangements in glass. J. Amer. Chem. Soc. 58, 3841.

Zackay, V. F., Mitchell, D. W., Mitoff, S. P. and *Pask, J. A.* (1953): Fundamentals of glass-to-metal bonding; I. Wettability of some group I and group VIII metals by sodium silicate glass. J. Am. Ceram. Soc. 36:3, 84–89.

Panel of Experts: Mr. *David Binns,* Dr. *Derek W. Jones,* Dr. *E. E. Jeansonne,*
Dr. *David Southan,* Dr. *David B. Lynn*

Chairman: Dr. *J. W. McLean*

Participant

Dr. *Jones,* with regard to your comments on the thickness of metal frameworks
did you take into account that the solder joint in fixed partials would be the same
size, therefore stronger and with less probability of fracture. Is that right?

Dr. Jones

No matter what the material is, the thinner the section, the greater the degree of
flexibility. The thickness of base metal alloy (or any other material) has a very
significant effect on flexibility; the modulus of elasticity has much less effect.
Failures in dental porcelain may occur because of the limited flexibility of the
porcelain, with fracture occurring at 0.1 % strain. If the metal substrate allows
greater flexibility, clearly there is a greater chance of porcelain failure. In the case
of aluminous porcelain, a reasonable thickness of porcelain is needed to obtain
the advantage of a realistic reduction in flexibility.

Dr. Miller – question

Despite the improvements in strength of porcelain systems, the flaw mechanism
continues to produce unpredictable failures. Can crack propagation be reduced
or eliminated by framework design? What are we doing to enhance the flaw
mechanism?

Dr. Jones

The limitations in strength are caused by built-in fabrication defects. These
defects cannot be reduced radically in the present system, but the situation may
be improved marginally. Clearly, other stresses, caused by the shape of the
substrate over which the ceramic is being fired, can be reduced as the presence

of the fabrication defects will, in terms of the failure mechanism, be enhanced by residual stresses that are present. If such stress works in the presence of moisture, it will produce static fatigue.

Published works indicate that certain oxides within the glass decrease the chance of static fatigue. For example, the incorporation of tin or some other element into the glass can cause the structure to be less prone to static fatigue. New dental porcelain formulations that are less prone to static fatigue may be derived. As to how flaws at the surface can be minimized, there really is little possibility of doing anything radical. To minimize the flaws, the ceramics would have to be fired to much higher temperatures to produce a very high glaze. This would not be particularly esthetic. To produce clinically realistic surfaces, we probably must accept a high proportion of faults at the surface.

Mr. Binns

Obviously, the framework design is going to have an effect on the crack. There remains the effect of technique, the effect of the application of the porcelain to the metal. When looking at the failure surfaces on bond test specimens, definite evidence of some variation of local adhesion in the properties of the porcelain can be seen at the interface—either more voids due to incomplete wetting or localized failures of adhesion.

Prof. McLean

Probably insufficient work has been done on sintered coatings on metal by employing very highly specialized layers, even much thinner than the current opaques, are used as a primer. Dr. *Southan* has studied the tin-plating system on platinum foil with Vitadur N and it didn't wet the foil very effectively. But as soon as the glass phase was increased, wetting improved. This is an area to which the manufacturers have not paid sufficient attention. We really need much better priming materials before even considering the opaque system.

Dr. Jeansonne

One of the problems of design of frameworks arises when using partially covered crowns or when the pontic is completely covered by porcelain with no free metal surface for cooling effects after it has been fired. I am sure this has a great deal of effect on some of the strengths and strains in the porcelains.

Participant

What are some of the problems associated with repeated firings (three, four, and five times) of porcelain that is formulated to be fused to metal, with regard to color stability, formation of cracks, and effect on strength? Would a crown in the oral cavity, seated with an unglazed occlusal surface after adjustment, be more likely to suffer static fatigue at an accelerated rate than a glazed surface?

Dr. Lynn

When Dr. *McLean* developed the bonded alumina system, he gave me the job of trying to determine the effect of repeated firings on both Vitadur N and VMK 68 porcelains, the latter being a highly fluxed porcelain and the other an aluminous porcelain. When these are fired repeatedly, the light transmission of aluminous porcelain was not affected by up to six repeated firings. Upon repeated firing, the VMK 68 enamels, because they have less of the coloring oxides, did show reduced light transmission.

Mr. Binns

There is a problem with color stability on repeated firings, and this probably depends upon the particular coloring system that is used. An optimum strength is reached in any firing process, whether it is a prolonged or repeated firing, and normally strength decreases thereafter. It should be noted that there is a possible increase in defects after repeated firings in vacuum.

Dr. Jones

Strength, in relation to repeated firings, does reach a point at which there is probably little variation. I think that the possibility of dramatic changes in strength are highly unlikely. The likelihood is that unglazed porcelain is more susceptible to static fatigue because of the much greater proportion of severe faults and flaws at the surface from the grinding process.

Dr. Southan

A glazed surface is not as smooth as it looks; it is deceptive. A glazed surface under high magnification shows a lacework of cracks, and these cracks in themselves can be detrimental. If the surface is ground and left with deep cracks, obviously it is going to be worse. However, the surface can be polished so that it is better than the actual glazed surface.

Dr. Miller

Is there a difference in flaw mechanisms when porcelain is applied to metal in incremental layers and in one–bake techniques?

Prof. McLean

I am absolutely certain that incremental building gives better density because grain boundary porosity is permitted to escape at the surface. This is why the glazed surface, if examined at depths of 20, 50, or 60 μm, has a higher density. I am therefore absolutely against bulk buildup of porcelain. I think you can leave large pores inside that can never be eliminated even under vacuum, and these are potential flaw areas.

Mr. Binns

When a layer of porcelain is applied, in effect, a porous layer is placed on what is virtually a nonporous layer. The inner surface of that layer is restrained from contracting while the surface is not. The surface will contract more. There will be a tendency to crack. The thicker the layer, the more tendency there is for crack formation. Thus, there is a case for applying the thinnest layer possible. The other question is whether you are obtaining perfect wetting and attachment of one surface to the other, and whether you get any discontinuities at the surface. If so, you may obtain the large voids described by Dr. *Miller,* which are difficult to eliminate.

Prof. McLean—written question

Would ultrasonic vibration provide significant improvement to the green porosity of the powder bed? It is claimed that it can reduce shrinkage.

Mr. Binns

In the case of vibration compaction, there is an optimum frequency and this, of course, depends on the powder itself. In the case of porcelain, I don't know whether this would be in the ultrasonic range. I imagine that an opposite effect would arise. If the frequency is higher than the optimum frequency, the compaction can be decreased. It is found to be critical, for example, when nuclear fuel cans are being filled with powder. Closely graded fractions and gap gradings are used. One is vibrated in, and then another, and they can get more than 90% of the theoretical density with three fractions. There, the frequency of the vibrations is critical, but I don't know whether it would be in the case of dental porcelain.

Prof. McLean

Mr. *Hughes* of the Warren Spring Laboratory and I found that only a very low vibration is needed on a slurry of porcelain powder because it is a comparatively coarse material.

Dr. Southan

Large pores in the slurry just will not be eliminated with vacuum firing.

Participant

In reference to comments about dentinoenamels, it was suggested that dentino-opaque could be used. Would the dentino-opaque be a combination of a paint-on opaque with a primary or secondary dentin, and if so, how would the introduction of dentin powders with opaque powder affect the opaque-to-metal-oxide interface?

Mr. Binns

You are describing an intermediate layer with lower opacifier content than the opaque layer. You might consider mixing dentins and opaques or try introducing less opaque in the first place. I don't think it is likely to affect the opaque-to-metal interface. In any case, the normal opaque, would be in contact with the metal, but even if the proportion of opacifiers in the opaque was reduced, this would not affect the interface much.

Participant

Dr. *Binns,* you mentioned the need for further study of rheology of the porcelain and the binding liquids—the type of fluid media that could be incorporated into porcelain to condense it much more easily to high density. What do you foresee as potential materials?

Mr. Binns

We know that you can increase the density of the powder layer by modifying the gradings of the powders to achieve much higher powder densities than in current dental porcelain. The point against this is the limitation to the behavior of the liquid powder slurry. In highly packed powders, there is a tendency for them to become what is known in rheology as dilatant, that is, a very small rearrangement of the powders will make them become very stiff because there is very little play in the free liquid that allows the particles to move around. This could be mitigated if one studies the liquid-powder system as a whole. That behavior can be changed by peptizing the powder surface by the liquids used. I don't know what liquids you would use, but you can change the nature of the liquid-solid surface by changing the ions in the liquid.

Participant

Dr. *Jones*–or perhaps Dr. *Southan*–, what is the effect of ion exchange on surface characterization? Does it preclude the use of extrinsic coloration of restorations?

Dr. Jones

I can't imagine that it would have a pronounced effect on coloration, although *David Southan* has more experience in this from a clinical viewpoint. It has been shown quite clearly that ion-exchanged glasses are less soluble and therefore less prone to static fatigue than materials having the same chemical composition at the surface. I think we certainly have a more stable surface chemically. I don't know that it should affect the color significantly.

There does not appear to be any significant variation in surface topography produced by ion exchange, that is, no chemical polishing of the surface or any change in the surface texture by any appreciable amount. But obviously, if you are using ion exchange, which is based upon modification of thermal expansion using salt bath treatments above the strain point, there is a greater danger of changing the surface texture.

Dr. Southan

Ion exchange by crowding the surface must be done after all other firing has been completed and after all characterizing with the surface colorants and pigments has been completed. The crown will be weakened by as much as it might be strengthened if it is fired after it has been chemically treated, because the crowded ions will migrate lower in the surface and create a tensile surface. Characterizing in the form of slight grinding or the like has minimal effects on the crown.

The use of extrinsic coloration depends on the composition of the frit supporting the pigment in the addition. It could be better; it could be worse. It's an unknown quantity, as far as I'm concerned. But when we know what is in the frit–what network-modifying ions are in the frit–then we could answer that question.

A way to approach this sort of thing might be to think of using a bath containing a salt with an ion much larger than sodium or potassium, e.g., cesium. This could overcome the problem. But without knowing what the frit contained, that is to say the proportion of sodium to potassium ions contained in frit, I can't answer. If you would like a personal view, I think it would have very little effect.

Participant

Dr. *Binns,* you refer to the "pinch effect" as a possible defect of the Shell-Nielsen shear test. If there is a significant difference between the metal substructure and porcelain, there is no escape—in any bond test because the residual shear stress at the interface also exists in the true shear stress test. As to interatomic strength, there is no effect of superimposed pressure on measuring pure interatomic strength. However, the bond strength is not that of interatomic forces but a measure of weaknesses from *Griffith* cracks, etc. Here, the residual shear stress owing to mismatch is far more serious than the normal residual stress effect.

Mr. Binns

Obviously the shear stress is something that cannot be avoided anyway, but there is an extra effect where the metal is completely enclosed by the porcelain, which is the effect of radial stresses on the adhesion between these two components. You might, for example, have a measurable bond strength with no bonding at all.

Participant

When fractures appear, what are the realistic methods to be used to produce a successful, permanent healing rather than just apparent healing to avoid delayed fracture? When crowns have been in the mouth for a period of time and need to be fired again, what would be the best method to avoid gas bubble formation?

Prof. McLean

If ceramic work is left in the mouth even for a trial period, it picks up plaque—probably proteinaceous debris—and when refired there is great risk of gassing. You cannot avoid this except by re-grinding the surface and re-glazing.

Dr. Jones

In answer to the first part of the question.
The possibility exists of having a balance between the corrosion at the crack tip and the stress which is present. Instead of these two phenomena acting conjointly to propagate the crack, there is the possibility, if we can in some way control the pH at the crack tip (e.g., by having suitable oxides present), to blunt the crack rather than to sharpen it by the corrosion process. Variations in composition may be able to achieve this.

To avoid the presence of bubbles in firing subsequent to the crown being placed in the mouth, I suggest a thorough cleaning in an ultrasonic bath with the appropriate cleaning agents. The carbonaceous products will not be burned off much below 500° C. Deposition of proteinaceous debris occurs as soon as the crown is placed into the mouth because the clean ceramic has a relatively high surface energy and readily attracts proteinaceous material.

Mr. Binns

With low fusing porcelain, when first firing it, all contaminants must be removed before the porcelain seals. When a restoration is being refired, all carbonaceous matter must be eliminated before there is a chance that the porcelain will seal over it. I wonder whether there is a possibility of a temperature hold at an intermediate temperature to assure this?

Dr. Jones

It should be possible. We should be able to burn off the carbon before fusion of the glassy phase seals over the contamination. Maybe a holding temperature just below 500° C might be appropriate for a suitable period of time.

Participant

Can pure aluminous oxide as a base material have high translucency and transparency?

Prof. McLean

Yes. G. E. C., for example, make one in the United States called Lucalox. They add magnesium oxide to form a spinel and slow grain growth, thus allowing pores to escape readily.

Participant

Is there a significant strength difference in firing of Vitadur N core for either 10 minutes or 30 minutes? Does this heat soak apply to bonded alumina crowns?

Dr. Jones

Yes, very definitely. There is no question that underfiring of any of these core materials is one of the problems that has not really been understood by many technicians. These porcelain materials must be fired much longer than most manufacturers recommend. Certainly 15 to 20 minutes would considerably improve the strength.

Participant

Dr. *Binns*, how many porcelains increase in expansion with subsequent firing? Is this body and/or opaque porcelain? How is this measured? Some data show inconsistencies between opaques and body porcelains and great differences between different brands.

Mr. Binns

We made specimens of the porcelains and measured thermal expansion; we reheated them and remeasured them. Variations in coefficient, of +1.5 to −1.7 x 10^{-6} were recorded. There is really no consistency. It must be a function of the stability of the Leucite-glass system at the normal firing temperature. With some materials, after 5–10 firings, a plateau may be reached at which there is no further change. Stability has been reached.

A Clinician's Interpretation of Tooth Preparation and the Design of Metal Substructures for Metal-Ceramic Restorations

Lloyd Miller

Tooth Preparation

Probably no other clinical procedure in fixed prosthodontics reveals to the trained observer the care, skill, and judgment used by a dentist than the quality of tooth preparation. This irreversible step in a complex series of procedures to restore teeth permits very little deviation from sound objectives. These objectives are:

1. Retention and resistance form;
2. Adequate reduction for restorative material;
3. Respect for tooth vitality;
4. Preservation of healthy periodontium;
5. Linearity of margin;
6. Ease in completion.

All of these objectives are governed by the mental stress and concentration required to produce them. Consider the first five as concentration factors. If all five are required at any stage, the stress level is high; reducing the number at any particular phase will minimize stress and improve ease in completion. Stress control in tooth preparation is an important

psychological objective, particularly for the operator. A high level of eye/hand coordination and skills enhances these desirable objectives.

Two of the most common failures measured in terms of clinical observation of completed intraoral restorations are inadequate space for metal and veneering materials (*Tylman*, 1970) and damage to the periodontal tissues (*Goldstein*, 1976). Bulky overcontoured porcelain veneers often reflect unskilled tooth preparation and, when compounded with unimaginative laboratory work, produce restorations recognized by even lay people as being too "fat" or too "big." Numerous means of measuring the success of restorative procedures remain controversial: form, composition, color, function, occlusion, longevity, and appearance. But the common denominator for all continues to be well accepted: the periodontal tissues must exhibit health. *Glickman* (1964) states that every dental restoration has a periodontal dimension: "in the final analysis, the periodontium is the ultimate testing ground of all restorative procedures."

A Logical Approach to Sequential Tooth Preparation

Effective tooth preparation requires the highest level of care, skill, judgment, and concentration that a dentist can offer. A logical approach should use definite stages in preparation and can dramatically improve reproducibility in technique. These are:

1. Depth guide channels;
2. Gross reduction;
3. Establishing margins;
4. Refinement.

The first two actions are supragingival; they should occupy less time than subgingival preparation (*Amsterdam*, 1974). Stress control in operative procedures is an important element in tooth reduction and will be evaluated as techniques are discussed. Division of operative procedure into supragingival and subgingival rationalizes the approach and also concentrates the operator's mind on the periodontium. Visualization of the completed geometric form at every step directs the operator in an orderly manner. *Contino* describes visualization by stating that "within the form of every unprepared tooth lies the perfect preparation."*

Depth Guide Channels

The purpose of depth guide channels is to establish an even depth cut in *enamel* surfaces. These measuring troughs should *not* be placed in root structure, even when roots are supragingival. The essentials are:

1. The depth cuts invade slightly beyond the dentoenamel junction.
2. The channels parallel the contour of the external surface.
3. Contact with the gingival tissues is avoided.
4. The channels restrict abrasion of adjacent teeth.

The depth cut tells you where you started and where you will finish at the very beginning of the procedures, and thus provides strategic references for meeting the six objectives in tooth preparation.
Instrumentation–the cutting tool of choice is a round diamond stone with a known diameter of about 2.0 mm., as introduced by *Stein* (Fig. 1).* This is a stress reducer instrument because the profile of the cut will always be the same regardless of the position of the handpiece and therefore the eye/hand coordination requirements are minimal. *The known dimension of every cutting tool is critical to the technique.* Pulp exposure can be avoided by observing the depth of the cutting tool in enamel (Figs. 2 and 3).
Other types of cutting tool configurations are useful. *McLean* (1979) recommends removing half the tooth at a time, leaving the remaining half as a guide. *Preston*

---

* Contino, R. Pasadena, CA (Personal communication, Jan. 1982).

* Stein, R. S. Boston, MA (Personal communication, Jan. 1982).

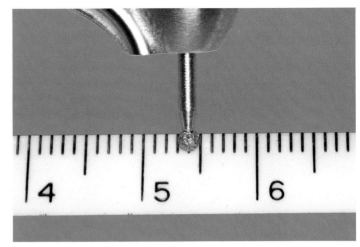

Fig. 1   Measurement of the depth guide diamond for predictable accuracy.

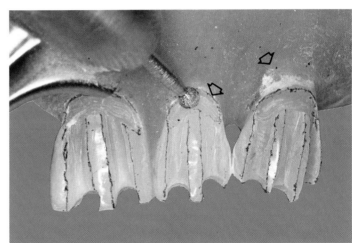

Fig. 2   Model   demonstrating channels placed in enamel and supragingival.

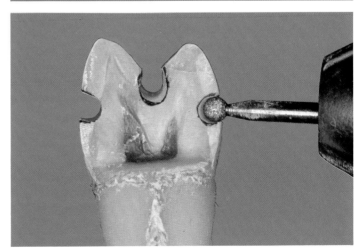

Fig. 3   Sectioned bicuspid showing relation of internal structure to guide channels.

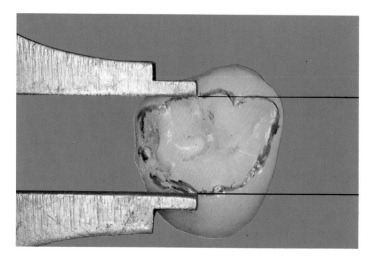

Fig. 4   The occlusal table is smaller than the bucco lingual width of the tooth.

(1977) prefers a "gauging groove" with a 170L burr. The important criteria are: (1) know the diameter of the cutting tool, and (2) leave uncut tooth structure in strategic areas to act as guides for determining the final size and form of the preparation.

Cooling.   In the hands of most operators, using copious amounts of water during vital tooth preparation is more likely to contribute to the inflammation-free status of the tooth than dry cutting. Additional spray from the water syringe by the dental assistant is effective insurance for coolant control (*Brown* et al, 1978).

Patient Safety.   Protective light weight plastic safety glasses are highly recommended for protection of the patient's eyes from the debris and bacteria of grinding (Palermo Sales, Co. Inc., Stratford, CT 06497).

Gross Reduction

The purpose of gross reduction is to remove remaining enamel and establish crude supragingival form with essentials of retention and resistance form. In addition, reduction of dentine to provide further space for restorative materials is normal when using cosmetic materials.

Instrumentation

Posterior.   An elliptical diamond is employed to shorten the occlusal of posteriors. This permits the use of shorter diamonds for the reduction of the remaining vertical walls. Improved concentric cutting and better cooling by water spray is thus achieved. The elliptical diamond is also useful for ensuring correct occlusal table width at this stage. Two single movements, buccal and lingual on posterior teeth, reduce the now wider occlusal table to its proper dimension (Figs. 4 to 7).

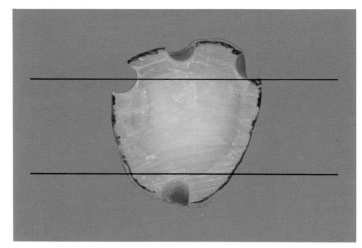

Fig. 5 Removing the occlusal enamel greatly broadens the occlusal table.

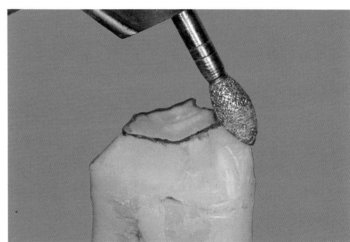

Fig. 6 Reduction of buccal and lingual enamel is simplified by the clear visibility of the dento enamel junction. The role of tooth preparation in form, function, and esthetics is beginning to emerge.

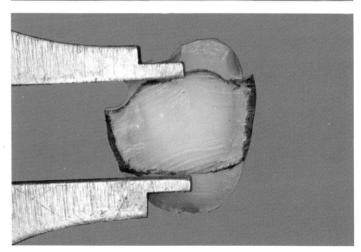

Fig. 7 The occlusal width is now programmed.

157

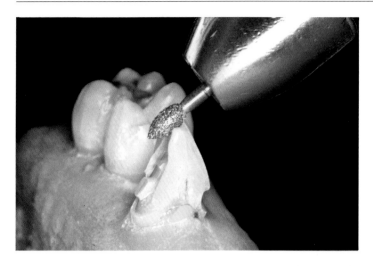

Fig. 8   The proper angulation for incisal table reduction. The same instrument removes lingual enamel.

Anterior. The reduction of length and lingual surfaces is rapid and efficient with the use of an elliptical tool. Its 2.0 mm. diameter facilitates visualization (Fig. 8).

Axial Walls

Posterior. The shortened teeth expose the dentoenamel junction and the residual islands of enamel present clearly defined dentinal walls. The proper cutting tool, namely, a tapered diamond round or square end, removes the remaining enamel (Fig. 9). At least two tangential confluent cuts are required on buccal and lingual surfaces. This produces even reduction of enamel conforming to the former external surfaces (Fig. 10). The proximal cuts are normally directed by holding the cutting tool parallel to the long axis of the tooth–the tapered diamond produces the proper angle.

The requirements of resistance and retention form often demand further alterations (*Gilboe* and *Teteruck,* 1974). Proper tooth preparation and a subsequent restoration should not permit rotation of a crown, as shown in Figures 11 and 12. Vertical rotation and subsequent tension in the cement may lead to loosening of the crowns. Alterations in geometry as shown in Figures 13 and 14 improve resistance and retention.

Anterior. A narrower tapered diamond is often required to avoid abrading adjacent teeth for proximal preparation. A lingual shoulder completes good retention on four sides of the tooth (Fig. 15). A chamfer may be substituted for the shoulder design.

Periodontal demands are avoided entirely by keeping all reduction at this stage supragingival. The visualization, stress control, and access are all improved if gingival contact is carefully avoided. The operator should be aggres-

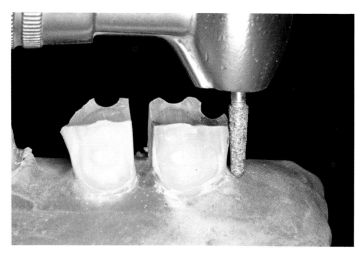

Fig. 9 Establishing early resistance and retention form by removing islands of remaining enamel with a tapered diamond.

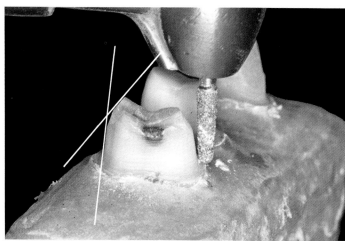

Fig. 10 Tangential lines demonstrate the necessary positions of cutting tools.

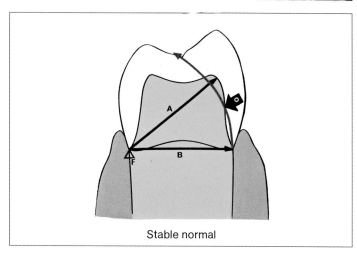

Stable normal

Fig. 11 Crown rotation is controlled around fulcrum F because hypotenuse A is longer than base line B. The arc of radius B should fall within the unprepared tooth. Binding will occur in the region of the arrow.

159

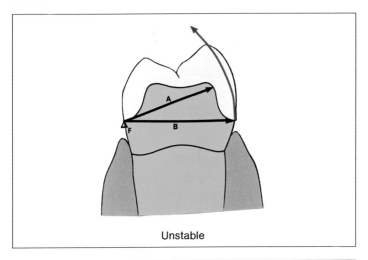

Unstable

Fig.12 The short tooth preparation frequently fails to have adequate resistance form. Rotation occurs when the radius B exceeds hypotenuse A. The arc of B passes outside the unprepared tooth.

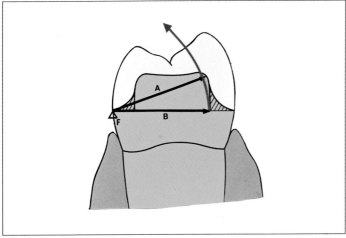

Fig.13 Correction of the unstable crown can be achieved by changing the lateral walls; the radius B is shortened.

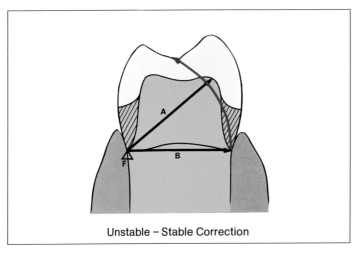

Unstable – Stable Correction

Fig.14 Another form of correction increases the length of the tooth preparation; the hypotenuse A is lengthened, the arc of B now falls within the unprepared tooth. Grooves and pin holes are also used to correct resistance and retention problems.

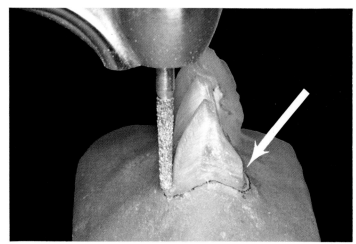

Fig.15 The lingual shoulder or chamfer makes a significant contribution to anterior crown stability.

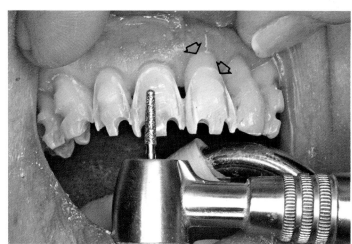

Fig.16 Preparation of teeth with supragingival roots confines depth cuts to enamel only.

sive with gross reduction to permit greater time and concentration for margins and refinement.

Cosmetic veneering materials require more space than metal castings to achieve optical quality and proper form. Therefore, esthetics place great demands on tooth preparation, requiring further alteration beyond basic resistance and retention form. *Providing room for porcelain is a key responsibility of the* *restorative dentist that must be met with unflinching authority.*

Teeth exhibiting supragingival root structure are prepared as above. Visualization is best achieved by confining gross reduction to the enameled areas only–as though the gingiva were the level of the cementoenamel junction (Fig.16). Subsequent to initial preparation, the prepared tooth is used as a guide to further reduce the supragingival root surface

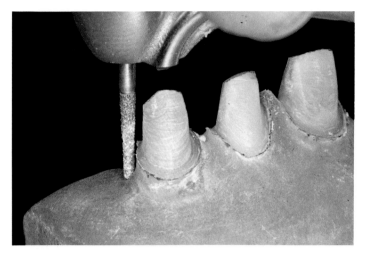

Fig. 17 Removal of enamel produces the basic preparation form; further reduction of root structure to the gingiva is restricted by this rough form. Excessive tooth invasion is avoided and tooth vitality respected.

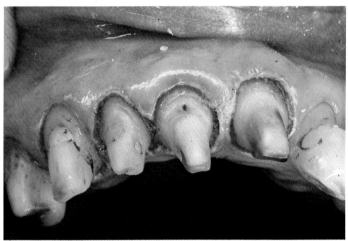

Fig. 18 Impressions of the cuspid and bicuspid preparation were taken with compound-copper band relined with black wax. Electrosurgery was used on the lateral and two centrals for access and visibility–followed by hydrocolloid impressions.

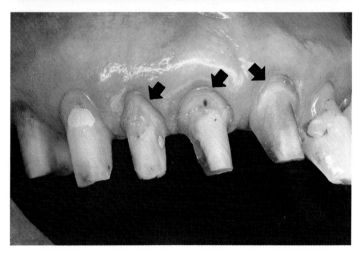

Fig. 19 Two weeks later the tissue appears normal. Note the regeneration of gingival tissue to cover the bevels.

(Fig.17). Resistance and retention form are rarely a problem with such "long" teeth, but undercuts, misalignment of abutments, pulpal abuse, and cosmetic demands complicate tooth preparation. Before any restorative treatment, it is wise to tell patients that endodontics may be required. Reassurance regarding the painlessness and high success level of vital tooth endodontics ensures patient confidence. If further invasion of the prepared tooth is required, then endodontic therapy may be incorporated into the treatment planning.

Establishing Margins

For supragingival margins, refinement of the preparations to this stage may be all that is required. Linearity of the margin between prepared and unprepared tooth structure facilitates subsequent laboratory procedures. Precise definition of tooth margins and their reproduction on laboratory casts is the hallmark of the meticulous dentist who desires the best for his or her patients. Subgingival invasion, when required for restorative margins, demands access and visability. Margins can be placed in the natural crevice without observing exactly the nature of the cut tooth structure; that is one reason why many forms of diamond stones have been designed to limit subgingival preparation. However, frank visibility vertically and horizontally presents far better control of the cutting tool tip and ensures the precise nature of the prepared surface. For that reason, the following approaches may be used to improve visibility and control subgingival preparation.

Access and Subgingival Depth Control

1. Electrosurgery in healthy tissue may be used to provide lateral and vertical space for visibility and movement of the cutting tool (Figs.18 and 19). It also provides space for subsequent placement of retraction string and/or elastic impression material. This last feature emphasizes the difficulty in capturing proximal margins with adjacent tooth preparations; the elastic impression materials can easily be displaced by interproximal gingival tissue. This tissue cannot be displaced mesially and distally simultaneously and frequently interferes with preparations and impressions unless some of it is removed (troughing). Therefore, electrosurgery permits controlled space requirements interproximally for undisplaceable gingival tissue. Buccal and lingual marginal tissue retraction is often possible by cord alone.

2. Another approach that appears to be gaining acceptance is the placement of the smallest retraction cord (size 0) in the bottom of the sulcus before any subgingival tooth preparation (Fig.20).* This not only improves access and visibility, but protects the sensitive epithelial attachment from abuse by the rotating cutting tool. The cord is cut and placed entirely within the sulcus (Figs.21 and 22). *Caution*–Do not forget

* Gingibraid–Van R Dental Products, Inc., L.A., CA.

163

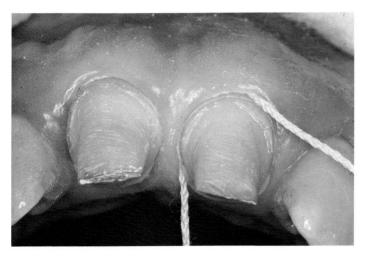

Fig. 20 Subsequent to gross reduction supragingivally, a small cord is placed to the bottom of the healthy sulcus. As shown, no chemical additives may be necessary.

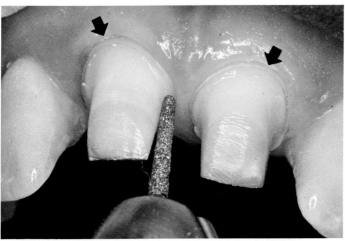

Fig. 21 The cord is cut to circumferential length and placed entirely in the sulcus. Arrows show edge of cord. For subgingival preparation the cutting tool can now be carried to the embedded string. Minor vertical displacement of the marginal tissue has occurred.

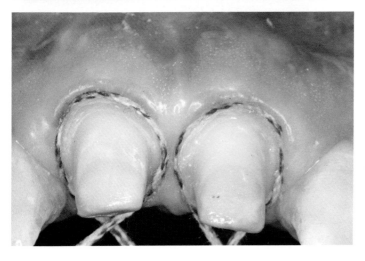

Fig. 22 After complete preparation lateral margin displacement is obtained with a slightly larger cord placed over the submerged initial cord. This second cord is removed just prior to the impression.

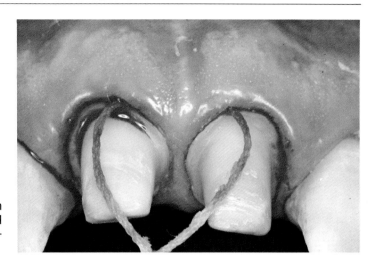

Fig. 23 Impressions have been completed. Removal of the initial submerged cord initiates immediate bleeding.

to remove the cord after taking impressions. Control of bleeding is also facilitated by this approach, even when the cord has no additive chemicals of any nature. Chemically treated cord should not be left in the sulcus for long periods of time; untreated cord should also be considered a biological irritant if left there too long (Fig. 23).

The extension of the basic preparation into the sulcus is now achieved with a tapered round or square end diamond stone with a tip diameter of no more than 1.0 mm (Fig. 21). These tools preserve the integrity of the preparation without lacerating the gingiva. An end cutting carbide can prove useful also (*Goldstein,* 1976). The depth can be limited by a small cord in the bottom of the sulcus; the lateral width is gauged by the previously prepared lateral walls of the tooth. Very small teeth and tipped teeth may require even smaller diamonds. The extension of a shoulder into the sulcus is primarily

required to ensure space for porcelain; sometimes short teeth need it for retention. If esthetics do not require subgingival porcelain, then only establishing a finish line is expected. If a metal collar is to be used, then the operator may choose to extend only a bevel subgingivally. A deep chamfer margin can be treated the same as a shoulder; a shallow chamfer should use a metal margin.

Refinement

The purpose of refinement of a completed preparation is: (a) to smooth and round all sharp edges and corners so that impressions and casts will be faithfully reproduced; (b) to check and redefine retention walls and resistance form and reduce minor undercuts; (c) to smooth coarsely ground dentine; (d) to sharpen and define the linearity of the margin so that a single junction between cut and uncut tooth structure can be clearly

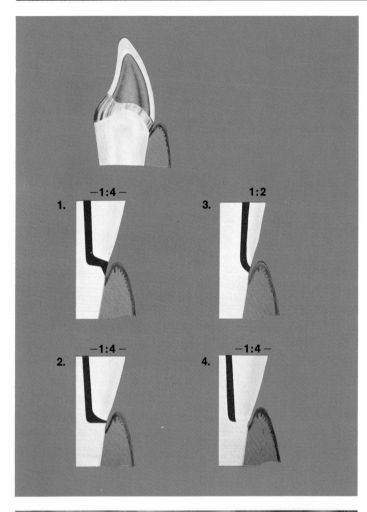

Fig. 24 Margin configurations.
1. Shoulder bevel.
2. Shoulder-metal margin may vary in thickness from 0 to millimeters.
3. Chamfer-metal margin sometimes reduced to 0.
4. Shoulder-porcelain butted.
The relative ratio of metal and porcelain indicated by the numbers 1:4, 1:2, etc.

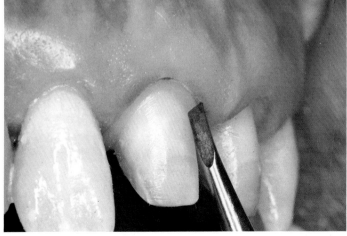

Fig. 25 Hand instrumentation of a shoulder preparation (ferrier 30–31) to remove loose enamel rods and improve linearity of the margin.

managed on the master dies and the impressions; and (e) to confirm adequate space for porcelain in critical areas.

Axial walls are normally refined by fine cut diamond stones the same shape as used for gross reduction. Sandpaper discs in a slow-speed handpiece work equally well. Margin refinement may take one of several configurations (Fig. 24).

1. Shoulder margins are smoothed at slower speeds, namely 50,000 rpm (author preference). Hand instrumentation (Ferrier 30–31 and P. K. Thomas 22)[1] removes loose enamel rods and improves linearity of the margins (Fig. 25). Chamfer margins are easily refined with comparable smooth diamonds. Some operators prefer a multifluted carbide of the same shape (chamfer) as the coarse cutting diamond stones.[2]

2. Bevels are smoothed and sharpened with: (a) steel flame shape burs No. 2 and No. 4,[3] or (b) multifluted flame shape carbides (40 flutes),[4] and (c) hand instruments (Ferrier 30–31). Refinement of vertical walls has become less significant in recent years due to the use of die relief materials that are programmed to provide room for cement. *Eames* et al. (1978) was able to show that die relief provided 25 % more retention because the castings seated better; this provided superior interface between prepared dentine and the casting. Die relief materials are commonly applied in thin layers 5 to 25 microns in thickness.[5] Some reduce the rough texture from coarse diamonds and minimize the need to polish preparations during refinement except for the margins.

Margin Location

The location of the gingival margin for extracoronal restorations continues to be controversial. The early tradition of placing all such margins subgingivally regardless of the patients needs was routine. Specific diamond stone designs were presented by innovative operators and manufacturers to permit guided subgingival preparation without visibility. Impression techniques, materials, and cements have at one time or another promoted the ease of subgingival management. Even the rubber dam is hailed for its control of marginal displacement. Mismanagement of the marginal gingiva, characterized by puffy, bluish, bleeding soft tissue (with slight provocation) remains the most obvious sign of failure of our restorative efforts. It is a multifaceted problem shared by dentist, laboratory technician, and patient.

Supragingival or Subgingival

The need to use subgingival margin placement revolves around one or more of the following factors:

1. Esthetics–as determined by the patient;
2. Resistance and retention form;

---

[1] Suter Dent., Chico, CA.
[2] Brassler, U.S.A. Inc., Savannah, GA 31405.
[3] Busch & Co. Germany.
[4] Midwest American, Melrose Park, Illinois.
[5] Belle de St. Claire, Van Nuys, CA, or George Taub Products, Jersey City, NJ 07307.

3. Control of cement dissolution;
4. Caries or previous filling material;
5. Anatomical defect such as erosion;
6. Root sensitivity.

The last three items above *could,* in many instances, be managed by conservative techniques such as fluoride treatments or specific filling materials. However, routine patient acceptance and dentists placement of a supragingival crown–visible to both–followed by a marginal restoration to correct a defect is unlikely to gain much popularity. For example, facial toothbrush abrasion on a root of a maxillary cuspid that is to receive a crown is a poor candidate for supragingival crown followed by a composite restoration of the facially abraded area. And when several adjacent crowns are placed, how do you convince the patient it is logical to place some crowns supragingivally, and some subgingivally? The essence of the problem then is the reluctance of the restoring dentist to prescribe supragingival margins and the resistance of the patient in accepting them when they are visible. Esthetics dominates the argument concerning supragingival versus subgingival, rather than the more important view that the subgingival placement of restorative material is a *biological irritant* and therefore indicated for only the most demanding situations. The fact that the patient pays the bill for elective esthetic restorations plays a major part in the decision not to display metal margins.

I propose the following regarding the biological implications. Supragingival margins on *enamel* present no mechanical or biological problem as long as the basic objectives of tooth preparation are met (page 153). However, the teeth with denuded root structure present a different set of needs. Root surfaces were not designed for the hostile environment of the oral cavity. The exposed dentinal tubules are particularly susceptible to further complications in maintenance, both personal (home) and professional (dental office). There is a credibility gap with the average practitioner who views this as a liability and the periodontist who considers it the perfect restoration for periodontal tissues. Even a cursory examination of teeth restored with metal-ceramic restorations demonstrates more crowns placed subgingivally than supragingivally. The following is proposed:

1. Supragingival margins on *roots* should allow maximum access for maintenance, both personal and professional. Simple homecare (toothbrush) will normally maintain these restorations on the labial, buccal, and most lingual *convex surfaces* having direct access to a toothbrush (Fig. 26). Restorative repair of these exposed root areas would also be definatively managed with simple filling materials should maintenance degenerate. The dentist cannot guarantee the longevity of the restorations; neither can the patient be expected to maintain teeth free of all plaque indefinitely. Is it fair to pass on to the patient all responsibility for crown failure?

2. Minimum access *root* areas for maintenance (personal and professional) should be covered by restorative materials; in other words, those requir-

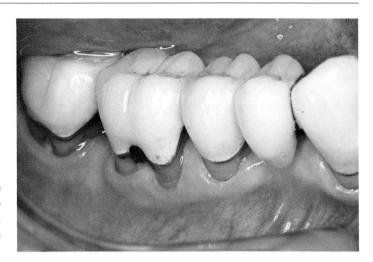

Fig. 26 A reconstruction of metal-ceramic restorations after 12 years. Oral hygiene has been excellent. Note amalgam repair in the furcation of the first molar.

ing complex home care procedures such as axial *concavities,* proximal areas, furcas, and difficult buccal or lingual areas. The root concavities harbor plaque deposits and interfere with adequate oral hygiene (*Sher* and *Vermino,* 1981). Further, studies by *Townsend* (1982) clearly demonstrate higher plaque levels on restorations with axial concavities, particularly those in proximal areas. Complex procedures require greater skill from the patient in plaque removal and often the use of complicated hygiene devices; a compromise in plaque control may jeopardize the susceptible patient. Basically, it's a trade-off on risk factors–a higher rate of iatrogenic periodontal irritation versus the risk of root caries or marginal leakage leading to early difficulties with full crown restorations. *Repair of major rehabilitation cases may be vexing, but replacement is prohibitive for all except the wealthy and the very tough.* Dentistry's credibility is chal-

lenged whenever extensive restorations fail after limited periods in the mouth.

All research and clinical evidence indicates that cemented full coverage margins are not sealing the tooth–imperfect on single units, and potentially disastrous on multiple splinted units. *Eames* concludes that the 24-hour test for zinc phosphate cement solubility is inadequate for clinical testing because the rate of solubility decreases after that short time span.* The cement appears to reach some equilibrium with the environment. It is possible to extrapolate from these conclusions that the rate and volume of liquids passing by cement alters the environment and enhances cement solubility. Therefore, the clinical observation that poor subgingival margins often resist cement washout for many years has

* Eames, W. B. (Personal communication, Jan. 1982).

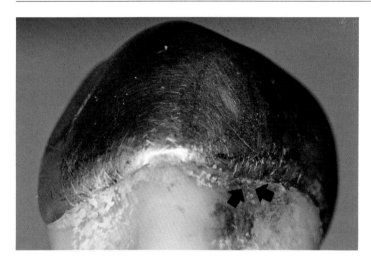

Fig. 27 Extracted tooth with full gold crown that has served many years in the mouth. A large opening on the distal approximating the thickness of a calling card has been plugged with calcified plaque.

some factual background (Fig. 27). Also, it can be observed clinically that irrigating devices may accelerate cement washout on less than superb margins (personal observation).

A personal communication with *Dr. Gerald M. Kramer** regarding this discussion of margin locations is quoted in the following. It merits serious consideration.

"1. The placement of the restorative margin depends on three things:
   (a) Esthetics
   (b) Caries or hypersensitivity
   (c) The inflammatory potential
   The first two are obvious; the third is a problem because each person reacts differently to the placement of a subgingival margin depending on his ability to react to the irritant. This relates to his antibody titers (his immune system), to the destructiveness or defensiveness

of his inflammatory response. It will relate as well as to whether he is a slow or fast plaque grower and, also, to his level of competence or motivation in plaque removal.

2. All research (in other words, *Silness, Waerhaug,* etc.) without exception, indicates any and every subgingival restorative margin is an irritant and that the natural tooth surface (cementum, dentin, enamel) is preferable to a foreign material.

3. Knowing the above to be true, what guidelines should a restorative dentist use? My own feelings are whenever possible (no esthetic problem, no caries problem, no erosions, no anatomic defect, etc.) all margins should be supragingival. I feel supragingival means from *at* the gingival margin to 2–3 mm coronal. This will allow the gingiva and its sulcus to rest against the natural teeth and also to have debridements executed regularly without the problems of catching (and possibly in-

* Kramer, G. M. (Personal communication, Jan. 1982).

juring) the restorative margin. Maintenance is, also, a lot easier without the presence of subgingival margins. If caries occurs (I, personally, do not believe it occurs more frequently with supragingival margins), its detection and correction is obviously easier. Just because more tooth structure is covered with a restoration does not mean that the tooth exposed below the margins (in the sulcus) will not decay. We know, in fact, that plaque bacteria do colonize subgingivally and cause decay (and periodontal disease). I do not think we prevent caries by root coverage, perhaps just the opposite.

4. The dilemma, of course, is what if one needs subgingival placement? If that is the case, the minimal subgingival margin placement, with the most defined margin, and without injury to the tissue (by tooth preparation, retraction, cement, etc.) is the optimum biological way to do restorative dentistry."

It is clear that the demands of restorative dentistry have grown immensely in recent years; our knowledge and skills can hardly keep ahead of patient expectations. The world of show-biz and the advertising media clearly influence the inordinate cosmetic demands of our patients to avoid any and all display of cast metal. In some cases the patient will forceably pull away the lips and cheeks in order to demonstrate their annoyance with visible metal margins. The desire for "white" teeth drives many anxious patients to seek correction (Figs. 28 and 29). Many dentists have difficulty accepting exacting patients' rigid requirements that they have the right to insist on their personal interpretation of dental esthetics with elective restorations. What the dentist considers a health service with functional comfort and longevity, the patient may interpret as an image improvement with overtones of youth preservation and vigor. *Rubin* (1980) in discussing our culture, notes that "our society is a glory-seeking, pride-oriented dynamic system . . . . We accept ourselves almost exclusively in terms of achievement and 'success,' as it is measured by money, prestige, power, sexual attractiveness, or youth." There is a price to pay for this image making and in dentistry it all too often means increased irritation to the teeth and investing tissues. Patient education and communication before treatment is highly advised to minimize these problems.

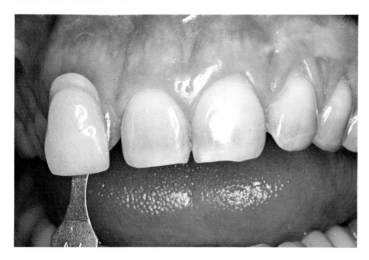

Fig. 28   Female, age 23, with dark teeth from tetracycline stain. Shade guide is Vita A 4.

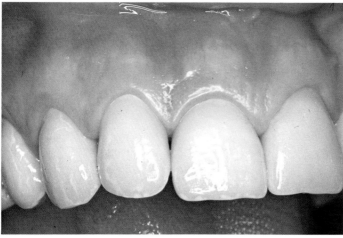

Fig. 29   Postoperative view. Incisors are aluminous porcelain jacket crowns. Marginal tissue reflects minimal irritation.

Metal Substructures for Metal-Ceramic Restorations

The potential of fused porcelain to imitate a natural tooth's optical quality is well recognized as being clearly superior to presently available plastics. Optical quality requires at least the following:

1. Color–in *Munsell's* term of hue, value and chroma;
2. Translucency–light transmission that permits *refraction* to occur;
3. Reflection and absorption;
4. Interpretation.

However, the superior optical quality of dental porcelain is counterbalanced by its poor tensile strength. Early efforts to improve this weakness usually involved some sort of metal backing for manufactured porcelain teeth. The major breakthrough occurred when techniques were evolved for specific alteration of the thermal coefficient of expansion for porcelain and metal–to harmonize the differences of these two dramatically different materials. When chemical bonding between the two was introduced, the two systems could be made compatible (*Shell* and *Nielsen*, 1963). Dentistry's major experience and research progress has been with gold-based alloys. Nonprecious alloys have assumed a large portion of full crowns being placed in some geographical areas; they deserve separate consideration and will not be discussed here. There is increasing evidence that certain nickel-chromium alloys are not only compatible with fused porcelain but offer certain superior qualities such as higher mechanical strength (*Weiss,* 1977; *Presswood* et al. 1980).

The design of the substructures has not changed greatly in recent years. A myriad of variables precludes reliable reproducible research. Design concepts for the metal substructures must include consideration of the following:

Principles in Design

1. Rigidity of support;
2. Control of tensile and compressive forces;
3. Shear resistance;
4. Marginal integrity;
5. Esthetics, form and function;
6. Access for maintenance.

Rigidity of Support

Two applications of this most important principle require consideration:

1. The metal substrate must be firm and unyielding to preserve precise abutment metal form while the porcelain is being fired (sintered). Distortion of this form can lead to:
   (a) Tensile strains within the porcelain, and
   (b) Potential porcelain fracture when seating the restorations that may bind on the abutment tooth. Marginal integrity and fit will also be compromised.
2. Frameworks for fixed partial prosthodontics, particularly those replacing missing teeth, require metal structures that withstand the forces of sintering

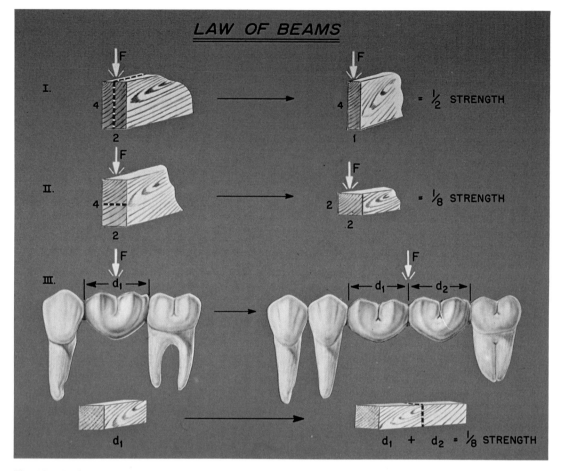

Fig. 30 A piece of wood, 2x4, is used to illustrate resistance to force.
I Changes in width   II Changes height   III Increasing length

shrinkage but also the functional and parafunctional forces of occlusion without fatigue or deflection beyond the limits of the porcelain or metal. Mechanical engineering principles govern basic design concepts.

The laws of beams apply (Fig. 30). Assuming a vertical vector of force, metal substructures will alter their resistance in the following manner.

(a) Doubling the height of the metal produces eight times the resistance of deflection because it is inversely proportional to the cube of the change in size.

(b) Doubling the width of the metal substructures produces twice the resistance—it is directly proportional to the change.

(c) Doubling the length of pontic space increases the deflection by eight times because the change in dimen-

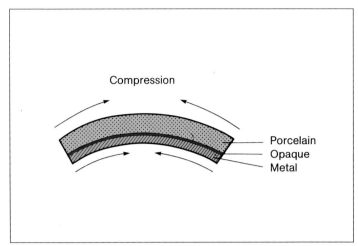

Fig. 31 The thermal coefficient of expansion is designed to allow the metal to shrink more than the porcelain veneer. This places the thin porcelain under compression.

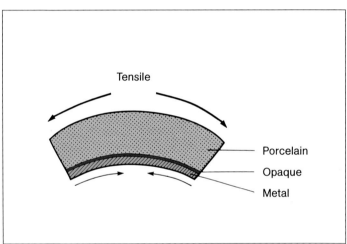

Fig. 32 Thick porcelain may demonstrate tension rather than compression. Such a composite is more likely to shear off some porcelain.

sion is inversely proportional to the cube.

Structural integrity is most efficiently controlled by manipulation of vertical dimension in connectors. Sound conceptual geometric forms still require skill and judgmental alteration for the myriad of diverse situations presented to the dentist and laboratory.

Control of Tensile and Compressive Forces

Dental porcelain is a brittle material of low fracture toughness. Tensile forces required to fracture porcelain in the mouth are easily achieved under many circumstances; but porcelain's resistance to breakage from compression is remarkably good. Therefore, design forms endeavor to emphasize metal support

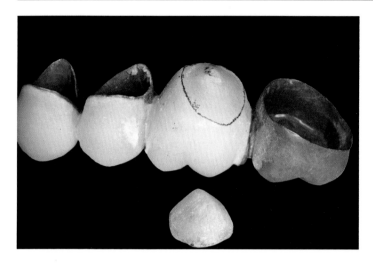

Fig. 33 The tip of a pontic that has sheared off in the laboratory–due to a tensile fracture. Probable cause is the thick porcelain, which was allowed to shrink on itself rather than metal.

wherever force is applied to the porcelain–preferably perpendicular to the major force vector.

The thickness of the porcelain veneer demands careful control–another problem in tensile and compressive forces (Figs. 31 and 32). Correctly applied, thin porcelain is stronger near the metal-porcelain interface because the mismatched coefficient of expansion is designed by the manufacturers to produce compression of the porcelain at the interface. This compressed porcelain possesses greater resistance to distortion. However, optical quality normally improves as the porcelain is made thicker; and the temptation to keep the metal thin and to thicken the porcelain for optimum optical quality is a constant threat to the integrity of the dual system. The optimum thickness for balance between the superior strength of thick metal solidus/thin porcelain and the improved optical quality of thin metal solidus/thick porcelain has not been clearly developed. Clinically, porcelain that exceeds 1.5–2.0 mm thickness develops more fractures when shear forces are applied. These fractures probably follow the flaw mechanisms, enhanced by tension or lack of compression in the thickened porcelain.

Another way of viewing this problem is to provide metal designs that permit porcelain to shrink on metal rather than on itself, for it will surely then produce a serious flaw (Fig. 33). Thick porcelain (greater than 2.0 mm) violates the basic concept of the manufactured metal-porcelain composite.

It should be noted that the reported shear strength of porcelain (*Craig*, 1980) is about 16,000 lb./in.^{2}, and tensile strength of about 5,000 lb./in.^{2} Both of these far exceed normal forces in the mouth. It is proposed that flaw mechanisms in the porcelain initiate failure. Rules for predictable control of these flaws are not yet available. Compressive strength, however, approaches 50,000 lb./in.^{2} and this

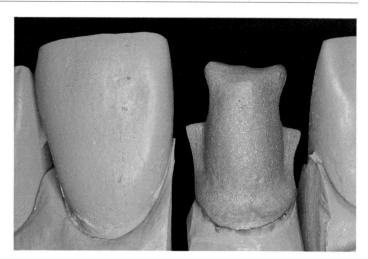

Fig. 34 Typical incisal corner support for superior strength.

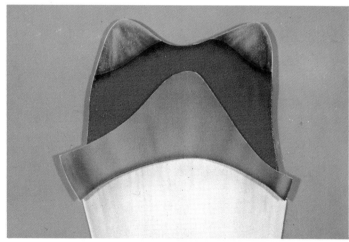

Fig. 35 Cuspal metal support for porcelain occlusion. A reinforcing collar enhances structural integrity. The proximal wing permits conservative tooth preparation, furnishes shear resistance to occlusal loading, and allows access for oral hygiene.

large margin of safety lends itself to greater flexibility in application. Good design in metal structure will incorporate this feature.

Shear Resistance

Without proper metal substructures the inherent shear resistance of the fused porcelain is inadequate to withstand intraoral forces. Three major areas deserve attention:

1. Incisal corners–the metal support limits porcelain to 2.0 mm or less in this critical area (Fig. 34).
2. Posterior porcelain cusps–the metal support maintains porcelain cusp integrity by limiting shear forces and increasing compressive resistance (Fig. 35).
3. Proximal posterior porcelain margins– the proximal metal strut provides superior support to preclude fracture

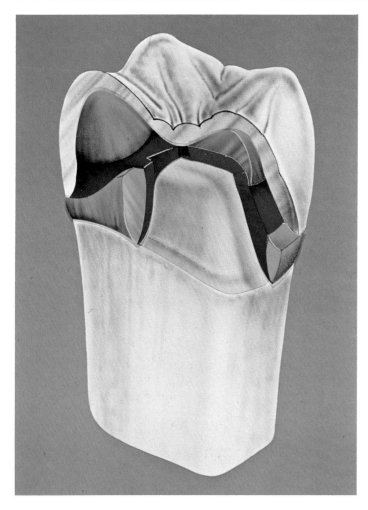

Fig. 36 A posterior ceramo-metal composite cutaway. Demonstrating principles in design.

in this crucial area when using porcelain occlusals (Fig. 36).

Marginal Integrity

The removal of sound tooth structure for crown preparation poses a critical consideration for the subsequent restorative phase. The finished restoration must:

1. Seal the denuded tooth structure from bacterial invasion;
2. Allow minimal cement dissolution;
3. Reproduce a normal emergence profile (*Stein,* 1977).

Full cast alloy restorations permit superior marginal adaptation. The cosmetic veneering materials such as fused porcelain introduce problems in controlling marginal integrity. Two aspects here require examination:

1. Seating of the finished restoration during cementation;
2. Avoiding metal creep (lifting of the metal margin during porcelain sintering and shrinkage).

Both problems could be limited if the need to hide the metal were less demanding. Further, a metal collar enhances control of contour at the gingival level; the emergence profile dictated by the wax-up is preserved in its original form.

Margin Design and Casting Seating

The beveled margin of castings has long been used to produce minimal cement lines in inlays and onlays. Some of those results depended upon finishing ductile gold alloys. The stiffness of alloys in metal-ceramic restorations ·precludes that possibility.
On the other hand, the bevel must be considered as a geometric form that can enhance marginal seal (slip-joint) (*Kashani* et al. 1981). It should be noted that the beveled cutting tool permits considerable vertical variation as it is guided around the tooth while still preserving *horizontal linearity* of the margin; this is an important quality of the beveled margin. The full shoulder preparation may not allow this luxury, particularly where the interproximal tissue is much more coronal than the buccal and lingual periodontal tissues. The full shoulder margin, good or bad, is usually more visible to the operator than the bevel margin. Secondly, before elastic impression materials became routine, copper band-compound impression were common. A beveled shoulder or knife-edge margin facilitated easy seating of the copper band when filled with soft compound. Shoulder preparations frequently catch the edge of the copper band, requiring repeated impression procedures. Hardened compound often locks in undercuts beyond the shoulder margin and resists band removal. A bevel minimizes this undercut problem. To some extent, hydrocolloid still retains some of this annoyance with severe margin undercuts because it tends to distort or tear off with impression removal. The question of the butt or shoulder preparation versus the beveled preparation centers around the open margin quality and quantity of the cemented cast restoration.

Rosner, 1963, notes four functions of the bevel in castings. These are:

1. Reduction of inherent defects in casting and cementation;
2. Protection of enamel rods at the margins;
3. Allowance for burnishing;
4. Development of circumferential retention.

The main thrust of the proposal argues that as the bevel approaches parallelism with the path of insertion of the restoration, the cement thickness is minimized between the tooth and the internal surfaces of the castings at the margin.
Pascoe (1978) found that the least marginal discrepancy was produced with a shoulder of the slightly oversized casting rather than a bevel.

Gavelis, et al. (1981) demonstrated in this study that the best seal comes from the feather edge and parallel bevel preparations, consistant with geometric considerations. The best seating, however, *during cementation* was produced with a 90° full shoulder and the poorest seating was produced with the 90° shoulder with parallel bevel. This is explained on the basis that shoulder preparations have poor seal prior to cementation, facilitating cement escape marginally.

To clarify the controversy, *McLean* and *Wilson* (1980) presented mathematical evidence indicating that bevels must be in the region of 70°–80° to produce significant improvement in marginal seal and decrease cement dissolution.

Joly (1979) in his study indicated that the presence or length and angulation of bevels has no effect on post cementation retention or seating of castings.

Consider the laboratory problem. The dies should be trimmed to the least amount of overextension that can be seen and managed by the technician. This permits overextension in wax by the same amount. It is too demanding to expect the technician to trim to the exact margin and then wax, cast, and finish to the same precise line. The casting overextension is maintained until the restoration receives the final polish (Fig. 37). The objective is to obtain optimum cement seal without introducing margins that are a biological irritant.

One design does not allow this liberty. The full shoulder preparation permits milling the casting to a knife-edge at the exact margin without overextension. Magnification of the work field is desir-able for this procedure. Porcelain is then fired to the same exact line. The luxury of slight overextension in the metal must be eliminated from this approach–otherwise reduction of the metal overextension in the final polish will produce a metal collar and opaque line. The proposed cosmetic achievement is therefore sacrificed. Fear of exposing the buccal metal margin while shaping the porcelain *intimidates* the technician or dentist, and overcontouring easily occurs. Where indicated, the substitution for this design with the all-porcelain buccal margin reduces this problem (Fig. 38).

Creep Problems During Sintering

Research by *Shillingburg* et al. (1973) shows that the chamfer produces the most distortion during the shrinkage of the porcelain. Their conclusions are supported in a study by *Faucher* and *Nicholls* (1980), who found that shoulder bevel designs exhibit significantly less marginal distortion than chamfer designs.

Controversy continues with a study by *Hamaguchi* et al. (1982), who found no significant marginal distortion when porcelain was fired regardless of marginal design. It was concluded that porcelain application and firing does not mechanically distort the facial margin because the layered porcelain "sandwich"–opaque, body, enamel, glaze–precludes metal creep.

I recommend controlling sintering shrinkage and potential creep by incremental layering of porcelain. Opaque is applied in two layers to obtain maximum wetting

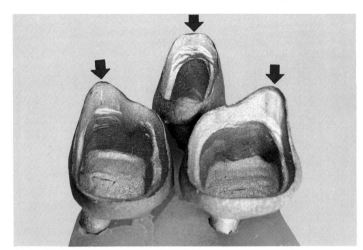

Fig. 37 Divested castings show-ing minimum overextension. This should be maintained until the final polish.

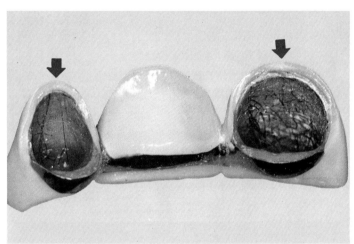

Fig. 38 Three-unit ceramo metal bridge utilizing full shoulder pre-parations and porcelain buccal margin.

with minimum thickness. Spraying tech-niques are highly effective. The first body buildup is kept away from the margin (Figs. 39 and 40). The subsequent body buildup is used to complete the under-contoured cervical area (Fig. 41).
Eliminating the gold collar labially intro-duces technical problems. Two popular techniques are considered.

1. The shoulder or heavy chamfer prep-aration, which permits grinding the metal to a knife-edge at the exact mar-gin as described previously.

2. The all-porcelain buccal margin is available by several techniques, after eliminating the buccal metal except for the vertical wall.

(a) The porcelain is applied to platinum foil, which is swaged to the die shoulder (*Goodacre* et al. 1977).

(b) A duplicate ceramic die is fabri-

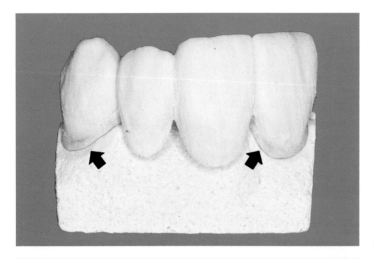

Fig. 39   First body buildup of porcelain. The knife edge metal margin is avoided.

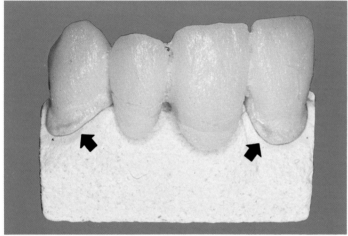

Fig. 40   After firing, porcelain shrinkage avoids marginal creep.

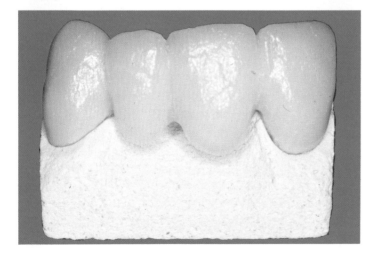

Fig. 41   Second bake to complete labial form.

cated with the metal coping and the porcelain is condensed and fired on this die (*Sozio* and *Riley*, 1977).

(c) A special separating medium* (Cerama Seal Sep Kit) is applied to the master die and the porcelain is condensed to this treated shoulder. The metal-ceramic crown can now be lifted and fired.

All these approaches require meticulous craftsmanship and normally more lab time than the all-metal collar margin. As the sintered porcelain shrinks from the margin it must be corrected by subsequent firings and fitting, a tedious task. Single restorations lend themselves to this technique with much more facility than splinted units (Fig. 38). Translucent glass ionomer cement may compliment the finished result.

I normally prescribe metal collars for all lower teeth and all areas of the upper dentition that do not show in a vigorous smile.

Amidst such confusion, how does one choose the correct margin? A single approach for all restorations is not appropriate. Priorities determine selection. Suggestions are:

1. Avoid deep subgingival margin placement. The closer the margin is to the epithelial attachment, the greater likelihood that severe gingival inflammation will result (*Newcomb*, 1974; *Silness*, 1970).
2. Use a metal collar whenever possible to provide control of emergence pro-

* Belle de St. Claire, Van Nuys, CA.

file and reinforce the collar. Terminating the metal margin *at* the gingival margin or *supragingival* will increase biological compatibility and access for professional and personal maintenance.
3. Eliminate or minimize gold collars for aesthetic priorities rather than going deep into the sulcus.
4. If bevels are used, avoid trying to hide the metal by covering with porcelain. In order to avoid overcontouring, *Kuwata* (1980) recommends a minimum margin angle of 50° if the porcelain is to be fused to the metal margin edge.
5. Recognize the skill limitations of your laboratory.

Basic Design–Single Units

The metal substructure should provide the following:
– Abutment seal,
– Reinforcing collar,
– Buttressing shoulder,
– Shear resistance.

Abutment Seal

The primary function of the metal design is to seal the restoration to the prepared tooth form. Optimum abutment seal requires meticulous attention to all procedures, including form of the tooth preparation, fabrication of the die, manipulation of the wax, investing procedure, casting methods, and finishing of the casting. The hardness of metal-ceramic alloys prohibits burnishing of marginal areas. The thin layer of metal also provides the mechanism for porcelain bonding–chemical, mechanical, and

183

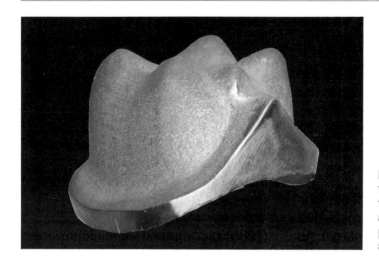

Fig. 42 Posterior coping ready for opaque application. Exit angle for the veneering area should approach right angles to the polished metal whenever possible.

compressive. It permits the porcelain to shrink against the metal matrix during sintering rather than upon itself.

Reinforcing Collar

The primary function of the metal collar is to maintain marginal integrity. Even at the wax pattern stage, it aids in avoiding distortion. Further, the collar is the beginning of the emergence profile and as such permits contour control *before* porcelain application. The final dimension of this critical area should be brought to a rubber wheel smoothness before veneering and thereafter remain free of porcelain (Fig. 42). Traditional techniques of waxing, casting, and finishing a metal collar maintain superior quality control over other metal-porcelain margin techniques.

Buttressing Shoulder

The metal coping is normally made more rigid by additional reinforcement. Proxi-

mally and lingually the collar is increased vertically to form a buttressing shoulder and augment the casting stiffness.

A continuation of the shoulder proximally with a vertical strut is designed to resist pressure in the direction of its length (occlusally) and provides support for marginal ridges. Also, the proximal design is conducive to conservative tooth preparation on the proximal aspect. Cosmetically, it is more desirable to stiffen the casting here. This specific coping design is biocompatible with interproximal tissues and facilitates access for oral hygiene (Fig. 35).

Shear Resistance

The metal cones supporting the posterior occlusal porcelain provide the important function of resisting vertical and lateral force vectors. As stated, the principle of compression rather than tension lends structural strength to the restoration. In addition, providing an even layer of the

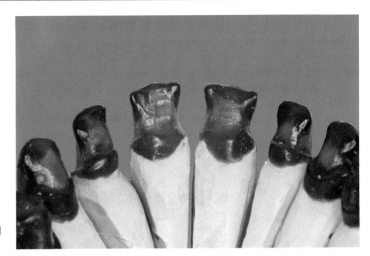

Fig. 43 Additional wax to incisal corners for porcelain support.

porcelain enables the ceramist to control the optical quality and minimize tensile stresses more easily (Fig. 36).

Anterior designs also require special attention to support incisal porcelain tables (Fig. 34). The temptation to use more than 2.0 mm of porcelain on incisal corners is evident from the occurrence of fractured edges. In particular, pontics present the possibility of inadequate incisal support. Pontic metal form should equal abutment metal size for predictable porcelain strength. Where single crowns or abutments are deficient in normal prepared tooth shape, the waxing techniques call for additional incisal support, as illustrated in Fig. 43. Single-unit design is illustrated in Figures 44 to 47. The gold occlusal design is esteemed by those who prefer metal occlusion to porcelain (Fig. 48).

Designs on Multiple Connected Units

The principles of design previously discussed for single units are also applicable to multi-unit (splint) prosthesis:

1. Porcelain support with metal substructures at right angles to force vectors permit porcelain compression rather than tension.
2. Designs that incorporate rigidity while conserving metal.
3. Even layering of porcelain and limiting thickness to 1.5–2.0 mm.
4. Pontic and connector design with consideration for strength, esthetics, and oral hygiene (Figs. 49 to 52).
5. Esthetic considerations.
6. Precise tooth preparations.
7. Access for daily home care.

Graphic representation of connected units incorporate the above principles (Figs. 53 to 57).

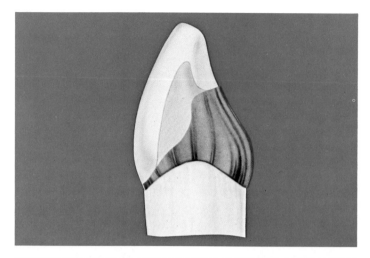

Fig. 44   Anterior   design.   The labial   porcelain   should   wrap around the incisal metal support.

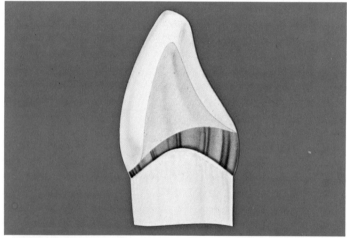

Fig. 45   Same basic design with more porcelain on the lingual.

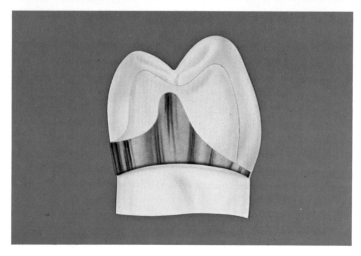

Fig. 46   Posterior design for porcelain occlusal.

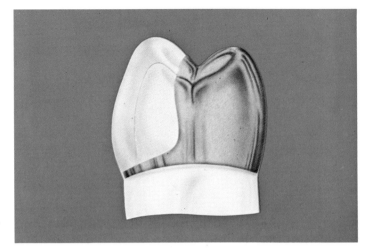

Fig. 47 Posterior design for metal occlusal.

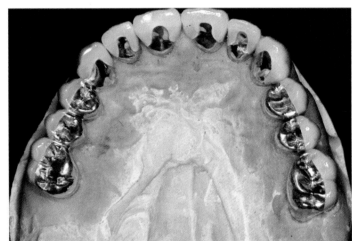

Fig. 48 Gold occlusion and emphasis on metal anterior guidance.

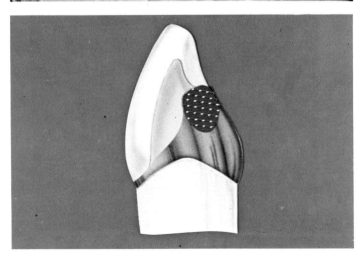

Fig. 49 Connector for anterior teeth with emphasis on vertical height, access for soldering and oral hygiene and lingual position for porcelain coverage.

187

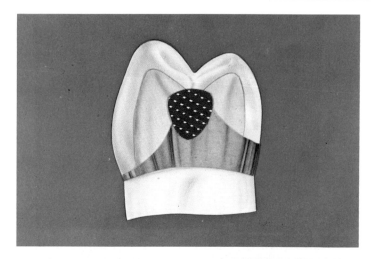

Fig. 50 Posterior connector "strawberry shape" permitting access for oral hygiene, vertical height and porcelain support.

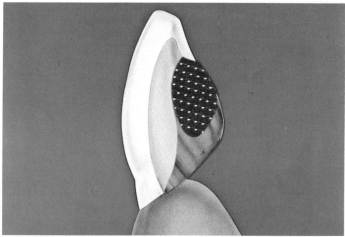

Fig. 51 Anterior pontic design. Ridge contact is minimal to permit floss cleansing.

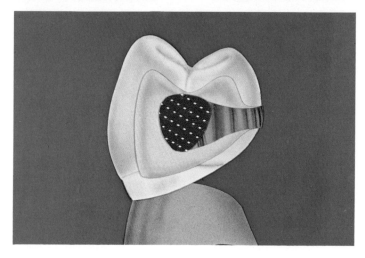

Fig. 52 Posterior pontic design. Ridge contact permits dental floss plaque removal.

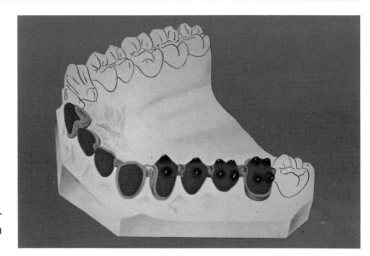

Fig. 53 Anterior and posterior sections are connected with an interlock.

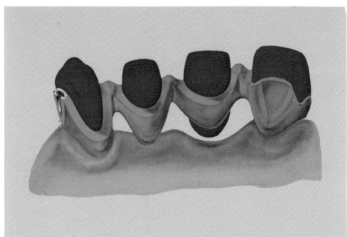

Fig. 54 Anterior section with trestle design. Variations in buttressing sections are permitted. Pontics should provide for even thickness of porcelain.

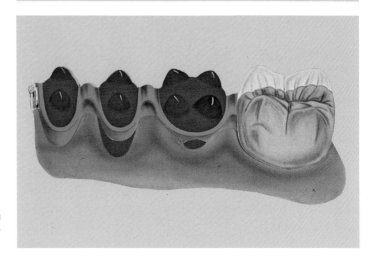

Fig. 55 Posterior frame design with gold occlusal on molar abutment.

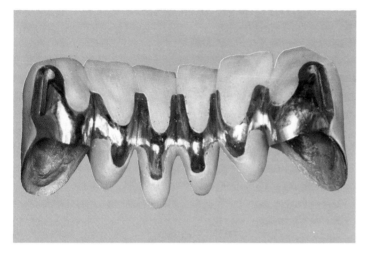

Fig. 56 Anterior pontics demonstrating good metal design. Small fingers of metal toward residual ridge permit porcelain to shrink on metal.

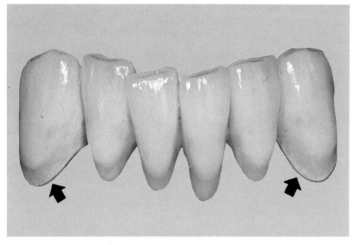

Fig. 57 Labial view of same fixed bridge. Note small gold collars.

Newer Designs

For the last three years, my private laboratory has produced little or no solid metal pontics to be veneered with porcelain. Instead, various custom designed "hollow" pontics have been used. At first it appeared to be a reasonable method to reduce the cost of using premium gold-based ceramic alloys (about 40% reduction by weight). Other advantages became evident.

1. Reduction in metal porosity because there was less metal in the pontics; the metal thereby achieves its cast strength potential. (See research report below.)
2. Easier soldering, when necessary, due to the absence of large heat sinks.
3. It can be hypothesized that there are potential improvements in strength due to the porcelain-metal composite "sandwich"; it presents high resistance

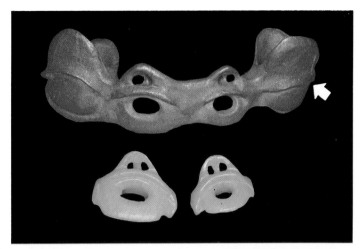

Fig. 58 Inzoma pontic designs with prefabricated forms. Note labial horizontal ridges designed to prevent flaw migration.

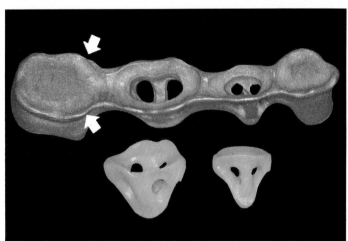

Fig. 59 Inzoma pontic design for posteriors. Note buccal and lingual ridges on abutments for porcelain support.

to tensile force. Were we in fact using the high compressibility of the porcelain "core" to improve the strength of the pontics?

Several pontic designs by other adventuresome people have been presented. J. M. Ney Co. (Technical Bulletin No. 110) advocates carving a solid pontic in wax and then hollowing the center of the wax pontic from underneath. Porcelain appli-

cation requires filling the hollow center with porcelain first in two or more firings. The Inzoma technique is an innovative approach to pontic design by *I. Shoher*, Tel Aviv, Israel and marketed by Ivoclar (Ivoclar AG, Liechtenstein). It also adds horizontal ridges external to the basic filigree design on abutments to reduce flaw migration (Figs. 58 and 59).

Belle de St. Claire (Belle de St. Claire, Van Nuys, CA) also markets wax forms that

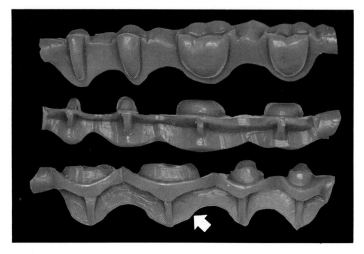

Fig. 60 Prefabricated wax forms by Belle de St. Claire. Note good vertical support and ridge bar to permit porcelain shrinkage on metal.

depart from the conventional solid form. They are available as a kit (Fig. 60).

Another approach utilizes a prefabricated porcelain core around which the wax form is fashioned and cast.

All such designs, however, would best be served by laboratory research as well as clinical testing. The cutting edge of scientific inquiry cannot be replaced by clinical examination alone. However, designing and fabricating reproducible geometric equivalents to clinical situations poses technical difficulties.

Thought Exploration:

(a) Metal design for most composite structures (e.g. concrete and metal) does not depend on sheer bulk of metal for strength, whereas most present pontic designs feature solid metal cores with a "skin" of porcelain. It has been said that the perfect form of ceramic-metal imitates an orange, with the edible part representing the metal and the skin representing the porcelain. Is there a better design? Is there a deleterious altered heating cycle of the porcelain veneer when fired on a solid metal pontic (heat sink) compared to a thin abutment metal coping?

(b) The high cost of gold-based ceramic alloys in recent years encourages the use of less metal rather than more. Will we be forced to abandon the traditional alloys because of cost? Is third-party payment based on least cost altering our laboratory prescription?

(c) The comparison of physical properties of dental porcelain demonstrates the impressive compressive strength compared to its other strengths (*McLean* 1979). How can we put this to better use?

1. Tensile strength	5,000 psi
2. Shear strength	12,000 psi
3. Compressive strength	50,000 psi

(d) Studies (J. M. Ney Co. Technical Bulletin No. 100) show that undisclosed poros-

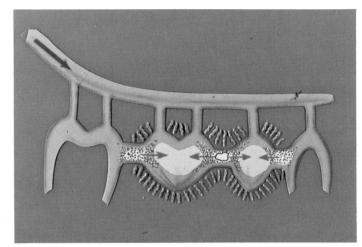

Fig. 61 Solidification Problems large all-metal pontics require molten metal to ensure dense castings much longer than thin sections. This can create porosity in the connectors.

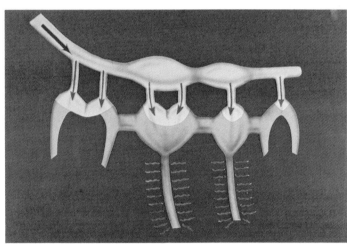

Fig. 62 Better spruing and the use of chill vents to cool the pontics aids in creating dense pontic castings. Chill vents are applicable to connectors also.

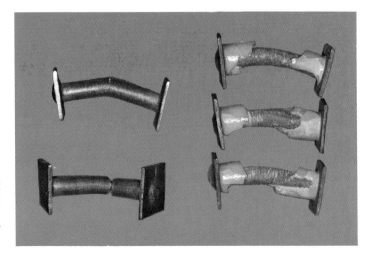

Fig. 63 Cast rods 3.0 mm thick become two to three times stronger to bend test when covered with 1.5 mm thick veneer of porcelain.

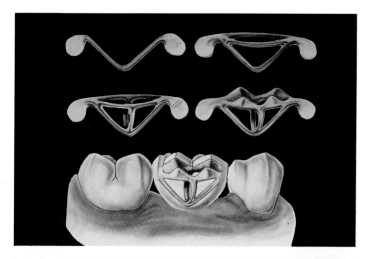

Fig. 64　Composite graphics of hollow design–from left to right:
1. "keel",
2. occlusal support,
3. vertical struts,
4. cusp support,
lower – "ghost".

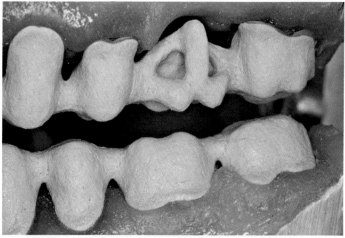

Fig. 65　Opaque applied to metal frame of practical case.

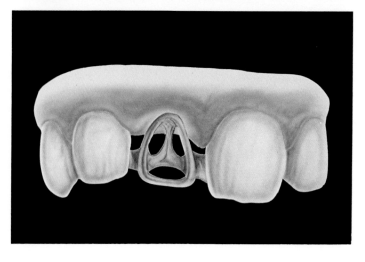

Fig. 66　Anterior hollow design. Lingual area has vertical and horizontal struts.

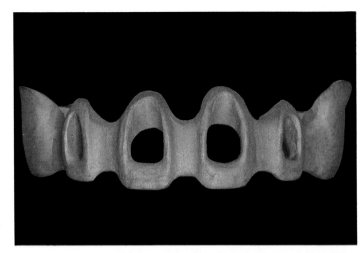

Fig. 67 Anterior design with four hollow pontics.

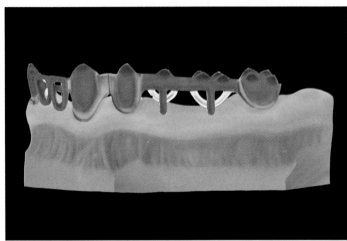

Fig. 68 Compare graphic representation with Fig. 53.

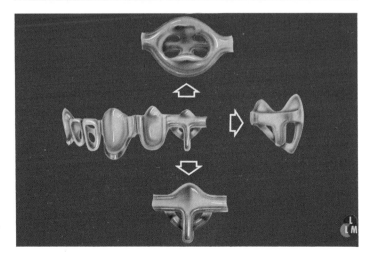

Fig. 69 Frontal, side, and occlusal view of metal framework.

ity in metal-ceramic castings may seriously lower yield points in otherwise normal appearing castings. These porosities easily occur when large, thick, all-metal pontics are cast; adequate spruing is problematic (Figs. 61 and 62).

(e) The difficulty in presoldering solid metal pontics is enhanced by the "heat sink" capacity of large amounts of metal.

(f) A preliminary study (Fig. 63) shows that a metal rod can increase its yield point two to three times when covered with a layer of fused porcelain 1.5 mm thick. Could a composite pontic be designed using these reinforced rods? A design was produced incorporating the following features and introduced into clinical practice in 1978.

1. A porcelain center "core" to be compressed between metal rods when external force is applied.
2. An open basketweave design using rods of metal surrounded by porcelain for improved strength.
3. Adequate support of external optical quality (translucent) porcelain by the composite core of metal and porcelain to maintain an even layer of external porcelain (anterior and posterior); this composite core would support the optical porcelain the same as an all-metal core.
4. Consideration for the laws of beams in metal design; connectors would be designed the same as tradition dictates.
5. Recognition of potential problems in reentry angles of porcelain fusion, which could produce porosities and flaw situations. This shrinkage is con-trolled by layered firing. It normally requires at least two extra firings for the core. Core porcelain is a mixture of 50% opaque and 50% body porcelain.

Hollow metal pontic designs for the porcelain core are shown in Figs. 64 to 69. These clinically tested forms have proven successful. While fabrication is simple, application allows adaptation to most pontic situations. Resistance to deformation and proper support of the porcelain indicate continued use. There is no interference with the esthetic requirements of the porcelain veneer. Continued success warranted laboratory research.

Research

An explorative pilot study was undertaken as follows (Figs. 70 to 72). Jelenko O[1] metal and Ceramco[2] porcelain were used for all test units. All modules were numbered, paired, and when porcelain was added, the unveneered metal mate was heat-cycled on the same sagger tray. Manufacturer's instructions were followed on casting (Thermotrol 2500), metal preparation, and porcelain additions. The rods and support mechanism were cast in one piece. Rod length was 17 mm ±.1.0 mm–a reasonable width of an upper first molar plus bicuspid; rod diameter was 2.0 mm–plastic sprues provided these dimensions. Porcelain application, where used, was 1.5 mm thick.

[1] J. F. Jelenko & Co., Armonk, NY 10504.

[2] Ceramco Inc., Johnson & Johnson Co., E. Windsor, NJ 08520.

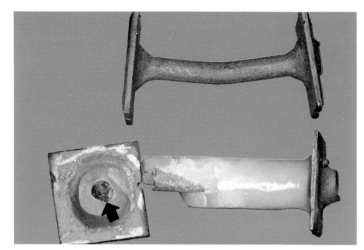

Fig. 70   Single rod after testing.
Porous casting.
Module #1.

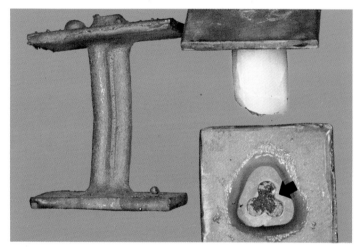

Fig. 71   Triple rod after testing.
Excessive porosity.
Module #2.

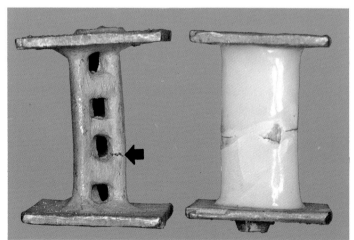

Fig. 72   Open design after testing. Poor tensile strength.
Module #3.

A compressive force was applied through a steel rod placed at the center and at right angles to the specimen. The load was supplied by an Instron testing machine at a crosshead speed of 0.02 in/min.* Graphic representation was recorded simultaneously with the force application and indicated when yield points were reached.

First Study–Modules

1. Single rod–5 samples.
   Single rod surrounded by porcelain 1.5 mm thick–5 samples.
2. Three single rods fused and cast as one–5 samples.
   Three fused rods plus porcelain 1.5 mm thick–5 samples.
3. Three single rods separated (simulated basket design)–5 samples.
   Vertical struts simulated support mechanisms used on posterior "hollow" pontics. A solid connector united all hollow specimens in the center where the force was applied. The space between rods was maintained at 2.0 mm.
   Three-rod basket design–5 samples– internal core 50 % body porcelain; external porcelain 1.5 mm thick.

The concept of design No. 2 to No. 3 was to attempt to keep the same mass of metal (at least in the horizontal rods). But this resulted in a much larger specimen cross section for No. 3. Comparing

compressive yield points for these two specimens does not appear as meaningful as anticipated.

Results

Several specimens reached a very low yield point and examination of the broken metal indicated large amounts of porosity (Figs. 70 to 72). Some units broke near the junction of the support mechanism and the rod–indicating poor sprue technique leading to porosity. The study was redesigned.

Second Study

A jig replaced the cast uprights of the previous specimens; it was cast in nickel-chromium alloy (Fig. 73). The distance between uprights remained at 17.0 mm. This design reduced the amount of metal needed for each test casting, an improvement in porosity control.

A new module (No. 4) was introduced by converting hollow module No. 3 to a solid bar (Fig. 74). New specimens of No. 3 and No. 4 were cast and prepared as before, with a porcelain veneer of 1.0 mm. Spruing was changed to reduce internal porosity (Fig. 75). Test specimens were loaded in the Instron to the yield point, crosshead speed 0.02 in/min. Paired specimens of metal and metal/porcelain were cycled together in the porcelain furnace. The modules tested were: (Fig. 76 and 77):

SOLID:
Metal–5 samples

* Instron Engineering Corp., Canton, MA.

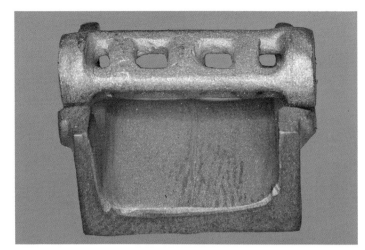

Fig. 73 Nickel-chromium casting to support test modules. Hollow model in place.
New Module #3.

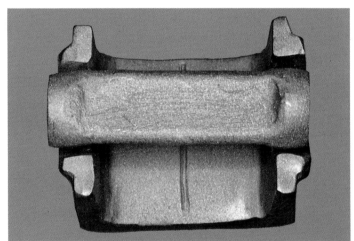

Fig. 74 Solid module on jig. Module #4.

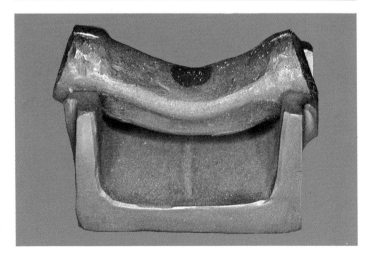

Fig. 75 After testing a solid bar exhibits excellent tensile (bend) performance. Improved spruing produced a dense casting.

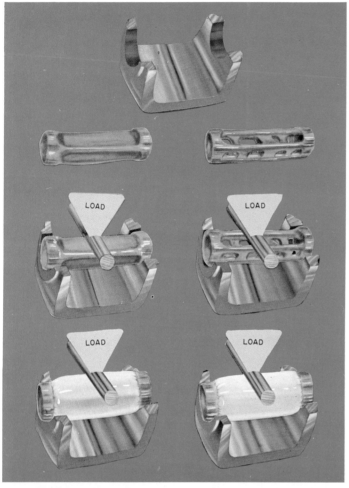

Fig. 76   Jig and test samples.

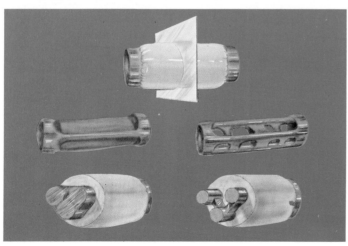

Fig. 77   Cross section of metal/
porcelain composites.

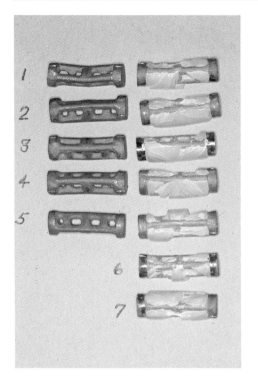

Fig. 78 Solid modules after testing. Each pair was heat-cycled through each stage.

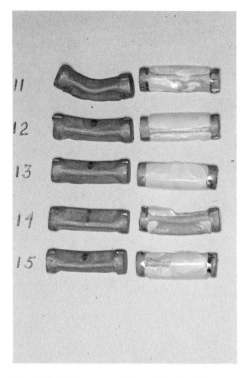

Fig. 79 Hollow modules after testing.

average weight 7.23 dwt.
Metal/porcelain—5 samples (Fig. 78)

HOLLOW:
5 samples
average weight 5.34 dwt.
Metal/porcelain—7 samples (Fig. 79)

Results

None of the specimens fractured through the metal as before. Cracks appeared in the porcelain composites well before the fracture point was reached; this proportional limit averaged 370 pounds for the solid metal/porcelain

and 331 pounds for the hollow metal/porcelain samples (Fig. 80). The strength figures are as follows:

SOLID:
Metal ave. 942
Metal/porcelain ave. 1177

HOLLOW:
Metal ave. 408
Metal/porcelain ave. 1058

A load-displacement curve typical of the metal specimens is drawn in Fig. 81. The curve can be divided into three regions, as follows:

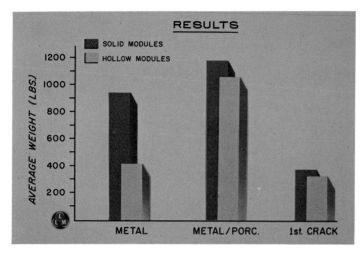

Fig. 80 Bar graph showing results of bend tests. Note dramatic increase in load resistance to hollow modules when porcelain is applied. First crack appearance is below load level of metal modules.

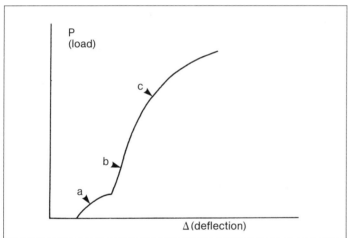

Fig. 81 Typical load-deflection curve for metal specimen.

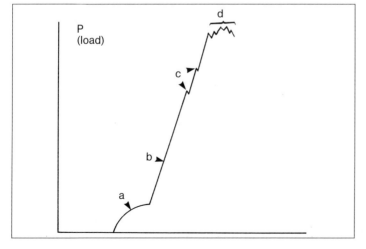

Fig. 82 Typical load-deflection curve for metal/porcelain.

202

a) Initial "setting" of specimen into constraints imposed by holder and load-transmitting rod.
b) Linear deflection, indicating elastic behavior (no permanent deformation upon unloading).
c) Nonlinear deflection, indicating plastic behavior (specimen has developed a permanent deformation).

The typical curve for a porcelain-coated specimen is shown in Fig. 82. The four regions distinguished are:

a) "Settling" of specimen.
b) Linear deflection. The first signs of cracking, including both the sounds of cracking and the appearance of a visible crack, occur here, usually in the lower end of this region, in most tests the tester was able to mark the first sign of cracking.
c) Small "hiccoughs," which correspond to fracture triangular crossection. This is probably attributable to shear stresses in the brittle porcelain coating.
d) The ragged uppermost portion of the curve indicates the fracture of the lower corner of the triangle, opposite to the applied load.

Discussion:

It is noted that in specimens with the porcelain layer, both solid and hollow, the metal was never strained beyond the yield point before the porcelain failed. Although the pressure on the specimen as a whole would have caused the metal to yield, the porcelain, in bending, was forced to stretch more than the metal.

This resulted in a higher stress in the porcelain, the metal remaining within its elastic region.

It appears that the very first instance of cracking is a more crucial measure of the performance of a porcelain specimen (especially from the patient's point of view) than is the highest load sustained by the piece. This can be compared in those specimens when noting an audible crack. The fact that the tested specimens produced this initial crack at a pressure level below the all-metal forms poses critical questions regarding metal stiffness.

Because this group of specimens had no end-plates, tests were more accurate these bend than the previous ones. The dimensions of the specimens were consistent, and the tests were quite reproducible.

Conclusions

The solid metal models are much stronger than the hollow (as expected). Veneering the two metal substrates with porcelain produced similar bend strengths. A dramatic increase in fracture strength of the hollow metal substrate occurs when the porcelain core is added (416–930). The increase in fracture strength of the solid metal/porcelain veneer was not as large as expected. The load limit of both metal/porcelain composites probably far exceeds normal requirements.

An enlightening observation regarding spruing and metal porosity demonstrates the need for better control over shrinkage porosity, particularly with bulky metal pontics.

Failure to achieve a dense casting will dramatically reduce the tensile strength of this premium gold alloy. Improved spruing and the use of chill vents should be used to control this problem (*Miller,* 1977; 1980).

The tests are not conclusive but add weight to the clinical observations that hollow pontics offer promise. Other types of testing are indicated, such as fatigue, thermal, impact, and shear tests.

The author wishes to acknowledge and thank technician Kathy Kaldenbaugh for specimen preparation and Jon Peltier of Mass. Institute of Technology for testing the research material.
Robert and Jane Ullrich contributed the artwork.

References

Amsterdam, M. (1974): Periodontal Prosthesis, Alpha Omegan. Dec., p. 29.

Brown, W. S., Christensen, D. O., Lloyd, B. A. (1978): Numerical and experimental evaluation of energy inputs, temperature gradients, and thermal stresses during restorative procedures. J. Am. Dent. Assoc. 96: 427.

Craig, R. G. (1980): Restorative Dental Materials, 6th Ed. St. Louis: The C. V. Mosby Company. 424

Eames, W. B., O'Neal, S. S., Monteiro, J., Miller, C., Roan, J. D., Cohen, K. S. (1978): Techniques to improve the seating of castings. J. Am. Dent. Assoc. 96: 432.

Faucher, R. R., Nicholls, J. I. (1980): Distortion related to margin design in porcelain-fused-to-metal restorations. J. Prosthet. Dent., 43: 155.

Gavelis, J. R., Morency, J. D., Riley, E. D., Sozio, R. B. (1981): The effect of various finish line preparations on the marginal seal and occlusal seat of full crown preparations. J. Prosthet. Dent., 45: 145.

Gher, M. C., Vermino, A. R. (1981): The Int. J. Perio. and Rest. Dent. Quintessence Pub. Co. 5/81.

Gilboe, D. B., Teteruck, W. F. (1974): Fundamentals of extracoronal tooth preparation, Part 1. Retention and Resistance Form. J. Prosthet. Dent., 32: 651.

Glickman, I. (1964): Clinical Periodontology. 3rd Ed. Philadelphia: W. B. Saunders Co., pp. 750–757.

Goldstein, R. (1976): Esthetics in Dentistry. Philadelphia: J. B. Lippincott Co., p. 338.

Goodacre, C. J., VanRoekel, N. B., Dykema, R. W., Ullman, R. B. (1977): The collarless metal-ceramic crown. J. Prosthet. Dent., 38: 615.

Hamaguchi, H., Cacciatore, A., Tueller, V. M. (1982): Marginal distortion of the porcelain-bonded-to-metal complete crown: An SEM study. J. Prosthet. Dent., 47: 146.

Hegdahl, T., Silness, J. (1977): Preparation areas resisting displacement of artificial crowns. J. Oral. Rehabil. 4: 201.

Joly, R. (1979): Effects of Preparation Design on Seating and Retention of Castings. Partial fulfillment for M.S, Tufts University School of Dental Medicine.

Kashani, H. G., Hera, S. C., Gulker, I. A. (1981): The effects of bevel angulation on marginal integrity. J. Am. Dent. Assoc. 103: 882.

Kuwata, M. (1980): Gingival margin design of abutments for ceramo-metal restorations. Quint. of Dent. Tech., 37–43.

McLean, J. W. (1979): The Science and Art of Dental Ceramics. Berlin: Quintessence Publishing Co., Inc. Vol. 1, 1979.

McLean, J. W., Wilson, A. D. (1980): Butt joint versus bevelled gold margin in metal-ceramic crowns. J. Biomed. Materials Research, 14: 239.

Miller, L. L. (1977): Framework design in ceramo-metal restorations. Dent. Clin. N. Am., 21: 699.

Miller, L. L., Shärer, P., Rinn, L. A. (1980): Esthetic Guidelines for Restorative Dentistry. Berlin: Quintessence Publishing Co., Inc.

Newcomb, G. M. (1974): The relationship between the location of sublingual crown margins and gingival inflammation. J. Periodontal., 45: 151.

Pascoe, D. F. (1978): Analysis of the geometry of finishing lines for full crown restorations. J. Prosthet. Dent., 40: 157.

Presswood, R. G., Skjonsby, H. A., Hopkins, G., Presswood, T. L., Pendleton, M. (1980): A base metal alloy for ceramo-metal restorations. J. Prosthet. Dent., 44: 624.

Preston, J. (1977): Rational approach to tooth preparation for ceramo-metal restorations. Den. Clinics N. Am., 21: 683.

Rosner, D. (1963): Function, Placement, and Reproduction of Bevels for Gold Castings. J. Prosthet. Dent., 13: 1160.

Rubin, T. I. (1980): Reconciliations; Inner Peace in an Age of Anxiety. New York: The Viking Press.

Shell, J. S., Nielsen, J. P. (1963): Study of the bond between gold alloys and porcelain. Bulletin of the S. California State Dental Lab. Society. Aug.–Sept.

Shillinburg, H. T., Hobob, S., Fisher, D. W. (1973): Preparation design and margin distortion in porcelain-fused-to-metal restorations. J. Prosthet. Dent., 29: 276.

Sillness, J. (1970): Periodontal conditions in patients treated with dental bridges II. The influence of full and partial crowns on plaque accumulation development of gingivitis and pocket formation. J. Periodont. Res. 5: 219.

Sozio, R. B., Riley, E. J. (1977): A precision ceramic-metal restoration with a facial butted margin. J. Prosthet. Dent., 37: 517.

Stein, R. S. (1977): A dentist and a dental technologist Analyze Current Ceramo-metal Procedures. Den. Clinics of N. Am., 21: 731.

Townsend, J. D. (1982): Coronal Contours: Periodontal and Restorative Considerations. Presented before The American Academy of Crown and Bridge Prosthodontics. Chicago, Feb. 1982.

Tylman, S. (1970): Theory and practice of crown and fixed partial prosthodontics (Bridge), 6th ed. St. Louis: The C. V. Mosby Co., pp. 225–229.

Weiss, P. A. (1977): New design parameters: Utilizing the properties of nickel-chrome alloys. Dent. Clin. N. Am. 21: 769.

The Porcelain Jacket Crown

David E. Southan

Dentine is the prime source of colour in a tooth and enamel envelops the dentine with a translucent, prismatic mantle. Highest light transmission occurs at the incisal one-third and in the proximal regions. A one-millimeter-thick section of enamel can transmit up to 70% light. A comparable slice of dentine only transmits up to about 30% light.

The chemistry and relatively low surface energy of the smooth surfaces of dental porcelain make it highly compatible with soft oral tissues. It also has a potential for aesthetic compatibility with the hard dental tissues. Nevertheless, providing an aesthetic single porcelain jacket crown on a maxillary central incisor can be an extremely demanding task.

Optical Properties of Dental Porcelain

The composition and structure of the phases present in dental porcelain and their arrangement all serve to regulate its properties. Differences in crystalline texture influence translucency and mechanical strength. The ratio of transmitted to diffused light can be used to describe the translucency of an object. Since diffusion of light takes place at boundary surfaces or interfaces, it follows that anything that reduces such irregularities increases translucency. As the indices of refraction of the various phases present in porcelain approach one another, so translucency is improved. The primary method used to increase the translucency of dental porcelain has been to increase its glassy content. Internal voids opacify dental porcelain markedly. Insoluble gases trapped within closed pores impose a limitation on the ultimate density that can be achieved during air-sintering. All things being equal, the extra porosity that vacuum-sintering eliminates is only about 2 to 3%. But this apparently small difference greatly influences the optical properties of dental porcelain. It does not have a significant effect on measured strength.

Fortunately, the eye is not as sensitive to colour, especially the numerous minute colour variations found in vital teeth, as it is to the outline form and surface texture of the teeth. The skill of the clinician is the only limiting factor in providing an aesthetic silhouette.

Matching translucency (or value) and "colour" optimally requires an informed consideration of the optical properties of the ceramic materials at our disposal. Too often we approach an aesthetic problem without weighing up the limiting factors associated with the various types of porcelain crown.

If artificial crowns are to simulate natural teeth, a depth of translucency is necessary. Colour must be seen in depth. Surface colorants cannot achieve this effect: their high covering power provides highly reflective surfaces.

Frequently, in crowns there is a need to mask undesirable ceramic or metal backgrounds. Accordingly, opaque porcelains were developed and it is from these that many of our aesthetic problems arise. Opaque porcelains are highly reflective and increase metameric problems (*Southan,* 1979).

Evolution of Dental Porcelain

Dental porcelain has evolved from the traditional triaxial whiteware materials. These were made from kaolin, feldspar, and quartz. Such porcelains show a heterogeneous microstructure (Fig. 1). A fine mullite-glass matrix contains feldspar relics of glass and mullite, quartz grains surrounded by their solution rims and pores (*Southan,* 1970a). Such porcelain is strong and relatively opaque. The kaolin content is the source of crystalline mullite. A great advance in the aesthetics of dental ceramics occurred when the formation of crystalline mullite was eliminated from the fired body by removing kaolin from the formulation (Fig. 2). This change resulted in a deterioration of their mechanical properties.

Modern dental porcelains differ from the older high-fusing and medium-fusing porcelains by being supplied as homogenized, fritted powders. The high-fusing types were more heterogeneous powders—not unlike some of the materials used today for the manufacture of porcelain teeth. Some had a relatively high kaolin content in the raw batch.

The introduction of vacuum-sintering in 1949 represented another aesthetic achievement: by this means color rendition and translucency were standardized. Such porcelains were dense, pigmented, quartz-bearing glasses (Fig. 3). They provided dentistry with a peak in aesthetics unequalled by today's materials. They allowed an appropriate diffuse transmission of light, which produced a natural depth of translucency. There were no dramatic changes in optical properties from the veneer porcelains to the "opaque" porcelains. The so-called "opaque" materials differed from the veneer porcelains only in their density of pigmentation. These opaques were still translucent enough to allow colored cements to influence the apparent shade of the crown (Fig. 4). Macrocrystalline quartz disrupted their glassy matrices. Unfortunately, because it was necessary

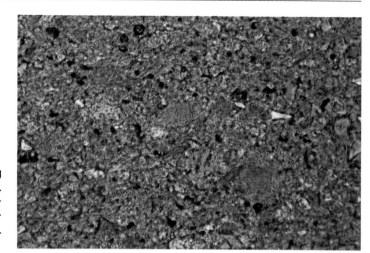

Fig.1 Triaxial whiteware showing hetereogeneous microstructure. Feldspar relics of glass and mullite, quartz grains, and pores reside in a fine mullite-glass matrix. Thin section, polarized light.

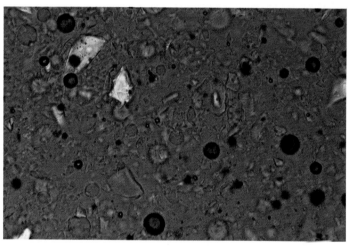

Fig.2 Air-fired, pigmented, quartz-bearing dental porcelain. Note homogeneity of vitreous matrix—no evidence of mullitization. Quartz grains are large and angular. Pigment is sparse. Thin section, polarized light.

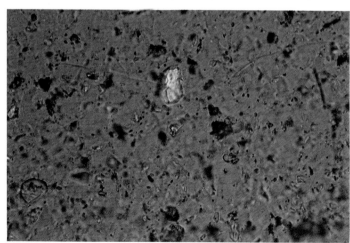

Fig.3 Vacuum-fired, pigmented, quartz-bearing veneer dental porcelain. Note absence of discernible porosity in matrix. Thin section, polarized light.

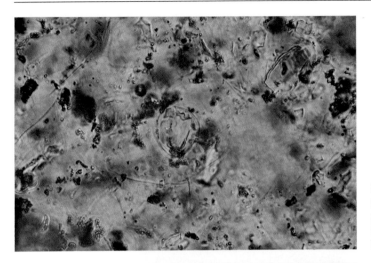

Fig. 4 Vacuum-fired, pigmented, quartz-bearing "opaque" dental porcelain. Note density of pigmentation in matrix. Thin section, polarized light.

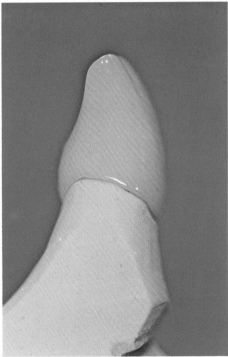

Fig. 5 Porcelain jacket crown constructed on platinum foil. Note poor adaptation at gingival margin. Tinner's joint in matrix on other side of crown.

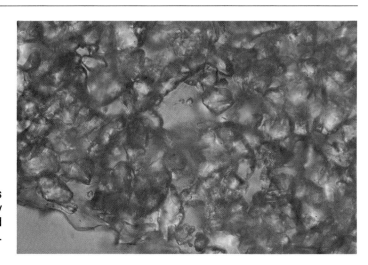

Fig. 6   High-fusing aluminous core porcelain. Note refractory framework of closely packed alumina crystals in glassy matrix. Thin section, polarized light.

to form such porcelains on platinum foil matrices, gross internal defects were encountered. Functionally unreliable crowns resulted (*Southan* and *Jørgensen,* 1972 b).

When a multiparticle-sized powder is mixed with a vehicle and condensed onto an impervious surface, a sporadic type of condensation occurs at this impervious surface. Good adaptation of the porcelain to the impervious surface is difficult to establish. Dental porcelain does not wet platinum, and the voids and vaults formed are too large to be eliminated by the normal driving forces during sintering (*Southan* and *Jørgensen,* 1973). Also, poor adaptation at the gingival margins is an inherent consequence of techniques that employ platinum matrices (Fig. 5).

In an attempt to remedy the unreliable serviceability of the quartz-bearing porcelains, *McLean* and *Hughes* (1965) introduced crystalline alumina into dental porcelain. The alumina grains (mostly 30–40 µm in size) are embedded in a low-fusing, high alumina glass. Pre fritting the mixture improves the bond between the alumina grains and vitreous matrix. Aluminous porcelain veneer crowns typically consist of a core material that differs markedly from the veneer materials. In the core porcelains, a pigmented, glassy matrix is heavily laden with refractory alumina crystals (Fig. 6), while the veneer porcelains consist largely of pigmented glass containing little crystalline material (Fig. 7). The core porcelains require higher temperatures and longer times to sinter to a dense body than do the veneer materials: they are also much less translucent.

A viscous liquid develops when dental porcelain is fired. The major part of densification results from viscous flow under the pressure caused by fine pores. This effect is due to surface tension. Viscous flow of the matrix is impeded by the closely packed crystals in aluminous core porcelains. These alumina crystals provide a refractory framework for the

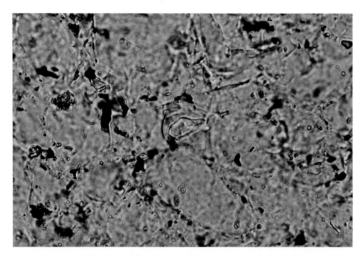

Fig. 7 Aluminous veneer porcelain. Pigmented glass matrix contains few crystals. Central grain is quartz, which is present as an impurity. Note prismatic effect in vitreous matrix. Thin section, polarized light.

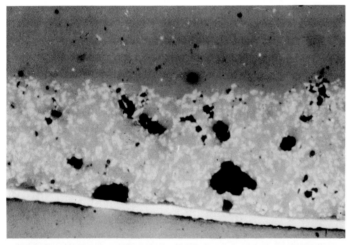

Fig. 8 Typical polished section of an aluminous porcelain jacket crown before removal of the platinum foil. Core contains many irregular voids. It has been underfired. Reflected light.

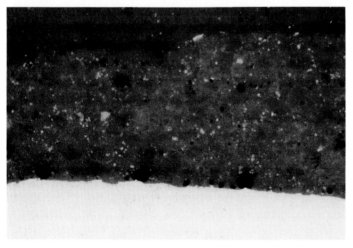

Fig. 9 Polished section of a metal-ceramic crown. Note the numerous opacifying particles in the core layers. Reflected light.

body. If these cores are not subjected to lengthy firing cycles at high temperatures their density, and hence optimal translucency and strength, may not be realized (Fig. 8). The veneer porcelains behave quite differently; no such refractory crystalline impediment to rapid densification during sintering is encountered.

One-millimeter-thick sections of core porcelains used in aluminous crowns can transmit 20% light if fired properly (*McLean* and *Hughes,* 1965). The veneer materials can transmit considerably more light.

The aluminous core and dentine porcelains are matched in hue, but any incorrect placement of the core porcelains can enhance metameric effects. If the core is built too thickly on the labial surface, increased specular reflection results. Optimal aesthetics are achieved only when the core is kept to about half a millimeter thick labially.

We have seen how aesthetic demands on the anterior veneer crown have influenced the evolution of modern dental porcelains from the triaxial whitewares. These empirical changes in formulation and microstructure enhanced the optical properties of dental porcelains but caused their mechanical properties to deteriorate. A compromise was needed. Perhaps this is embodied in the aluminous porcelains. But overcompensation has occurred and has resulted in a loss of optimal aesthetics. Routine use of the metal-ceramic crown in the incisor region is an example of such overcompensation.

The metal framework in the metal-ceramic crown dictates the use of opaque porcelains with high covering power. Light transmission through the opaque porcelains used to mask the metal coping is very low indeed. One-millimeter-thick specimens transmit about 0.2–0.5% incident light. By way of contrast, opaque core porcelains used in the aluminous crown transmit up to 100 times more light.

A natural tooth always allows diffuse transmission. Aluminous porcelain crowns permit some diffuse transmission of light, while metal-ceramic crowns, except at the incisor region, do not. The aesthetic limitations of metal-ceramic crowns stem from these facts. They show an increased reflectance. Opaques for the metal-ceramic crown contain minute particles of opacifiers that have an index of refraction far different from that of the vitreous matrix (Fig. 9). Opacifiers used in dental porcelain include tin oxide (SnO_2), zirconium dioxide (ZrO_2), and titanium dioxide (TiO_2).

The veneer porcelains used in the metal-ceramic technique are generally more opaque than comparable aluminous porcelains. Unfortunately, this also causes an increase in surface reflectance (*Eissman,* 1977).

Metal-ceramic crowns tend to look less vital because they have little depth of translucency. The metal-ceramic crown can be used successfully when the teeth happen to show an optical density in themselves. To compensate for the higher reflectance in metal-ceramic crowns, it is popular to select shades with a higher chroma: dull and unattractive crowns result. To reduce brightness, the value of the shade should be decreased.

In metal-ceramic bridgework, because the metal framework encroaches into the proximal areas, a depth of translucency is impossible to achieve in these regions. Naturally, such stringent aesthetic demands are almost nonexistent in posterior teeth.

The term "devitrification" refers to any crystalline precipitation in the glassy matrix of porcelain. Repeated firings make this process more likely to occur, and some materials are more inclined to devitrify than others. Devitrification opacifies porcelain. Both quartz-bearing and aluminous porcelains show little tendency to devitrify. Of course, repeated firings affect the pigmentation. Porcelains formulated to match metal frameworks are much more inclined to devitrify during repeated firings.

The Fracture Mechanism in Dental Porcelain

Dental porcelains are brittle materials, but one should not regard their brittleness as being synonymous with weakness. Because of the strength of the silicon-oxygen bond and the absence of grain boundaries, the glassy matrices of dental porcelains should have high intrinsic tensile strengths.

A strain of approximately 0.1 to 0.2 is required before a plane of atoms is completely removed from the attractive force of its neighbors. Rupture, then, would be expected at a maximum stress of 0.1 to 0.2 E. Since the measured strength is about one-hundredth of this theoretical stress, it becomes necessary to explain this weakness.

At room temperature, dental porcelain is almost perfectly elastic, and fracture occurs in tension and is due to the stress-concentrating action at the tip of a surface flaw. Classical stress release in metals at the crack tip is by glissile dislocation. This is not possible in vitreous materials. Fracture occurs in porcelain when the applied stress produces a stress at the flaw tip equal to the intrinsic strength of its matrix. Naturally, this would occur at the most severe flaw present in the stressed region. Once initiated, the extension of the crack is ensured by the applied stress and increasing stress-concentration factor of the growing crack. The presence of surface flaws in dental porcelain is by far the most important factor in determining its observed strength.

At the tips of surface cracks, where stresses are high, a stress-enhanced chemical reaction between glass and water is responsible for delayed failure in porcelains. Porcelain jacket crowns must function in the presence of moisture; externally from saliva and internally from the cementing agent (*Southan* and *Jørgensen*, 1974). A time factor is involved in this fracture process of porcelain jacket crowns. *Lehmann* (1967) observed that about 5% fail after an average time

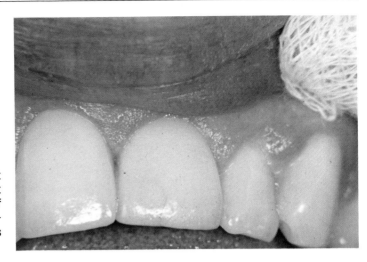

Fig.10 Crack detected in intact porcelain crown on upper left central incisor after two years of service. Crown had been fabricated on platinum foil. Six months later, the crown fractured.

of two years of service. Indeed, clinical experience indicates that most of these fractures represent examples of delayed failure (Fig.10). The presence of surface flaws, macroscopic or microscopic, on porcelain crowns can have a devastatingly weakening effect, especially if they occur where the tensile stresses are high.

Figure 11 shows the type of internal surface produced by forming porcelain jacket crowns on platinum foil matrices. These can be classified as serious macroscopic polymorphic surface defects. They are more numerous at the gingival shoulder-fitting surfaces of crowns, especially at the axio-gingival angle. In these regions the defects can be as large as half the crown's thickness (Fig.12). One of the ways microscopic flaws form is by matrix disruption by macrocrystalline quartz. All quartz-bearing porcelains whose glassy matrices are rigid at the inversion temperature of quartz (573° C.) demonstrate this phenomenon. The matrix surrounding the quartz grains is stressed enough by the volumetric change that accompanies their inversion to cause microcracking during cooling from the firing temperature, regardless of the rate (Fig.13). Quartz grains occur as impurities in some aluminous porcelains (Fig.14).

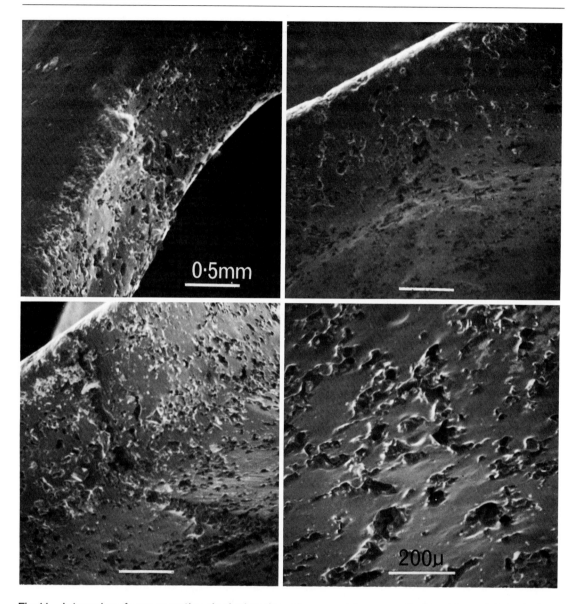

Fig.11   Internal surfaces near the gingival region of a porcelain crown that had been fabricated on platinum foil. Scanning electron micrograph.

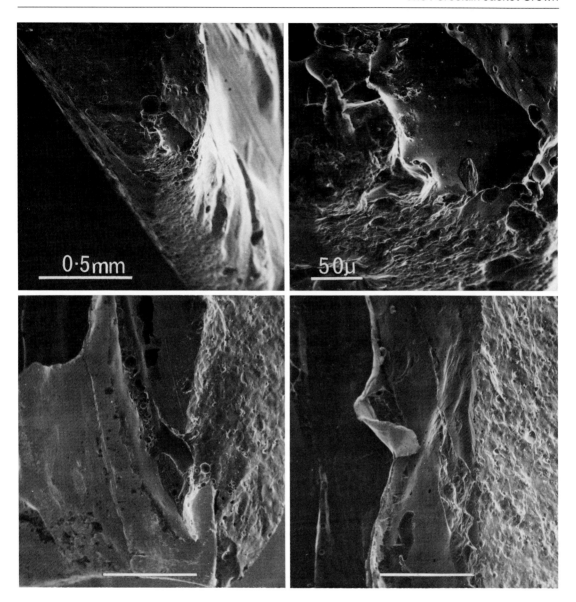

Fig.12   Fracture surfaces of porcelain crown that had been fabricated on platinum foil. Note position and size of defects at axio-gingival angle, upper left and right. Large area defects, lower left. Tag of platinum foil, lower right.

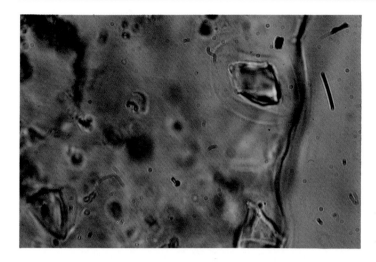

Fig. 13 Quartz grain near the surface of a quartz-bearing porcelain. Note the microcracking around the grain. Thin section.

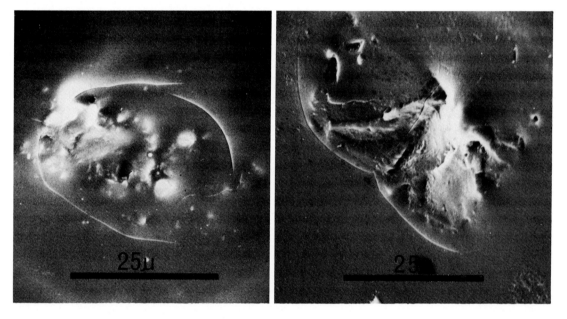

Fig. 14 Left: Cracks at the surface around a quartz grain in a quartz-bearing porcelain crown. Right: Cracking around the occasional quartz grain found in some aluminous porcelain crowns. Scanning electron micrographs.

Service Conditions for the Porcelain Jacket Crown

Porcelain in a porcelain veneer crown serves constantly as a thin shell in a moist environment and it undergoes intermittant stress over long periods. The crown (E = 57–99,000 MPa) functions mostly on a preparation of dentine (E = 14–28,000 MPa) and the intervening cement film (E = 9,100 MPa). Because of its relatively low elastic modulus, the supportive role played by the preparation is limited. A strain of only 8 to 10 μm per cm is required in dental porcelain before it fractures (*Southan,* 1975a). This inability to deform permanently without fracturing appears to have attractive clinical implications–this, perhaps, combined with porcelain's low surface energy. Carious involvement around even poorly adapted gingival margins is not a common finding.

It seems that bending stresses are of major importance in crowns, and in order to increase their reliability in service they need to have surfaces that are flawless and they need to be stiffened.

ent upon their elastic moduli (*Frey* and *Mackenzie,* 1967). But opacity is a feature of all heterogeneous systems and this presents a severe practical limitation for this method of strengthening.

All successful methods of strengthening porcelain without interfering with its translucency to any notable degree have involved the introduction of a compressive stress at the surface to offset the tensile stresses developed under a load. Chemical strengthening has been applied to dental porcelain (*Southan,* 1970b). This is an example of low-temperature ionic crowding at the surface. The strengths of existing aluminous porcelains can be trebled by chemical treatments. Chemical treatments are lengthy and need to be carried out when no further staining or fire-finishing is contemplated. The core material of at least one brand of aluminous porcelain differs slightly in thermal expansion from the veneer materials. These facts make chemical treatments less attractive at this time. However, formulation of the materials could be modified to overcome the second objection.

Strengthening Dental Porcelain

Two methods have been employed to strengthen dental porcelain: (a) dispersion strengthening and (b) chemical strengthening. Aluminous porcelains are glass-crystal composites and behave as constant strain systems. Amongst other things, their rupture strength is depend-

Tooth Preparation for the Porcelain Jacket Crown

Much has been written on the form of tooth preparation for the porcelain veneer crown. We have seen what a poor support dentine provides. It is flexible and gingival shoulders cannot support a crown that is poorly adapted to them.

Aesthetic considerations dictate that the depth of tooth structure removed from the labial surface be such as to accommodate at least 1.25mm thickness of porcelain, and that a space of about 2 mm exists between the incisal edge of the crown and that of the preparation. On the lingual surface, 1 mm clearance from the opposing incisors is required in all movements of the mandible. If there are no biological or functional disadvantages, retain enamel on the lingual surface wherever possible. This provides a stiffer support for the crown. There is no necessity to accentuate the cingulum in the preparation. The lingual surface may follow a gentle curve from the gingival shoulder to the incisal edge. Retention has never been a problem for the porcelain jacket crown. It generally has to break before it comes away from the preparation.

The shoulders should be at right angles to the long axis of the tooth and should be at least 1 mm wide with no bevels. Try to keep the levels of the shoulder in one plane. The proximal levels should approach those of the labial and lingual shoulders wherever practical and acceptable to the periodontium. A crown with its gingival margins approaching the same horizontal plane is the aim. There is absolutely no need to sharpen the axio-gingival line angles on the preparation. Since intimate adaptation of a crown built on platinum foil to such sharp internal line angles is impossible to achieve, this procedure is completely ineffective as a supportive measure for the crown and unnecessarily injurious to the pulp.

The preparation should be as wide mesiodistally in incisors and buccolingually in canines as is practical, and rounded. Except for the cavo-surface angle there should be no sharp external or internal angles on the preparation. Wherever possible, bear the crown on a hard gold alloy thimble, core, or shoulder. This provides a stiff support.

Requirements of a Porcelain Jacket Crown Technique

We have seen how aesthetic demands have influenced the formulation and densification of dental porcelain. These efforts produced quartz-bearing, vacuum-sintered materials that depended upon the platinum foil matrix for their fabrication into crowns. By now it must be obvious the influence the platinum foil matrix has on the serviceability and adaptation of porcelain crowns.

This heretofore inexplicable and unpredictable behavior of such restorations instigated the unreasonable and indiscriminate use of metal-ceramic crowns on anterior teeth. Nevertheless, it is only reasonable to look for a technique to replace the highly aesthetic, but easily fractured porcelain crown.

A porcelain veneer crown technique for anterior teeth should possess the following requirements:

1. Porcelains designed for the technique should not be opacified to compensate for and cover dark backgrounds.

2. These porcelains should not contain quartz and the light transmission of the body and veneer porcelains should approach that of dentine and enamel respectively.
3. The production of gross internal sub-surface and surface defects in the crowns must be reduced or eliminated.
4. The technique should reliably produce accurately adapted crowns at the gingival margins. It would be preferable if hard stone dies could be used to achieve this.
5. Provision of about 50 µm relief for cement on all parts of the die except on the gingival shoulder should be possible.
6. The porcelains should have a coefficient of thermal expansion comparable with that of alumina.
7. A method of stiffening or reinforcing the crown without providing an optically dense background should be available.
8. The technique should provide for good cement retention of the crown.
9. The crown produced should not totally obscure the outline and position of the coronal pulp in a radiograph.
10. In the event of root therapy being necessary, it should be possible to penetrate the lingual surfaces of the crowns produced without requiring their replacement.
11. The technique should be easily modified to produce accurate and aesthetic splints and bridges.

Providing more serviceable porcelain crowns is not without its aesthetic cost. Our objective is to employ an acceptable compromise.

A Survey of Porcelain Crown Reinforcing Techniques

Techniques employed to reinforce porcelain jacket crowns include:

1. The metal-ceramic crown technique
2. The alumina-reinforced porcelain crown technique
3. The technique of further reinforcing aluminous crowns with sintered high alumina profiles
4. The platinum-bonded alumina crown technique
5. The electroformed gold matrix porcelain crown technique
6. The gold-coated platinum foil porcelain crown technique
7. The pervious refractory die technique

It is appropriate to examine these techniques in the light of optical and physical requirements for anterior porcelain crowns.

The Metal-Ceramic Crown

The metal-ceramic crown technique is well known. Meeting the optimal aesthetic requirements imposed in the anterior region should make selection of the metal-ceramic crown often improbable.

The metal framework dictates the use of opacified porcelains with high covering power. These porcelains do not contain quartz and their translucency is less than ideal for anterior teeth.

Usually, there are no gross defects at the metal-ceramic interface. Using the appropriate tooth preparation and framework design, well-adapted crowns with relief for cement can be made very acceptably on modified stone dies.

These porcelains have been fluxed to match the thermal expansion of the metal framework–not that of alumina. The reinforcing metal framework provides an optically dense background.

Cement retention is good. While these crowns can be penetrated lingually without great detriment, they are radiopaque. This technique can be modified to produce accurate splints and bridges with less than optimal aesthetic properties.

The Alumina-Reinforced Porcelain Crown

The alumina-reinforced porcelain crown technique represents the first attempt made to replace quartz-bearing, vacuum-sintered porcelains with relatively aesthetic reinforced porcelains (*McLean* and *Hughes,* 1965). The materials designed for this technique have not been opacified to cover dark backgrounds and contain little or no quartz. *When the core porcelains are sintered to achieve optimal density, their translucency approaches that of dentine.* The veneer materials possess a prismatic translucency that resembles enamel. Best results are achieved when the core is formed to match the silhouette of dentine for the tooth.

These crowns are fabricated on platinum foil and are affected with the internal defects and unreliable accuracy that result from such a method. For best results in gingival adaptation, metal or metalized dies are necessary. Aluminous core porcelain is more resistant to deformation than the quartz-bearing opaques. The fit of alumina jackets is more easily maintained during firing of the veneer porcelains because the core will not shrink or distort after its final firing. Provision of relief for cement is difficult to make in this technique.

The thermal expansions of these porcelains do match that of alumina. The aluminous porcelains represent examples of dispersion strengthening. They should behave as constant strain systems. In the thin shells that are porcelain jacket crowns (1–2 mm thick), surface defects are far more influential in determining measured strength than are the available dispersion strengthening techniques (*Southan,* 1968). This is not necessarily true for thicker sections of porcelain (> 5 mm). These facts explain the relatively poor clinical performances shown by such crowns.

Cement retention is high in these crowns and they are radiolucent. One cannot reliably penetrate their lingual surfaces without subsequently needing to replace them.

Because these porcelains match the thermal expansion of alumina, this tech-

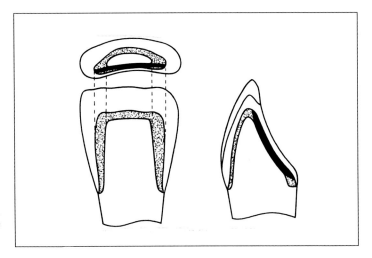

Fig.15 Diagrams of an aluminous porcelain crown with high-alumina reinforcement. Speckled areas represent core porcelain. Black areas represent the high-alumina profile. (a) Note the form required to achieve optimal aesthetics. (b) Note distribution of porcelains.

nique can be modified to produce splints and bridges. Although they are aesthetic, achievement of acceptable accuracy is unpredictable.

Aluminous Crowns with High-Alumina Profiles

All the points made for the alumina-reinforced porcelain crowns apply here. High-alumina reinforcements that are about eight times stronger than dental porcelain can be used within the core porcelain on the lingual surface. The high alumina profiles that are available* are translucent and have little effect on the color and depth of translucency of a crown. A curved 0.5 mm thick high-alumina bite pad is cut out and embedded in and bonded to the core porcelain (Fig.15). For best reinforcement and aes-

* Vitadur Profile M, Vita Zahnfabrik, Säckingen, W. Germany.

thetics, always extend the profile past the mesial and distal axial walls of the preparation. To allow for platinum foil reburnishing, the profile must be cut short at the gingival lingual margin.

Such translucent ceramic reinforcements stiffen crowns and act as crack stoppers. They are radiolucent. They can be reliably penetrated without failure and increase the clinical performance of aluminous crowns markedly.

In the past, uranium compounds have been used to simulate the fluorescence of natural teeth. This practice has been discontinued and accounts for the change from Vitadur to Vitadur-N porcelains.

The Platinum-Bonded Alumina Crown

The Vita-Pt® platinum reinforced crown was introduced to overcome the development of internal defects in porcelain crowns (*McLean* and *Sced*, 1976). This involves a twin foil technique whereby a platinum matrix, plated with 0.2 to 2.0 μm of tin, which is subsequently oxidized, is left within the finished crown (*McLean, Kedge*, and *Hubbard,* 1976). The platinum foil that has been coated with oxidized tin provides a dark background; and this has influenced manufacturers to formulate a core porcelain (Vita-Pt core*) that will cover this greyness optically. Aesthetically, it is a retrograde step from the other aluminous materials. However, there are times when this effect can be used to advantage. Vitadur N veneer porcelains cover the Vita-Pt cores. The metal is no more than 0.025 to 0.05 mm thick, but aesthetics dictate that it finish short of the labial margin. Here there is a porcelain butt fit.

The glassy phase in the porcelain wets the prepared metal surface during sintering, and chemical bonding occurs where intimate adaptation of the core porcelain to the foil has been achieved in the build-up. In areas of poor adaptation, the rate of wetting would be impeded by the crystalline alumina phase and the size of the defect. Crowns made in this manner perform well under clinical conditions. The bonding of a thin layer of platinum to dental aluminous porcelain can increase breaking stresses by up to 80 % (*Sced, McLean,* and *Hotz,* 1977).

As with all platinum foil techniques, the fit of the crown is determined by the re-adaptation of the foil at the cervical margin at the second core porcelain application. For this reason, metalized

dies are to be preferred. When the crown is completed, the unplated inner foil is stripped out to leave a space for the cement lute. Polyacrylic acid-based cements will bond chemically to the tin-plated platinum foil.

The porcelains are aluminous and can be further reinforced with high-alumina profiles. The crowns do not totally obscure the outline of the pulp on a radiograph. They can be penetrated lingually without great risk.

Achieving acceptable accuracy with the modifications to this technique that are advocated for bridgework is unpredictable.

The Electroformed Gold Matrix Porcelain Crown

This technique is based on the procedure used for forming a gold matrix for indirect gold inlays (*Rogers,* 1970). In two hours, twenty gold matrices can be electroformed simply and accurately.* A flash coating of electrodeposited tin on the gold matrix ensures good wetting of the matrix by porcelain (*Rogers,* 1979).

The coefficient of thermal expansion and firing temperatures exclude aluminous porcelains from use in this technique. Porcelains designed for the metal-ceramic technique must be employed. The electrodeposited gold is 0.15 to 0.2 mm thick. When the tin coating is oxidized, a deep gold metal background results. This is an optically mellow and

---

* Vita-Pt core porcelain, Vita Zahnfabrik, Säckingen, W. Germany.

* E. G. M. Electrodent System, Electro-Ceram Pty. Ltd., 70 Gymea Bay Road, Gymea, N.S.W., 2227, Australia.

chemically reactive surface. Aesthetically, such a metal background is preferable to dark oxide surfaces that are characteristic of silver grey alloys. The production of internal defects is greatly reduced and the discrepancies introduced by the tinner's joint in platinum foils are eliminated.

If an apron of matrix is left, adaptation to the die and/or tooth is possible to ensure optimal adaptation of soft gold to tooth margin. Marginal correction is possible before, during, and even after cementation. *Rogers* (1979) advocates this technique for lower incisors with shoulderless preparations. Relief for cement can be accommodated, as can venting the lingual surface. Internally, the tin-plated surface of the matrix is receptive to polyacrylic acid-based cements. Stresses required to fracture the porcelain are as much as doubled by this technique (*Rogers,* 1981).

The crowns are reasonably radiolucent. Penetration of the lingual surface is possible without great detriment. To produce splints and bridges, separate metal frameworks would be necessary.

The Gold-Coated Platinum Foil Porcelain Crown

Porcelains formulated for the metal-ceramic technique can be built over platinum matrices coated with a thin layer of gold* (*Dorney,* 1978). The gold coating

* Deck-Gold, Degussa, Germany.

provides a mellow, ductile background for the metal-ceramic porcelain formulation. The fluidity of the porcelain results in good adaptation to the matrix with few gross defects (*Southan,* 1979).

Of course, the use of platinum foil limits the technique's accuracy. Cement relief can be provided.

Such a procedure has distinct advantages, especially when one is faced with repair to metal-ceramic bridgework. However, from an aesthetic point of view, it retains the limitations of the ceramic materials it employs.

Cement retention would not be enhanced by this technique. The crowns are radiolucent. With care it should be possible to penetrate their lingual surfaces without fracturing them.

Separate metal frameworks would be necessary to produce splints and bridges.

The Pervious Refractory Die Technique

Some aluminous porcelains furnish us with relatively refractory cores. This property is utilized when the refractory die technique is employed for the manufacture of porcelain crowns (*Southan* and *Jørgensen,* 1972a). Such porcelains have not been opacified and contain little or no quartz. Indeed, when correctly sintered, the light transmission of the core and veneer materials approach that of dentine and enamel respectively.

Phosphate-bonded investments can be mixed with distilled water to make accurate and pervious dies that have a thermal expansion comparable with aluminous porcelain. Since the dies are pervious, the production of internal defects in the porcelain is greatly minimized (Figs. 16 to 18).

Space for cement can be provided by forming readily removable resin copings over the stone dies of the master cast. Erkopress spacer material 0.15 millimeters thick[1] is admirable for this purpose. When heated and pressed[2] over the die it forms a coping about 50 μm thick. The coping is trimmed to leave the cervical shoulders of the die uncovered.

Record the modified die in a low viscosity elastomeric impression material. Vinyl polysiloxane is excellent for this purpose.[3]

Pour a phosphate-type investment that contains no carbon into this impression.[4] Use distilled water in the proportion of 3.5 ml to 25 gm of investment powder. Subject this set die to a firing cycle of up to 1150° C at reduced atmospheric pressure.[5]

Like the aluminous crowns with high-alumina profiles, translucent alumina reinforcements are prepared to be incorporated into the core porcelain. If need be, this technique allows the profile to be placed right on the lingual gingival shoulder.

Mix the appropriate core porcelain* with distilled water and condense it onto the moistened, pervious die, embedding the profile in the process. Moisture can be absorbed through the die, condensing the core porcelain intimately onto its surface. Form the ceramic framework to provide a suitable optical and mechanical base for the veneer porcelains.

The dried framework is sintered slowly from 850° C to 1100° C in a partial vacuum. Break the vacuum and raise the temperature to 1150° C at atmospheric pressure. Hold the temperature at 1150° C at atmospheric pressure for five minutes. Cool and remove from the furnace.

A well-condensed framework will display wide cracking. Fill these cracks carefully right down to the pervious die with thin core porcelain slip and subject the body to a firing cycle similar to the first one. When 1150° C is reached, hold the work there for ten minutes under atmospheric pressure. Cool and remove from the furnace.

Break the investment die material away from the framework and sandblast it from the internal surfaces. An ultrasonic scaler can be used for this purpose, also.

Locate the trimmed ceramic framework onto the master die. Accurate adaptation at the gingival shoulder areas should be accompanied by a loose fit due to the predetermined cement space around the vertical walls of the preparation.

[1] Erkopress–Material UZF 0.15 mm ∅ 70 mm, Nr. 531715.

[2] Erkopress ES2002–Erko Dent Erich Kopp, Dental-fabrikation D-7293 Pfalzgrafenweiler, P.O. 1140, W. Germany.

[3] Permagum, Espe-Fabrik Pharmazeutischer Präparate GmbH., D-8031 Seefeld/Oberay, W. Germany.

[4] Whip-Mix Hi-Temp Casting Investment. Whip-Mix Corp., P.O. Box 17183, Louisville, Ky. 40217, U.S.A.

[5] Vita-Inframat–Vita Zahnfabrik, Säckingen, W. Germany.

* Vitadur S–Vita Zahnfabrik, Säckingen, W. Germany.

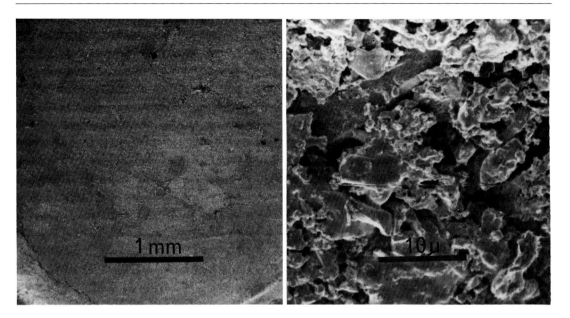

Fig.16 Scanning electron micrographs of pervious refractory die.

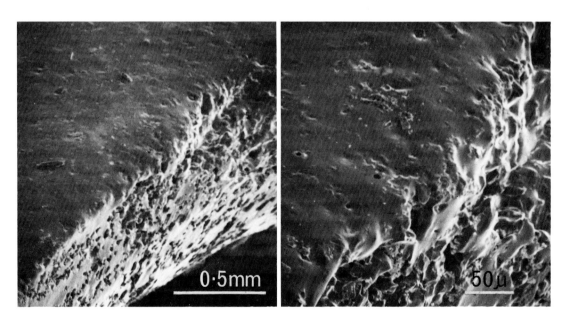

Fig.17 Scanning electron micrograph of cervical margin of porcelain crown fabricated on platinum foil. Note the abrupt change in surface condition where contact with the matrix finishes.

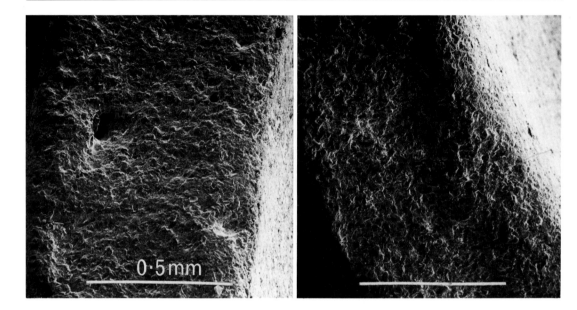

Fig.18 Scanning electron micrograph of the cervical shoulder and internal surface of a crown fabricated on a pervious refractory die. Note the relative absence of defects compared with Figure 17.

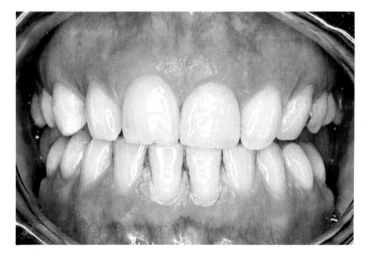

Fig.19 Aluminous porcelain jacket crown on upper left central incisor. This crown was fabricated on a pervious refractory die and has been in service for five years.

Finish the lower-firing veneer porcelain build-up. Fire the assembly using the ceramic framework as an accurate and stable base.

These crowns provide for good cement retention. They are radiolucent and can be perforated lingually without serious risk. Accurate and aesthetic splints and bridges can be made readily using this technique (*Southan,* 1975b; *Southan,* 1981).

Over the last eight years 435 porcelain crowns have been made in this manner on incisors and canines with aesthetics as the criterion for selection, not low functional demands. Only 0.68% have fractured and most of these failures can be related to identifiable traumatic incidents (Fig.19).

Conclusion

Providing aesthetic restorations is the ever more demanding taskmaster of modern dental practice. It is only when we fully appreciate the extent and nature of a particular problem and the limitations of the solutions that are available that we can plan the appropriate course of treatment.

References

Dorney, L. S. (1968): Alternative reinforced jacket crown construction. Information Bulletin. Sydney, Martin Halas Dental Co. Pty. Ltd., June/July.

Eissman, H. (1977): In Dental Porcelain–The State of the Art. Edited by H. N. Yamada, Los Angeles: University of Southern California School of Dentistry, pp. 297–301.

Frey, W. J. and *Mackenzie, J. D.* (1967): Mechanical properties of selected glass-crystal composites. J. Mater. Sci. 2 (March): 124–130.

Lehman, M. L. (1967): Stability and durability of porcelain jacket crowns. Br. Dent. J. 123: 419–426.

McLean, J. W. and *Hughes, T. H.* (1965): The reinforcement of dental porcelain with ceramic oxides. Br. Dent. J. 119: 251–267.

McLean, J. W., Kedge, M. I. and *Hubbard, J. R.* (1976): The bonded alumina crown. 2. Construction using the twin foil technique. Austral. Dent. J. 21 (June): 262–268.

McLean, J. W. and *Sced, I. R.* (1976): The bonded alumina crown. 1. The bonding of platinum to aluminous dental porcelain using tin oxide coatings. Austral. Dent. J. 21 (April): 119–127.

Rogers, O. W. (1970): The electroform gold matrix inlay technique. Austral. Dent. J. 15 (Aug.): 316–323.

Rogers, O. W. (1979): The dental application of electroformed pure gold. 1. Porcelain jacket crown technique. Austral. Dent. J. 24 (June): 163–170.

Rogers, O. W. (1981): Personal communication.

Sced. I. R., McLean, J. W. and *Hotz, P.* (1977): The strengthening of aluminous porcelain with bonded platinum foils. J. Dent. Res. 56 (Sept.): 1067–1069.

Southan, D. E. (1968): The physical properties of modern dental porcelain. Ph. D. Thesis, University of Sydney, p. 317.

Southan, D. E. (1970a): The development and characteristics of dental porcelain. Austral. Dent. J. 15 (April): 103–107.

Southan, D. E. (1970b): Strengthening modern dental porcelain by ion exchange. Austral. Dent. J. 15 (Dec.): 507–510.

Southan, D. E. (1975a): In Scientific Aspects of Dental Materials. Ed. Von Fraunhofer, J. A. London: Butterworths, pp. 277–305.

Southan, D. E. (1975b): Precise porcelain bridges. Austral. Soc. Pros. Bull. 5 (June): 8–11.

Southan, D. E. (1979): Aesthetic limitations of dental ceramics. Ann. R.A.C.D.S. 6 (Nov.): 117–126.

Southan, D. E. (1981): All-porcelain bridges–a ten-year study. Proc. Int. Congr. Biomats. Stom. (Sept.), p. 43.

Southan, D. E. and *Jørgensen, K. D.* (1972a): Precise porcelain jacket crowns. Austral. Dent. J. 17 (Aug.): 269–273.

Southan, D. E. and *Jørgensen, K. D.* (1972b): Faulty porcelain jacket crowns. Austral. Dent. J. 17 (Dec.): 436–440.

Southan, D. E. and *Jørgensen, K. D.* (1973): An explanation for the occurrence of internal faults in porcelain jacket crowns. Austral. Dent. J. 18 (June): 152–156.

Southan, D. E. and *Jørgensen, K. D.* (1974): The endurance limit of dental porcelain. Austral. Dent. J. 19 (Feb.): 7–11.

State-Of-The-Art Metal Ceramics

Utilizing Nickel Chromium Superalloy Frameworks

Peter A. Weiss

Background

The development of esthetic veneer restorations based on precious metal substructures reached its zenith in the early 1970s with the acceptance of the porcelain-fused-to-gold system as the industry standard. However, the use of gold alloys as structural components in dental restorations has always been plagued with problems because of the inherent weakness and poor fatigue resistance of gold: the dental industry is the only one in the world where gold is used in a structural application. In order to ensure freedom from structural failure, which is anathema to all concerned, substructures were traditionally overcontoured with such regularity that eventually the distortions became institutionalized in the educational literature available to technicians. Also, the unique economics of gold: "you have it–you sell it–you still have it," provided an enormous incentive to maintain the status quo.

Compounding the problem was the increasing distancing of the dental profession from dental technology and vice versa. This was nowhere more in evidence than the manner in which the technician's training was defaulted to the manufacturers. The result was that clinical dimensional parameters were set by people three times removed from the recipient of the service. Added to all this was the fact that most dentists were unfamiliar with the basic engineering principles that determined the success or failure of their restorations, and most technicians were utterly uninformed regarding the relationship between periodontal health and contour, neither one receiving sufficient feedback from the other's perspective to produce anything resembling optimum results.

It is not surprising that this milieu has produced a substantial amount of iatrogenic disease. It was to address these problems that I embarked on the twin course of establishing a private laboratory and then, with my own team, researching and developing the technology for nonprecious ceramics.

The purpose of this paper is to present an overview of the nickel chromium technology, highlighting its outstanding features and identifying critical areas of the clinical and laboratory technique.

Nickel-Chromium Alloys

The premier alloys under the general heading *nonprecious* are nickel-chromium-beryllium systems. They are characterized by three properties: resistance to oxidation, great strength, and superior flow. It is this triad of properties that is responsible for the elegant features we have come to recognize as "state-of-the-art."

Other alloy systems that fall under the broad heading of nonprecious are nothing more than responses to areas of market resistance. For example: alloys without nickel and/or beryllium to assuage those who espouse a selective environmental concern; alloys that are softer (via the addition of highly toxic gallium) for those who believe hardness is synonymous with difficult processing; or alloys that melt like gold (via the addition of toxic boron) for those who believe force of habit is a terminal limitation. Most of the alloys in this group oxidize badly and require special treatment to ensure bonding of the porcelain. Since the bond between porcelain and metal is paramount, it is foolhardy to go with systems that oxidize in an uncontrolled fashion, especially if desirable features must be given up in the process. The nickel-chromium-beryllium systems are best by a wide margin. Of these, Jeneric Industries' Rexillium III sets the standard.

Rationale

The purpose of replacing the gold alloy framework with one made of a nickel-chromium alloy is to enhance biocompatibility and esthetics by reducing the thickness of the coping and the cross-sectional area of the interproximal connection. Nickel chromium based ceramics, properly executed, allows superior esthetics, maintenance access, biocompatibility, and structural integrity to coexist routinely within the same restoration.

Overcontouring and miscontouring produce degenerative soft tissue changes and pocketing. Bacterial activity in these iatrogenic moats spews out toxins and enzymes. The presence of these noxious bacterial effluents in apposition to highly absorptive oral tissue is anathema when one considers that a few seconds after the blood courses through this region, it is traversing the heart valves.

Features

1. Reduction in coping thickness from 0.3 mm to 0.1–0.2 mm. Very small areas can be 0.05 mm. These are "as cast" dimensions (Figs. 5 and 6).
2. Reduction of the cross-sectional area of the interproximal connection from 4–8 mm^2 to 1–2 mm^2 (Figs. 18 to 20).
3. Reduction of the width of the interproximal strut/lingual collar to 1 mm (Fig. 18).
4. Full circumferential porcelain coverage for superior aesthetics and individual repair capability (Fig. 30).

5. Complete resistance to sag and deformation at temperature (Figs. 14, 15). Super-thin coping sections will not be deformed by porcelain firing (Figs. 5, 6, 26).
6. Thermal insulator. Thermal shock is virtually nonexistent.
7. Corrosion resistance. Maintains a lustrous polish in vivo (Fig. 12).
8. Facial and interproximal porcelain margins are routine (Figs. 26, 27, 28, 29).[1]
9. Casting accuracy sets a new standard (Figs. 7, 8, 9, 16).
10. Fourteen unit spans can be cast accurately in one piece (Fig. 13).
11. Framework repair, correction, and addition capability.[2]

Tooth Preparation

The basic preparation is a deep chamfer configuration that is made in very direct fashion with the Brasseler RCB 14, 15 torpedos. A frequent modification of this preparation consists of cutting a shoulder just above the finish line, creating a "beveled" shoulder in reverse (see Figs. 1 to 4). If necessary, standard retentive features can be added either with the primary cast or the secondary cast.

[1] International Journal of Periodontics and Restorative Dentistry, 1/81.

[2] Quintessence of Dental Technology, June, July, August 1980.

Gingival Retraction

Exposure of the finish line is via electrosurgery using a .012″ tungsten tip. This straight tip is modified by bending the last ½ mm at a 45 degree angle. Four such modifications, to each of the four compass directions, allow the required "V" shaped trough to be executed in 90 degree sectors, with the tip of the probe always directed toward the tooth. Facial areas and delicate, friable tissue are treated with a shortened straight probe that has also had its diameter reduced to .008″. Success of this procedure is dependent upon moisture control, by interaction between high-volume suction and a spray from the three-way syringe.

Impressions

The material of choice is hydrocolloid, the only aqueous compatible system. The advantages are many and outstanding:

1. No custom trays need be fabricated.
2. Associated cold and pressure combine as an innocuous yet potent hemostatic.
3. There is no dessication of tissue.
4. A wet field precludes bubbles, especially in internal line angles.
5. Excess material extruded beyond the posterior borders of the tray can be evacuated with the high-volume suction system. The danger of aspiration, therefore, is close to nil.
6. Hydrocolloid is extremely accurate; patterns and castings transfer freely between independent models.

7. The technique is noncritical. It can be taught to ancillaries.
8. Hydrocolloid is very cost effective.
9. As the material can be softened before model separation, there is no danger, whatever, of breaking the model.
10. The material will not deform beyond its elastic limit, tending rather to tear. This is a major advantage that makes distorted models unlikely.
11. Impressions can be taken at the rate of one every four minutes. This, together with modest cost, allows multiple models to be taken for every case. Distorted materials are thereby identified in the laboratory by transferring the pattern and/or casting to an independent model.

The light blue, heavy bodied material by Van R is best. There is little advantage gained by injecting the syringe material around each abutment. The syringe material should be discharged quickly on top of the tray material. Center the tray over the arch, and bring it "home" with a single, determined motion, generating as much hydraulic pressure as possible. The amount of pressure generated is a function of: (1) the height of the tray material, which determines the length of the seating path (overload trays vertically), (2) the difference in viscosity between syringe and tray material, and (3) the length of time it takes to seat the tray in the patient's mouth.

Models and Dies

Impressions are poured at once in Whip Mix "Super Die." When the models are dry, they are parallel-pinned using a Pindex machine. Do not use the Pindex dowel pins. They fit tightly and do not allow passive removal of the dies from the model base. Medium brass dowel pins are cemented into the parallel-placed holes with cyanoacrylate cement. An annulus of wax is placed around the base of each pin using the electric wax pen. The underside of the model is lubricated, and a base is poured.

Dies are sectioned, after drying, with a .007 jeweler's saw. Care must be taken not to peen the ends of the dowel pins with the model trimmer.

The dies are ditched below the finish line, which is highlighted with the side of a pencil lead.

Die Spacers

Paralleling the general deterioration of values, a school of thought has emerged that advocates restorations "seating" rather than "fitting." Any restoration will seat so long as it is larger than the die. This is what perpetuates copper band technique. It has, however, nothing to do with "fitting." The worst misfit can "seat" beautifully. Of course, it won't "fit." Fitting and seating aside, however, one of the strongest elements of retention is an intimate fit. It is a shame to degenerate it by default because we lack confidence in our ability to make the casting "fit."

Waxup

No die spacers are used. The simple expedient of using a thyxotropic cement (such as Caulk's Fynal or a glass ionomer cement) obviates the need for relief within the crown for cement. The dies are coated with a very thin film of Lubritex No. 12. An electric wax pen is used for all waxup procedures. If the words "technique sensitive" have any place at all in describing laboratory materials, they should be reserved for wax. Only its familiarity makes its many negative idiosyncrasies tolerable. For example, the use of a Bunsen burner with an 1800 degree flame to build up a wax laminate (the pattern) is frought with the risk of introducing internal stresses into the fabrication. And, as wax melts at around 150 degrees, it is hardly necessary that we continue with it. Using, instead, an electric wax pen set at a temperature somewhat above that of the wax's melting point obviates the problem.

The bright, reflective die stone (Whip Mix "Super Die") allows a visual estimation of the wax thickness (Figs. 5 and 10):

$$\text{yellow} = >0.1 \text{ mm}$$
$$\text{yellow green} = 0.1 \text{ mm}$$
$$\text{green} = 0.2 \text{ mm}$$

Each coping is released immediately after the wax has been applied. Margins are left slightly (0.1 mm) thickened to allow for finishing procedures.

Framework Design

There are a number of considerations beyond porcelain support that should be considered in designing a ceramo-metal framework, especially with the added versatility afforded by the nickel chromium technology:

1. **Removability.**–At some point, the best restoration will have to be redone. To facilitate removal, either the facial or the lingual surface should be cast to no more than 0.2 mm thickness. At that dimension, the alloy can be cut with the greatest of ease.
2. **Repair Capability.**–If each unit is designed for full circumferential porcelain coverage, beginning with the preparation, then each unit is individually repairable by merely removing the porcelain and replacing it with a ceramo-metal repair unit.
3. **Endodontic Access.**–If an endodontic encounter can be projected, a portion of the occlusal (lingual) surface should be cast thin enough to allow easy penetration by a round carbide bur.
4. **Maintenance Access.**–If the restoration is not maintainable then its service time becomes a function of host resistance. Esthetics and root proximity permitting, all embrasures should allow passage of an interproximal cleaning instrument (ProxaBrush) (Fig. 20).
5. **Processing Ease.**–Interproximal struts should be located in such a way (toward the lingual) that they are accessable for polishing procedures (Fig. 16).

A general rule is that if maintenance access (biocompatibility) and esthetics are in conflict, then the former is deferred to in the way of a metal display. Such occasions will be relatively infrequent with the premier nickel chromium systems.

The interproximal areas of nickel chromium substructures should resemble "gothic arches." This form best meets the demands of maintenance access and natural, gingival level tooth contours. The inferior aspect of the interproximal connection should be rounded. A sharp line angle in this area predisposes to breakage.

Spruing, Single Units

A standard sprue configuration is made using three 8-gauge hollow plastic sprues connected to each other at one end, and to an 8-gauge hollow, plastic runner bar at the other. This creates four positions on the runner bar at which copings can be mounted. One or two single copings can be attached to each site, using the shortest possible length of 14-gauge hollow plastic sprue material. Connections are made with sticky wax. All surfaces should be super smooth. If two sprues are attached at one position, they should form a tight "V" so each is as close to the orbital plane as possible. All thin, facial margins should face the direction that trails the motion of the casting machine.

There should be a "long throw" from the pattern area to the sprue base. This allows the melt to cool slightly and drop off debris before entering the pattern end of the mold. Close inspection of the castings confirms that most of the inclusions stay behind near the sprue base. The closer we get to our casting, the cleaner the surface appears (Fig. 8).

The sprue system is affixed to the sprue base with periphery wax, and this connection is shaped into the form of a venturi. It is secured with a minimum of sticky wax. All surfaces below the runner bar are then coated with a film of low-fusing wax (1:1 red baseplate wax and petrolatum).

Spruing Multiple Units
(Sequential Spruing Technique)

To begin spruing a multi-unit pattern, place an imaginary arch above and concentric within the pattern arch. Locate the first of a series of Surgident reservoir sprues at the midpoint of the pattern on top of the interproximal connection, with the other end "touching" the imaginary arch. Secure with sticky wax. The sticky wax connection should be spherical and smooth. Locate the second reservoir sprue at the top of an adjacent interproximal connection so that there is a three-point contact between the ends of the two sprues, their reservoirs and between the tip of the sprue and the interproximal connection. Join the contacts between the two sprues only. Repeat for the other adjacent interproximal connection. Now make a "tack" joint with a minute amount of sticky wax where the tips of the reservoir sprues touch the interproximal connections. Complete the joint with a very low-fusing wax. Repeat this sequence. If three-point contact cannot be maintained, alternate the reservoir sprues with plain hollow plastic sprues or use a hollow plastic sprue shim between two reservoirs. Always maintain contact between the tip of the sprue and the top of the interproximal connection, between the two adjacent reservoirs, and between the ends of the adjacent sprues. Do not allow the angle between the reservoir sprue and the occlusal plane to become too acute. If it threatens to, insert a plain hollow plastic sprue between two reservoir sprues and/or shim the ends of the reservoir sprues.

When finished, allow the temperature of the sprued pattern to stabilize. Remove the pattern from the model with minimum pressure. Either the copings will come off their dies or the dies will come out of the base. In the latter case, carefully remove the dies individually from the pattern. Secure the sprued pattern to the sprue base with periphery wax, molding the wax into a venturi shape. All surfaces below the runner bar are coated with the red wax/petrolatum mixture. The basic idea in centrifugal investment casting is to have no sharp changes in direction and no rough surfaces, i.e., nothing to produce turbulence within the incoming molten alloy.

Investing

The investing procedure is the heart of a precision casting technique. The investment expands in a manner that is controllable, compensating the contraction of the alloy as it cools to room temperature. There are two types of dimensional casting errors: distortion and over/under compensation. The former enters during waxup or spruing and is related to the relative ease with which stresses can be built into the developing pattern. The latter is a function of the investing parameters:

Increased Expansion

$<$ liquid concentration
$<$ spatulation time
$<$ burnout temperature
   hygroscopic technique

Decreased Expansion

$>$ liquid concentration
   expansion impeded

Manufacturers have difficulty maintaining consistency in the investments they sell due to the vagaries of their raw material supply. They do not standardize their investments. But it is evident from the chart above that virtually any combination within the range of the investment is possible.

In order to access the available expansion of a combination, it is necessary to arrange that the expansion is not impeded. Traditionally, varying numbers of wet asbestos liners provided the necessary "give." This technique has limitations. We have for some time and with excellent results used rings lined with a very low-fusing wax (1 : 1 red baseplate wax/petrolatum). As the investment begins to react, heat is generated, softening the wax and allowing the ring to be lifted off. Expansion can now proceed, unimpeded. The investment block is burned out without benefit of ring. Expansion is unimpeded, elimination of exhaust gases facilitated, and the lighter load in the casting machine increases the very important initial thrust.

Large patterns are invested using a slight dilution of the investment to increase working time. Small patterns may need an assist via the hot water tap to remove the ring.

The best, most consistent results by far are with investments made by the BEGO Company in Bremen, West Germany.

Burnout

For very smooth-surfaced castings a stepped burnout is effective (Fig. 8). A typical schedule is:

Pyrometer Setting (Fahrenheit)	Set Timer (Minutes)
300	30
600	30
900	until smoke stops
1560	15–120 minutes

Casting

Since the alloy is very light compared with gold, it needs a higher initial thrust from the casting machine. The best machine we have found to date is a vertical centrifugal machine from the Dick Ells Company in Los Angeles, California.

Heat transfer from torch to alloy is poor. It will therefore take longer to melt the metal. The end point is somewhat difficult to judge but occurs when a "shadow," which recedes gradually from the flame tip, disappears. Melting can be with oxy-acetylene or propane/oxygen, but the torch must have a large, multi-orifice tip to bring a large quantity of heat to the alloy in a short period of time.

Devesting

Non-recycling airbrasive equipment is mandatory. For devesting, 50μ optical grade alumina at 100 pounds pressure will work rapidly. Rather than chance a commercial compressed air source, we use "extra dry" bottled carbon dioxide. To free large cases, a small pneumatic mallet is a great convenience.

Occupational Health

A dental laboratory is a noxious environment unless adequate measures for the evacuation of airborne particulate are in force. In general, the smaller the particle size, the more dangerous the contaminant. Abrasives, in whatever form, pose a special hazard. They should, if possible, be evacuated outdoors. Suitable equipment is inexpensive and can even be made by simply mounting a commercial kitchen fan in an outside wall near the floor and boxing it in with a counter unit. A grating, 12″ to 16″ in diameter, in the countertop produces a vortex that will bend an air turbine exhaust at a 90 degree angle.

If the evacuated air has to be recycled, a multi-stage system with several hundred square feet of filtration area would be minimal.

The alloy, although it contains beryllium, is a lesser danger because of the substantial particle size. Only two rotary instruments are required for processing nickel chromium ceramo-metal frameworks: (1) a high-speed lathe with a 2″ cutoff wheel for sprue removal. This piece of equipment has a suction port built into its housing that should be exhausted outdoors; and (2) an air turbine handpiece (such as a Star "Concentrix") with a No. 6 or No. 8 carbide bur for contouring the substructure. This instrument produces a very large size particulate but should still be used over a suction grate (see above).

The laboratory (and dental office) ambient air should be monitored for nickel, beryllium, silica, and alumina on a regular basis. In our State this service is provided free of charge by the Department of Public Health. In all their visits they have yet to detect even a trace of these substances.

Nickel Sensitivity

There has been much concern about "nickel sensitivity." Some individuals are indeed sensitive to nickel, such sensitivity being manifested as a contact dermatitis. However, there is no oral equivalent to the skin reaction. After a 14-year experience spanning some 50,000 units I have yet to see an oral lesion attributable to the restorative work. This is a substantial number. Either there is no such entity as an oral lesion related to nickel sensitivity, or it is so exceedingly rare as not to warrant limiting the use of nickel-containing alloys. The tissue response in Figs. 12, 20, 28 and 29 speaks for itself.

As with most situations, it is well to put things into perspective: We live in a nickel intensive society. From the coinage to the "stainless" steel knives and forks, to the hydrogenated vegetable oil (over a nickel catalyst), to the desalinated sea water (through nickel pipes), nickel is all around us. Its removal from the dental scene would accomplish next to nothing.

The position of the anti non-precious forces is almost wholly without merit. That this concern is selective and transparently selfserving should be apparent to anyone acquainted with the subject.

The same verbiage used to frighten people away from the new technology could easily be turned around to describe the precious metal systems. For example: Ceramic "golds" do not have elemental gold active on their surfaces. Gold is a ceramophobe. It has great disdain for porcelain. The only way to make porcelain adhere to gold is to alloy the gold with nonprecious components that will oxidize. It is these oxides to which the porcelain bonds. The alloying elements used for this purpose are tin and indium. Indium has a low-to-moderate level of toxicity. Tin is found primarily in the mineral *casserite* together with sulfur and arsenic. Some tin compounds are powerful toxins and are used as biocides!

This is not to suggest that gold alloys are a hazard, but only to underscore the absurdity of making projections in such a simplistic fashion. Unfortunately, the end result of such activity is to give some of the people who are using gold, without benefit of dust control equipment, a false sense of security by thinking that they are "safe," when, in fact, their health is in jeopardy from breathing the submicron abrasive particulate emanating from their grinding wheels.

> "There is nothing more difficult to plan, more doubtful of success, nor more dangerous to manage, than the creation of a new system. For the initiator has the enmity of all who would profit by the preservation of the old institutions and merely luke-warm defenders in those who would gain by the new ones."
> —Machiavelli (*The Prince*, 1518)

Surface Preparation

A bond is formed when the vitreous elements in the porcelain opaque "wet" the prepared surface of the substructure. Such preparation has as its goal the rendering of a chemically clean surface with a high degree of capillarity. There are basically two steps to this process:

1. Airbrasive Treatment

Function:

(a) Increases area of the surface.
(b) Increases the capillarity of the surface.
(c) Buffers the interface against shrink stresses.

Equipment:

A non-recycling airbrasive unit such as is manufactured by Comco, and others.

Abrasive:

50μ optical grade alumina.

Carrier:

Bottled extra dry carbon dioxide.

2. Degreasing (Ultrasonic)

Function:

(a) Decreases contact angle.
(b) Removes surface reactants.

Equipment:

Ultrasonic cleaner.

Solvent:

Reagent grade ethyl acetate.

The surfaces of oxidized nickel chromium alloys are "getters" for airborne organic contaminants. The opaquing should, therefore, proceed without delay.

Spray Opaquing

Applying the opaque porcelain with an airbrush (Figs. 21 and 22) produces a coating of dead even thickness and with no tendency whatever to pool on inside line angles or at the margin. The carrier has a very low vapor pressure, ensuring that the opaque impacts the surface of the casting dry. A basic formulation is as follows:

reagent grade ethyl acetate 90%–95%
U.S.P. collodion* 5%–10%

Two coats are applied, the first of which is ultra-thin (5μ) and visually transparent

---

* collodion acts as a "binder," allowing the sprayed coping or framework to be handled. It is cellulose nitrate dissolved in an ether/alcohol mixture and is obtainable from a local druggist or from a chemical supply house. Do not use "flexible" collodion.

(Fig. 23). As the firing temperature is reached, glazing elements in this opaque (Williams or Ultratek) melt and "wet" or flash over the surface of the casting. The opaque used for this coat has greater amounts of glazing elements in it. This coat, when fired, establishes the bond (Fig. 25).

A second, covering coat, is applied to hide the color of the metal and provide a reflective base for the body porcelain. This coat has an opacifier (tin oxide) in it. When fired, the minimum, total metal/opaque thickness should be 0.2 mm (Fig. 24).

Porcelain Breakage

Porcelain breakage can occur in the laboratory, operatory, or post-cementation. It can be precipitated by technique errors occurring during preparation, impression taking, casting, porcelain buildup or combinations of the four. Breakage of porcelain can involve a fracture (1) within the body porcelain, (2) at the interface between body and opaque porcelain, (3) at the interface between the 2 opaque layers, (4) at the interface between metal and opaque, or (5) within the metal. Innumerable suggestions and rigid routines have been suggested to overcome it. A popular remedy is to build the framework (pattern) to full form and contour, and then cut back for a very even thickness of porcelain. A monumental waste of time.

The two most relevant factors in porcelain breakage are: (1) dimensional errors in the dies and/or models and (2) inept porcelain buildup technique, especially as regards condensation.

Errors in the die can produce breakage under the best of circumstances. Preparations have low taper angles. Downward pressure against these inclined planes can multiply the lateral forces, resulting in breakage. Similarly, errors in the master model from die to die or occlusal prematurities all act as multipliers, making the basic tolerable forces destructive. The best insurance against this category of breakage is to use the hydrocolloid technique and make multiple models. Laboratory transfer of the patterns and/or castings will flush out inaccurate material before expense is generated. This routine will also save endless hours of chairtime spent in frustrating "fitting" procedures.

The second category of breakage is laboratory related. Each of my technicians who trained in porcelain sustained a substantial percentage of breakage as a novice which promptly disappeared as the medium was mastered and proficiency developed. In general, rapid buildup with large incremental additions and excessive shrinkage is synonymous with breakage. Buildup involving a number of laminations (as with an internal staining technique) and small additions, well condensed, produces breakage close to nil.

Metal breakage with properly designed and executed nickel chromium-based ceramics should be close to zero. Porcelain breakage with an experienced ceramist and a clinical input from multiple hydrocolloid impressions should be close to it.

In the end, however, everything we make for a patient can be broken. It is unrealistic, therefore, to proceed as if it cannot. Fixed bridgework must have reasonable repair capability. The full porcelain coverage so characteristic of nickel chromium-based metal ceramics resists breakage on the one hand (full coverage with porcelain is the strongest possible configuration for the porcelain/metal sandwich), and allows repairs on the other. The best of both worlds.

Porcelain Margins

The esthetic demands of patients must be considered and given weight. Few patients today will tolerate gold collars and other metal displays. After experimenting with a number of different techniques, both old and new, we settled on a rather simple and straightforward approach: The casting margin is feathered to a knife edge. Before the second coat of opaque is fired, it is cut at a 45 degree angle to the margin. This results in a feathered configuration. Body porcelain is now applied in normal fashion, but with the aid of magnification. Minimal optical aid consists of a pair of three diopter loupes. Preferred is a Bausch and Lomb Stereo Working Microscope with 10–25X zoom. An ideal result occurs when metal, opaque, and body porcelain meet at a common line angle. When the emergence angle has a positive value, the effect is the visual equiva-

lent of a porcelain jacket (International Journal of Periodontics and Restorative Dentistry, 1/81, pp. 34–44.

Porcelain margins allow the supragingival placement of restoration margins without attendant degradation of esthetics (Fig. 27). They can be so placed by design or the configuration can develop slowly as tissues recede for a variety of reasons.

The Secondary Cast Technique

Soldered joints rarely attain their theoretical strengths or the strength of a cast joint. The reason is twofold: (1) the strength of a solder joint is strongly related to the gap distance, or the separation of the two parts from each other. Any deviation, in either direction, results in rapid degradation of the strength of the joint; (2) the strength of a solder joint deteriorates as a function of time/temperature. Beyond these basic limitations, nickel chromium alloys simply cannot be soldered to the same standards as precious alloys.

A system was needed that superseded soldering, allowing additions, corrections and repairs to be made to nickel chromium frameworks. The system we developed was simplicity itself. The framework is prepared by providing it with mechanical retentions. The new area is then waxed, invested, and recast. The result is not a welded joint and success is most definitely dependent upon sound mechanical retention being established. However, if results are what count, this system is an unqualified success.

That triad of distinctive properties— strength, oxidation resistance and superior flow—imparted to the alloy by the beryllium allows a straightforward solution to a difficult problem. The types of repairs that can be made are limited only by the imagination of the technician. Corrections, and additions include: retrofitting interlocks; extending short margins into the sulcus; enhancing retention with grooves, pins, and shoulders, and making routine connections.

Type of Repair	Preparation
extending margins	No. 4 carbide bur (air turbine), *internally* bevelled
adding units	No. 4 perforations *internally* bevelled
retrofitting interlocks	No. 4 perforations *internally* bevelled
adding internal retentions	No. 4 perforations *externally* bevelled
connection (through pontic)	section; place two undercut grooves at right angles to each other and in register on the two facets

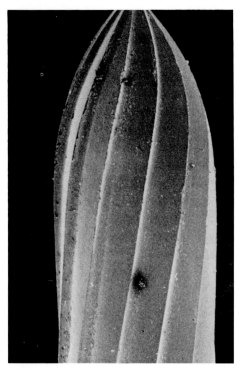

Fig. 1　The RCB 15 "torpedo" showing the fluted carbide blades. This instrument, preceded by its mated diamond, RCB 14, produces, in very direct fashion, the deep chamfer preparation shown in Figure 3. Scanning electron micrograph 20 X.

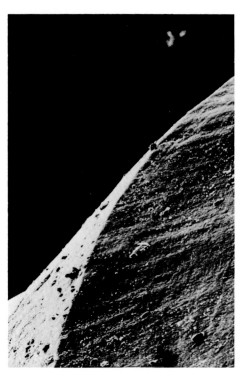

Fig. 2　Deep chamfer finish line produced by RCB 15 enlarged 100X by the scanning electron microscope.

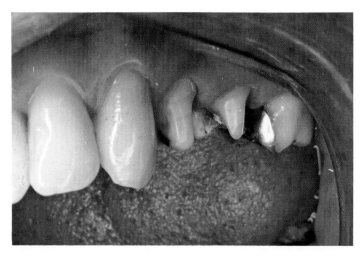

Fig. 3　Deep chamfer preparations made with RCB 14, 15. Note the bloodless field and the mirror-smooth surface.

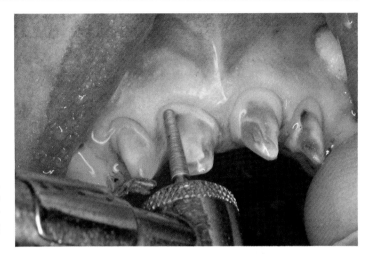

Fig. 4   Applying a round end taper instrument such as the Star 772-8P above the deep chamfer finish line produces a beveled shoulder modification.

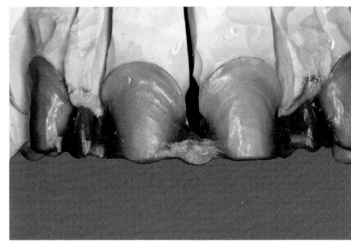

Fig. 5   The bright, reflective Whip Mix "Super Die" stone allows a direct reading of the wax thickness. The extensive thin area on the facial aspect of this framework will require auxilliary feed sprues.

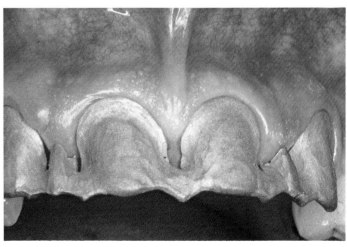

Fig. 6   The superior flow of the Rexillium III alloy allows such thin sections to be cast successfully. Note the placement of the margin about ½ mm into the sulcus.

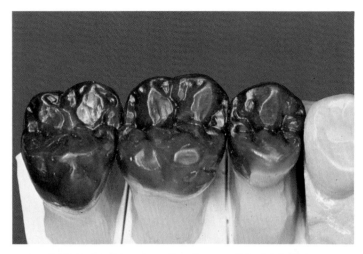

Fig. 7   The wax pattern should be advanced as far as possible in surface finish.

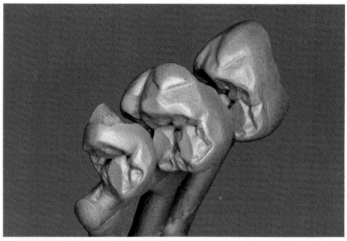

Fig. 8   All delicate margins face the same direction and trail the motion of the casting machine. Note the smooth surface texture of the casting.

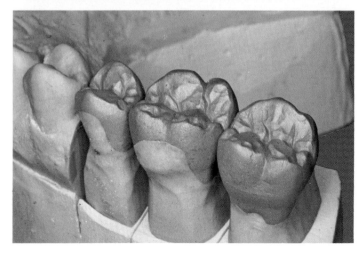

Fig. 9   Understanding the factors that increase or decrease the expansion of the investment will ensure accurately fitting castings.

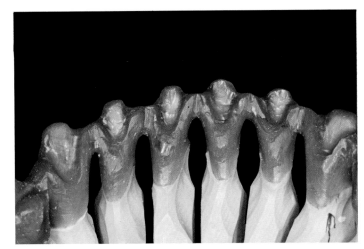

Fig.10 The architecture of the interproximal connections is that of a gothic arch. The thin lingual areas (yellow) measure less than 0.1 mm.

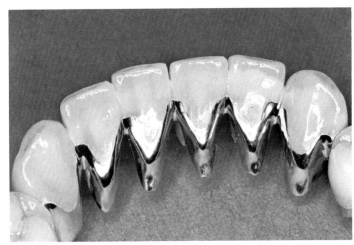

Fig.11 Note the natural gingival third contours facilitated by the reduced dimension of the interproximal connection.

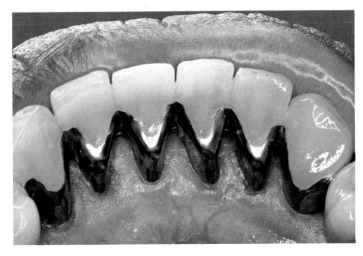

Fig.12 The tissue response to the premier nickel chromium alloys is uniformly good if the restoration fits and if the contours are biocompatible (Rexillium III).

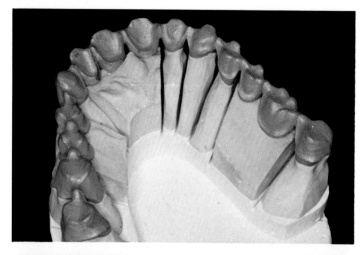

Fig.13 Fourteen unit castings can be executed if indicated.

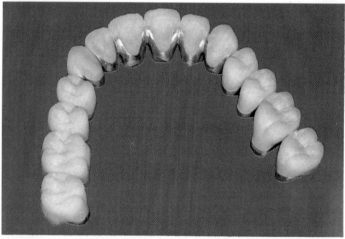

Fig.14 The nickel chromium alloys are sag resistant. The framework will not deform during porcelain firing.

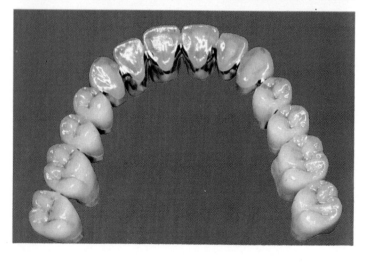

Fig.15 Each unit of this upper splint is repairable because the format is full circumferential coverage with porcelain.

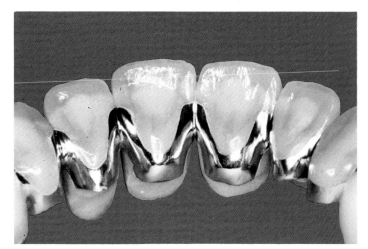

Fig.16 The Rexillium III alloy takes a lustrous polish. Note how the interproximal struts have been driven lingually to make them accessible for polishing procedures.

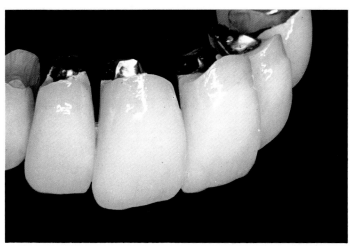

Fig.17 The reduced cross-sectional area of the interproximal connection allows the ceramist freedom to develop natural contours.

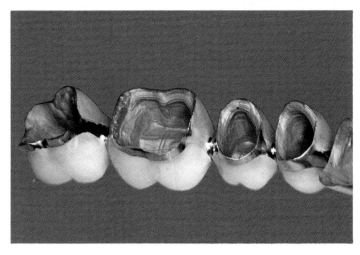

Fig.18 A typical framework. Note the greatly reduced dimensions of the lingual collar and the interproximal struts. The internal surfaces indicate that spacers were not used on the dies resulting in an intimately fitting restoration.

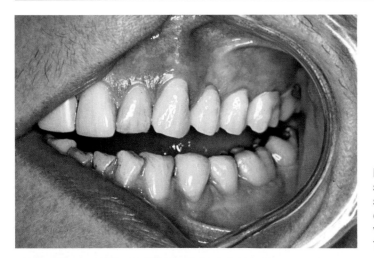

Fig. 19 The upper cuspid has strong gingival and incisal embrasures. Unless the interproximal connection is held down in size it will be impossible for the ceramist to create contours such as this.

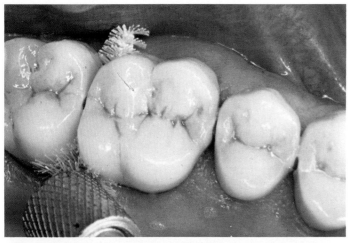

Fig. 20 The interproximal brush is the key to effective maintenance. As far as is possible, every posterior embrasure must be opened sufficiently to pass one.

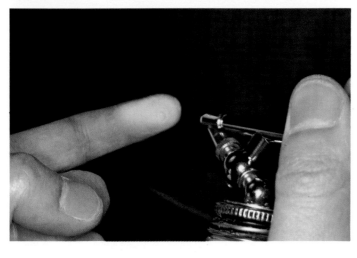

Fig. 21 Adjusting the Paasche Airbrush. Sprayopaqued deposits are dry on impact avoiding marginal puddling.

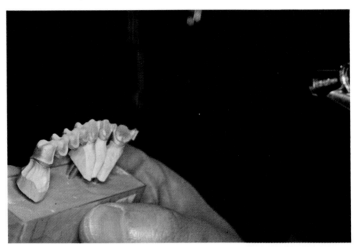

Fig. 22 The casting to be sprayed is mounted on its dies to avoid internal overspray.

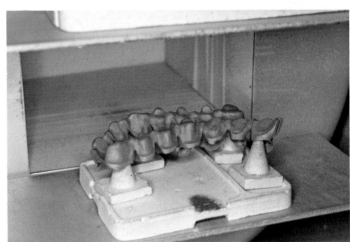

Fig. 23 The first opaque coating is thin and transparent. It establishes the "bond."

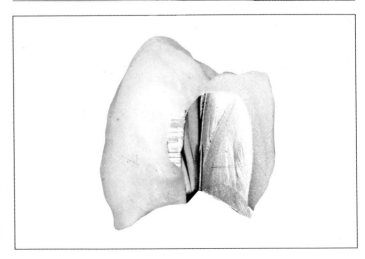

Fig. 24 A cross section through a pontic showing the reduced interproximal connection area. Note the dense casting and the thin opaque covering.

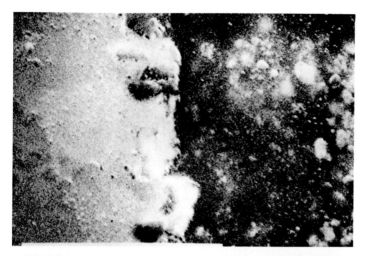

Fig. 25 The porcelain/metal interface. Note the intimate relationship between porcelain and metal. There is no sign of delamination or chemical activity at the surface. Metal is at left.

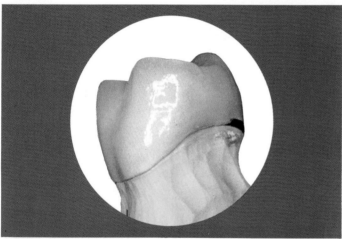

Fig. 26 There is no tendency for the alloy to distort when the porcelain is fired to it, even though it has been feathered to a knife edge.

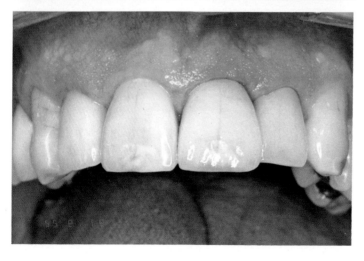

Fig. 27 Porcelain margins allow supragingivally placed margins even in this difficult upper central incisor area.

252

Fig. 28 Open embrasures and natural contours combine to produce this tissue response three years after placement.

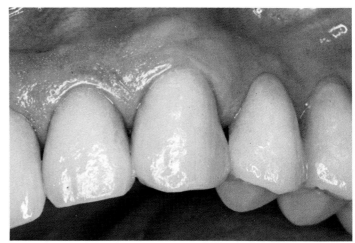

Fig. 29 This anterior restoration has subgingivally placed porcelain margins. Note the response of the tissues.

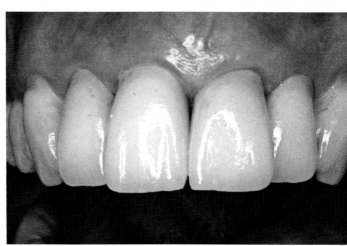

Fig. 30 Four single porcelain to metal (Rexillium III) crowns. For the first time dentists can remove tooth structure with reasonable assurance that the results will rival nature.

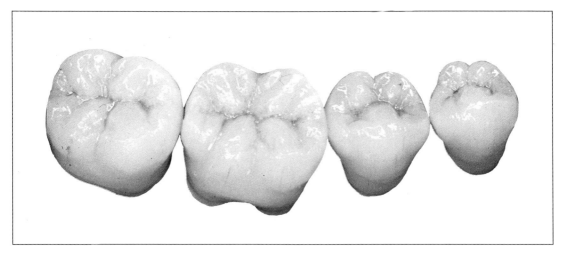

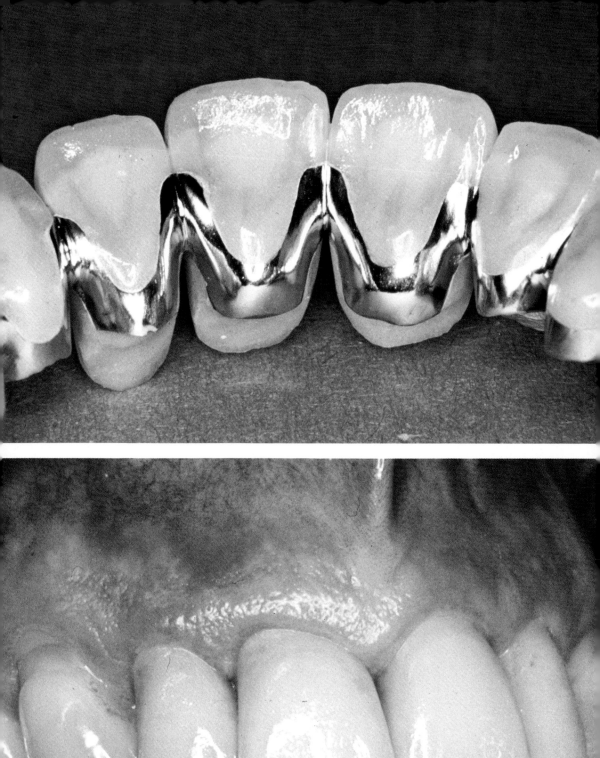

Conclusions

With the elegance, finnesse, and versatility of nickel chromium based metal ceramics firmly in place, dentistry has reached a major plateau. This marks the first time in the history of the profession that we can remove tooth structure with full confidence that the restoration will be the esthetic equivalent of the original. Collars and metal displays are a thing of the past. Frameworks can be altered in any number of ways so that virtually any technical problem can be dealt with.

The technology, mislabelled a decade ago as "technique sensitive," has become a model of simplicity. The casting accuracy, long criticized in the early 1970s is now the standard of the industry. Porcelain bonding is automatic. Virtually any clinical situation can be accommodated.

New Horizons?

Despite the beauty and effectiveness of this system, there has been a flurry of activity to find an "improvement." Nothing in this world is beyond improvement, but this time we have a difficult act to follow, indeed.

Porcelain fused to metal came to us from industry. But it was an aberration. In industrial processes hundreds of thousands of copies are run off a single master mold. In dentistry every "mold" is unique. The demands of dentistry as regards customization, fit, and structural specifications of multi-unit restorations are so high, that very few industrial processes can be considered for transfer. What the future holds, no one knows. But for the present, we have a great system. Let's use it.

laboratory work by:

ESTHETICS INCORPORATED
1253 Highland Avenue
Needham, MA 02192

Peter A. Weiss, D.M.D.
Isamu Hasegawa, Ceramist

Friday Afternoon, April 23, 1982

Panel of Experts: Dr. *Howard Bruggers,* Dr. *Lloyd Miller,* Dr. *David E. Simmons,* Dr. *David Southan,* Dr. *Peter Weiss*

Chairman: Dr. *J. W. McLean*

Participant

What is the source of discussion of the so-called toxicity of beryllium? Is it toxic to the technician or to the patient?

Dr. Weiss

I have to take credit for drawing attention to the beryllium in these alloys. I started it in 1968 by subjecting one of the alloys I was using to a spectrographic analysis. The assay revealed that one of the components was beryllium ($>1\%$).

The problem with beryllium is only with the air-borne particulate. I understand that some work has been done recently which indicates that the particle size of the alloy is so large as to constitute little danger. The real danger is from the submicron particulate emanating from the grinding wheel (alumina, silica, and the ceramic binders).

The danger for anybody who runs a reasonable laboratory operation with adequate exhaust equipment is nil. Exhaust equipment is essential in the dental laboratory. Mine is rather minimal, yet the Massachusetts Department of Public Health has yet to find any beryllium in the air of my laboratory or office environment. For the patient, there is no problem. Passivated beryllium-containing dental alloys, if toxic at all, are toxic only as a $>10\ \mu m$ air-borne particulate. The problem, if any, is restricted to the laboratory.

Participant

Dr. *Weiss,* does your casting technique for nonprecious alloys involve centrifugal torch casting or induction?

Dr. Weiss

We use centrifugal casting, mainly because the induction equipment that I have tested is deficient with regard to the centrifugal mechanism, although I'm impressed with the Shofu apparatus.

Participant

Do you find long-term bluish changes in the sulcular areas after electrosurgery? How do you stop the loss of the tip of interdental papillae? I find that in all my complete dental crown work, the very tip of the interdental papilla is lost.

Dr. Miller

Yes, I sometimes get long-term bluish changes in the sulcular area, but not from electrosurgery. How can one ascribe blame to electrosurgery six months, a year, or three years later? That's like saying electrosurgery causes recession. Time after time, when I see recession, it is caused by cement and acrylic, both biologic irritants, being maintained in tissue contact.

Dr. Bruggers

I agree with Dr. *Miller.* I think that probably the temporaries cause more damage to gingival tissue than anything else. However, I think that with anterior teeth, less damage is done with carefully placed cords than with electrosurgery.

Dr. Simmons

It is a function of careful technique. Certainly I would hesitate in using electrosurgery with thin tissue in the anterior region. As Dr. *Miller* has noted, the emergence profile is important with regard to future recession, in addition to the way the sulcus is handled.

Participant

Dr. Weiss, how do you cast to a tenth of a millimeter and polish your alloys?

Dr. Weiss

The only difficulty with casting these alloys is that they are extremely light. The ratio to gold being 2.2 to 1. Therefore, to make thin castings the casting machine requires a higher initial thrust. There is no difficulty if a machine that has adequate initial thrust is used as well as a correct spruing, burnout, and melting procedure; under these circumstances castings can be made to 0.1 mm quite easily. As to polishing away the margin, care is required at that dimension (0.1 mm). For example, we don't polish until we have the external staining checked and approved by the patient.

Participant

What is your view of the relative clinical strength of presoldered joints and post-soldered joints? Is there a best way to presolder for the strongest joint?

Dr. Miller

Postsoldered joints are much better, even in the hands of unskilled persons. Soldering will always be a hazardous procedure.

Participant

Does acidulated fluoride etch dental porcelain surfaces?

Dr. Weiss

Yes, acidulated fluoride does etch enamel and porcelain, and in my practice, it is used only in the control phase at the beginning of a reconstruction and while temporary restorations are in place. Patients with porcelain restorations use a neutral fluoride gel such as Therafluor-N.*

Participant

Dr. Miller, do you feel that there is a potential for improving the quality of porcelain butt margins by using burnished platinum foil during fabrication and removing it just before cementation, rather than using the separating media of which you spoke? Your concept of direct porcelain shrinkage would appear to support the foil method. Many of the castings that you showed appeared to be cast of white alloy, yet the margin color appeared to be yellow, as if electroplated. What is your rationale for this process?

Dr. Miller

We gold-plate our gold alloys before we put them in the mouth. I deny that the so-called white gold, as sold by the manufacturers, looks better because it imitates the color of white teeth. Polished white silver-colored alloy in the mouth reflects the darkness of the mouth and appears black to the patient. That is one of the things I don't like about it.

* Manufactured by the Hoyt Company, Norwood, Massachusetts.

As for using the porcelain butt margins, one of the reasons we started doing them more often is the introduction of a separating medium, one of which is made by Belle de St. Clair. We had been using a duplicate die in the ceramic material. I have no complaint about the foil technique except that shrinkage problems are not avoided. Porcelain shrinks, no matter what it is fired on.

Now consider reducing the visible metal collar to a knife edge.

A technician machines a metal margin down to a knife edge and does it under magnification, carefully, as perfectly as possible. Then the technician starts to build porcelain on it and at some point it becomes necessary to overbuild the porcelain slightly to compensate for the shrinkage to get the correct contour. Later, the technician must take a diamond or a stone and, holding it against the margin, begin to bring the excess porcelain back to the proper contour. It's *intimidating* to the technician to reduce that margin to the perfection that was present in the metal, because if the metal is contacted, a little black line becomes visible, and the esthetic control is lost.

Prof. McLean

In looking for the ultimate in esthetics, many people today are looking at porcelain butt fit in the metal ceramic crowns. How, in your experience, do you find obtaining a porcelain butt fit with the pure alumina and the metal ceramic?

Dr. Simmons

I have found that it is very difficult to get a good porcelain metal butt fit. Technicians prefer the all porcelain margins.

Dr. Bruggers

In teaching dental students and laboratory technology students, we have found that the students are better able to produce fine fitting margins with porcelain butt fit with aluminous porcelain than make the castings and then developing the close fits with the metal.

Dr. Southan

It is my experience with the metal, that vision is the limitation, while the aluminous porcelains provide the opportunity for using refractory dies whose properties enable one to get a very accurate butt fit.

Participant

What is the error in impression technique to which you alluded? It involved semilunar defects at the margins?

Dr. Weiss

Any negative error in an impression will have a tendency to produce such defects, especially in feather type preparations, which are the most vulnerable. The safest thing to do is to eliminate all the impression errors by taking multiple impressions and doing a laboratory transfer of the pattern or the casting, or both on the independent models.

Participant

Is the new Coors aluminous ceramic material opaque and available only in three colors that do not resemble dentin in any way?

Prof. McLean

The final formulation of this material is of course, a magnesium aluminate spinel; it is not a crystal/glass solid like the alumina porcelains. A fired ceramic of the Coors type would be considerably more opaque but could be stronger.

Dr. Miller

For matching a vital tooth crown to an adjacent vital tooth, nothing else on the market will duplicate the all aluminous jacket crown without the foil. The Coors unit does not provide the 20% light transmission of that crown; it is very, very opaque.

Dr. Simmons

Speaking about the 20% light transmission of the tooth, you mentioned the vitality of the tooth. That's important, too, as the patient ages. There is more secondary dentin and the pulp chamber is eliminated. As such teeth are more opaque, one may get by with a more opaque material.

Participant

Do you find hemorrhaging of the sulcus upon removal of the initial cord if you wet that cord before removal?

Dr. Miller

When dry string is put in the sulcus, it always becomes wet during manipulative procedures. When the string is pulled out, it is always wet and there is usually some bleeding unless vasoconstrictors or some other mechanism is used.

Participant

Does spruing to the connector areas in the nickel-chrome alloy eliminate the suck-back porosity described by Dr. *Miller* in his gold castings?

Dr. Weiss

I have not seen any suck-back porosity, at least not with the spruing technique that I showed you.

Occlusal Restoration in Dental Porcelain

William Comcowich

Clearly, the restorative dentist wants to be successful; and perhaps the measure of that success is how well the dentist can fulfill both his or her expectations and the patient's, relative to the finished case. Fortunately, I think that there is substantial agreement between patient and dentist as to what the treatment goals should be. The criteria for success should include aesthetics, function, longevity of service, and practicality from both clinical and economic standpoints. We all know, but should remind ourselves daily, that many potential areas of patient dissatisfaction could be obviated by really learning to listen so that we might better understand a patient's expectations, and, indeed, his entire perception of his role in the dental health rehabilitative process. If the patient wants to take little or no responsibility for his oral health, even in the hands of the best clinical dentist (and technician), this restorative case is surely doomed to failure. The tragedy here is that ultimately when the case does fail and the patient is unhappy and perhaps recriminating toward the dentist, many fine dentists feel that they somehow failed when the reasons for the failure were totally beyond their control.

Candid discussions of aims, goals, and expectations are necessary, and a clear understanding must be reached such that the role of the reconstructionist is simply as the therapist, and the patient ultimately assumes responsibility for his own health. Usually, this will require some education; sometimes it will require a near total reorientation of a patient's attitudes; and very seldom an impasse will be reached where the patient either can't or won't accept responsibility, in which case the reconstructionist would be well advised to refer the patient elsewhere.

Clearly, the use of porcelain can fulfill the four criteria for successful restorative dentisty:

1. good aesthetics
2. good function
3. outstanding longevity
4. practicality both clinically and economically.

When its use falls short of ideally attaining these goals, failure, in my judgment, can be attributed to two major factors:

1. preparation design
2. adverse forces of occlusion, primarily in parafunction.

If this is true, the conscientious dentist can more easily acquire the necessary skills to assure successful ceramic metal restorations by beginning modestly. The use of porcelain in restorative dentistry is surely not limited to cases restoring or replacing "28 new tops of the teeth." My understanding of reconstructive dentistry involves everything from a single unit to quadrant dentistry, to opposing quadrants, to mouths rebuilt in segments, and, finally, to the few we call full mouth reconstruction. The principles of preparation and occlusal considerations apply to all and are so much easier to sort out and perfect on the more modest cases. It is common for the "talented young dentists" who want to move their practices toward more aesthetic reconstructive dentistry to ask questions about how to do the 28-unit bite opening case with joint pathology, i.e., the "big case." My response to this is that there are so many things that can go wrong (technically) on the "big case," why not really learn all the necessary critical clinical steps (occlusion, tooth preparation, impression technique, centric relation bite-registration technique, mandible manipulation, provisionals, aesthetics, and phonetics, and TMJ considerations) on the "little cases." First, learn to do fine restorative dentistry by segments: perhaps posterior reconstructions by quadrants on patients with healthy joints, then opposing quadrants. Finally, after technical proficiency is garnered, an ideal full-mouth case where

"all the parts are there" in some semblance of order.

Parenthetically, from an economic and practice-building perspective, this approach also makes eminently good sense. There are many, many patients who really want full dental care but who feel overwhelmed by the cost of total restoration. If they could have their mouths properly restored in segments (fourths or halves or anterior, then posterior) rather than all or nothing they would accept the treatment plan and buy dentistry.

Understand, if they want and can afford the entire dental reconstruction at once, fantastic! But, I'm less than enamored with the "all or none" neuroses many dentists seem to have. Then they wonder why their case acceptance rate is low and naturally get quite discouraged with their profession.

Does this segmental approach mean a "compromise" in the final result? Nonsense! Even when I am doing a "full case," I prefer to do it by segments, where possible, to make it simpler and therefore better. I will address this more thoroughly later. Now, let's address in detail the reason ceramo/metal restorations are sometimes less than optimum in fulfilling our criteria and what we can do clinically to achieve better success.

The main factors over which we have control are, as noted earlier: (1) preparation design, and (2) occlusal stress considerations. In my judgment, *each* of these clinical considerations has a very direct effect on some or all of the criteria. For example, poor preparation design can surely be the reason for poor aesthetics, poor function, poor longevity, (porcelain fracture), and, therefore, economic impracticality.

Preparation Design

So, let us begin with preparation design first for anterior teeth and then for posterior teeth. Really, this is not all that complicated. However, we should reason conceptually, rather than have hard and fast rules. Be a "thinking dentist!"

Unquestionably, the biggest deterrent to natural looking porcelain aesthetics is insufficient removal of tooth structure. The classic example of this problem is well illustrated by the young lady for whom we are to do a cuspid restoration (either alone or as an abutment). We timidly cut our preparation with less than 1 mm of enamel structure removed and then send it to the laboratory with the instructions that we want a small, feminine cuspid, just like the precut model, with nice, natural, vital-looking porcelain. This is an obvious contradiction! We know there must be room for the metal framework, the opaque, and then sufficient bulk for vital translucent porcelain. But, our instructions said, don't make it bigger or bulkier than the original tooth.

Obviously this cannot be done in 1 mm. We remember that in the movie "The Godfather" when they wanted a more masculine, tough, or sinister-looking actor, they made him larger, longer, more prominent cuspids. So, if you want nice, tough-looking ladies in your restorative practice, continue to do grossly insufficient removal of tooth structure on your cuspid preparations so that the laboratory must make big prominent cuspids! More positively, if you really want the crowns to be small and feminine, give your skilled technician half a chance: the labial surface must have a very minimum of 1.5–2 mm of tooth reduction for proper vital aesthetics.

Next, the labial tooth reduction must not be done in one plane. The tooth curves to the incisal and thus for the preparation to have sufficient reduction in the critical incisal area for nice vitality and translucency, it, too, must be prepared in a curved manner (Fig. 1).

An often neglected area in anterior tooth preparation is the lingual concavity. Once again, let us assume sufficient reduction of tooth structure, but respect must also be paid to the curvature. If the lingual is simply prepared flat in one plane, it is extremely difficult for the technician to restore a pleasing, harmonious anatomical contour with a cingulum, ridges and grooves, and still get good functional anterior guidance. If the anterior guidance is to be changed in the final restoration, it must be planned for in the preparation stage.

Margins! There is absolutely nothing more critical to anterior aesthetics than marginal integrity, regardless of the margin design selected or even the position of its placement. This, of course, has many ramifications. Perhaps the biggest mistake we consistently make is "jumping into the restorative phase" too soon! In a moment, we will discuss in depth the absolute necessity of stabilizing the case

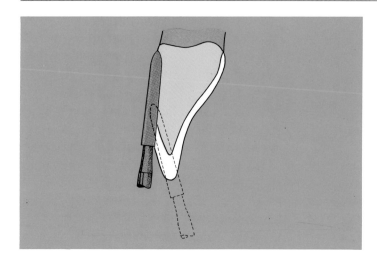

Fig. 1   Labial preparation done in two planes for sufficient reduction at the incisal third for proper contour and incisal translucency.

from the occlusal aspect prior to restoration. Equally important, we must establish optimum health in the periodontium, especially the gingiva, if optimum aesthetics is to result. Where do we want the margins relative to the sulcus in this case? Perhaps it may even be a different judgment on different teeth, but at least we have a concept of what we would like to attain in the finished case. Prior to restoring anterior teeth, where obviously aesthetics are critical, we like to have the gingiva in the very best condition possible. How sad it is when we do technically nice restorations, placed in a non-optimum sulcus, only to find that six months later our patient has accepted our health responsibility message and has finally attained beautiful, healthy, stippled gingiva–with our margins now well exposed. Good margins, to be sure, but not what we had planned. We require a healthy gingiva first and then maintain it with our restorative dentistry.

In any event, if we have poor marginal fits subgingivally, there will be local irritation and a predictably attenuated gingival aesthetic result. Poor marginal adaptation where we elect to be super-gingival also diminishes aesthetics with a cement margin. We can stain and glaze and characterize forever, but it will in no way overcome the basic deterrent to vibrant vital anterior aesthetics–unhealthy gingival tissue. Firm, healthy, natural gingival tissue with good papilla of proper color and texture is achievable only with meticulous attention to detail in fine restorative techniques of tooth preparation, impression-taking and concern for marginal integrity. It is then maintainable only by similar dedication to home care by the patient.

But what kind of margins? This is surely no place for dogmatic pronouncements, since many outstanding operators favor various designs with consistently acceptable clinical results. And, as new materials become available, more progress will be made to respect both

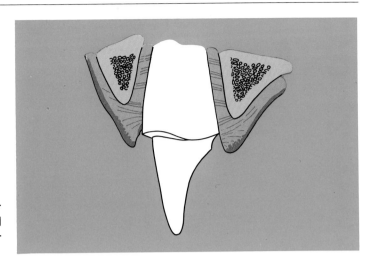

Fig. 2 Minimum 1.5 mm shoulder on the labial, and well–defined chamfer on the lingual with a well–rounded incisal area.

aesthetics and periodontal integrity. Personally, at present, I prefer a definite chamfer with an unmistakable finish line on the lingual and proximals. Sometimes, particularly on individual maxillary units, and more especially on virgin teeth where I have "the first go" at the preparation, we prefer the labial shoulder prep where the porcelain is baked directly to a treated stone dye without an intervening matrix as has been done in Australia for at least ten years and described by *Peter Vryonis* (1980). Note, however, that we need a shoulder of at least 1.5 mm width for this technique to be successful (Fig. 2).

Other times we use a deep chamfer labially, attempting to show as little metal as possible, and cover as much of the collar as possible with porcelain without excessive bulk and associated periodontal insult. Admittedly, this is a compromise. *Monginni's* work (1977), where he allowed the glaze to cover the gold collar, seemed to indicate clearly that tissue response with the glaze over the gold

was far superior to a restoration where the gold collar was simply polished and left unglazed. The improved tissue response to glaze clearly enhanced the overall aesthetic quality of the restoration.

The obvious dilemma, however, with trying to "hide" precious-metal collars is that if the collar is thick enough to resist bending (even in cementation) and subsequent chipping of the overlying porcelain, it is too bulky from a periodontal consideration in this critical area. If the contours are thin and proper, we indeed experience bending, chipped porcelain, and poor marginal adaptation. The use of premier nickel-chromium alloys for the substructure seems to hold great promise, since they can be thinned to .1 mm with no compromise in strength and can still properly support aesthetic opaque and porcelain for a total bulk of .25 mm at the chamfer junction (*Weiss,* 1981).

It should be noted that often in repreparing anterior teeth from previous dentistry, our options for "ideal" preparation are

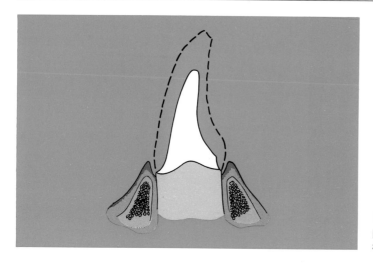

Fig. 3 Mandibular incisors prepared with full chamfer to preserve tooth structure.

unrealistic. Good clinical judgment must always be exercised and a balance reached between our conception of an ideal preparation and respect for the limited amount of tooth structure remaining. This concept of concern about severely weakening the tooth is invoked in design for lower anterior preparations also. Can we get a 1.5 mm shoulder here without substantially weakening the small tooth? I think not, and thus nearly all of our lower anterior preparations are chamfer preparations where, fortunately, aesthetics are not as critical and a metal collar, even if it shows, is not as detracting (Fig. 3).

Surely, I have nothing against the shoulder-bevel design concept either, except that its proper utilization presents the ultimate difficulty to both the operator and the technician.

Next, a few comments about a concept I refer to as "instant orthodontics". Aesthetic near-miracles can no doubt be accomplished by either repositioning or rotating the final restoration relative to the tooth position prior to the restorative procedure. But there are obvious limits, and the results are nearly totally dependent upon what can be accomplished in the preparation. If a protruding tooth is to be moved lingually, nearly all the preparation must be done at the expense of the labial, and it must be gross. Additionally, spaces may be closed, midlines moved, crowns placed "off center" over the tooth, but only within the limits of what we can do with the preparations, understanding that indeed a vital pulp does reside within the tooth. There are realistic limits as to what we can do orthodontically with preparations, but outstanding things certainly can be accomplished and should be attempted.

There are limits as to how much framework and subsequent bulk of porcelain can be built. It is very difficult indeed (or impossible) for a technician to "move" a tooth millimeters by simply bulking out the porcelain. The failure here occurs very early: as the unit is cooling from the bake!

Many people seem to worry excessively about the resultant loss of axial loading in this "instant orthodontics" by restorations, particularly on posterior teeth, where, for example, we might wish to correct a single-tooth crossbite in the bicuspid area. As long as one of the preparations can be done mostly at the expense of the labial and the other at the expense of the lingual, such that we can get realistic centric stops and eccentric disocclusion, the lack of perfect axial loading is not a problem, as we will discuss more fully under "Occlusion", relative to the magnitude of functional versus parafunctional loads.

Finally, to conclude our major thoughts on anterior preparations, it is absolutely essential to round the incisal area of the preparation well, in order to make the technician's job of waxing and casting possible; but it is far more important to eliminate (or reduce) the propensity for porcelain fracture, which, to a great extent, can be attributed to stresses set up by the sharp incisal angles (Figs. 1 to 3).

Most of the concepts described for proper tooth preparation for anterior teeth apply as well to the posterior teeth, with some modification. Once again, the biggest single problem is insufficient reduction of tooth structure (or base buildup), this time occlusally. I love enamel as much as any dentist alive, but, in order to properly fashion an occlusal scheme in keeping with the proper criteria of occlusion, which are soon to be addressed, there must be adequate room interocclu-

sally. If we intend to use full porcelain occlusion, obviously there must be room for cement, metal, opaque, and finally porcelain–all with cusps, fossa and supplemental grooves. This requires at least 2 mm of occlusal reduction.

Just as provision for proper anterior guidance must be made at the tooth-preparation phase in the anterior part of the mouth, so, too, provision for posterior occlusal considerations must be made while preparing posterior teeth. If, for example, our final occlusal scheme demands posterior disocclusion in eccentric movements, particularly in the orbiting or balancing excursion, it would seem essential that the "prepared tooth" be reduced enough such that at very least it does not touch its antagonist with no wax or restoration on it! How can the technician build a case free from posterior interferences if there was so little tooth removed in the preparation that these prepared teeth themselves touch each other in an excursive movement prior to the wax up?

The other place where sufficient tooth reduction is important is on the buccal surfaces, primarily for aesthetic considerations. If there is too little buccal reduction, we end up with bulked out or fat teeth, usually much larger-looking than the uncut natural teeth. Unless there is an important reason to make the teeth larger, purposely, good aesthetics would dictate that the restorations be the same size as the teeth were prior to restoration. So, once again there must be room for cement, framework, opaque, and sufficient thickness of porcelain for vitality. I prefer to use a deep chamfer preparation

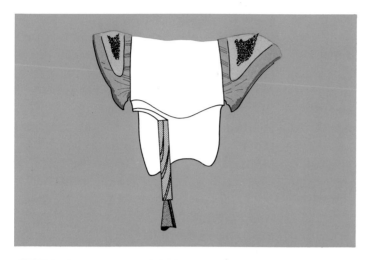

Fig. 4 Labial shoulder prepared above the chamfered finish line, well into the interproximal embrasures for added bulk of porcelain and thus a more vital appearance.

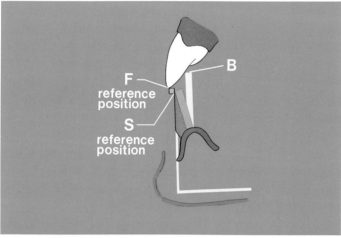

Fig. 5 Position of incisors is dependent upon proper function in speech.

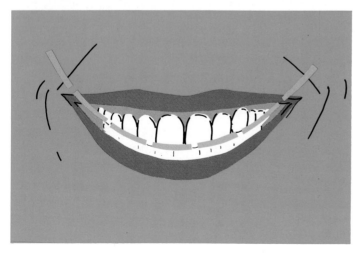

Fig. 6 Smile line of maxillary anteriors and the buccal cusp tips of bicuspids approximates the smile line of the LOWER lip.

totally circumferentially and to remove an extra millimeter in the buccal to a shoulder design that ends above the buccal chamfer line (*Ingraham,* 1981). For vital-looking porcelain interproximally, this shouldered buccal tooth removal must be carried well into the inner proximal, (Fig. 4). Here, too, the preparations should not be in one plane. Buccal tooth reduction done in one plane generally has the tendency of sufficient tooth reduction at the gingival third but insufficient reduction at the area of the cusps, where proper contour and bulk of porcelain are necessary for the finished crowns to be vital and to look like teeth. Posterior preparations, like anterior preparations, must have all angles well-rounded to minimize the potential of stress fracture (Fig. 4).

Preparation design is a vitally important consideration for successful ceramo/metal restorations that fulfill our essential criteria of aesthetics, function, longevity, and practicality. It goes without saying that learning proficiency and improving our skills in tooth preparation are hardly predicated on the necessity of doing full-mouth cases. Unquestionably, our learning curve will improve dramatically as we apply these preparation design criteria to routine, everyday dentistry, be it single-unit or quadrant restorations, without the inherent distractions that accrue to the big complicated cases.

There are several other important aesthetic considerations, none of which relate directly to preparation design: the length of anterior teeth, consideration of the smile line, shades and staining, and soft-tissue consideration. All, however, require excellent communication (a two-way process) between dentist and technician.

The position of the anterior teeth is not as arbitrary as once presumed (*Pound,* 1973). For example, the position of the incisal edges of maxillary anterior teeth belongs on the vermillion border (wet/dry line) of the lower lip in enunciating the "F" sound (*Pound,* 1973). Further, the maxillary incisors should be of sufficient length to show perhaps 1–2 mm of incisal edge with the lips at rest, while the pitch of these teeth labially is a function of support for the upper lip. Lateral incisors are generally 1 mm or so shorter than the central incisors and the cuspids are either more or less prominent, depending on our desire to create a more masculine or feminine effect.

Similarly, there are some constants in the placement of lower incisors (*Pound,* 1973). The incisal edges of lower incisors should make their closest approach to the maxillary incisors in enunciating the "S" sound, and this should ideally miss the incisal edges of the uppers by approximately the diagonal of a 1 mm square. That is, the incisal edges of the lower incisors should be down and to the lingual of the maxillary incisors by this distance. The pitch of the labial surfaces is nearly always at right angles to the mandible as viewed from the sagittal plane, while the long axis of the root remains at approximately 20° to the mandible (Fig. 5).

The smile line or curvature created by the length of the incisal edges of maxillary teeth is of critical importance for optimum aesthetics. Contrary to common belief, the incisal edges of maxillary anterior teeth and, indeed, the buccal cusp position of posterior maxillary teeth, should be harmonious with the curvature of the *lower* lip. If, the lower lip is relatively straight or flat, the incisal edges of the maxillary teeth should be similarly straight or flat. If, however, there is a well-curved lower lip, the incisal edges (and posterior buccal cusps) must manifest this same curvature (Fig. 6).

For one interested in enhancing aesthetic sensitivity, I would simply suggest making a concerted effort to look at beautiful people and note those things which seem to enhance aesthetics and harmony, and also note that which seems distracting and detracts from pleasant aesthetics in those with less pleasing smiles. You, will, of course, quickly verify the above comments.

How, then, do we convey this essential information to the porcelain technician? Actually, we can run the entire gamut from very unsophisticated aids to the most sophisticated. The least sophisticated method of communicating this information to your technician would be to check out the "F" and "S" sound tooth position of the unprepared anterior teeth prior to restorative procedures, take a study model, and then verbally describe the changes that would improve aesthetics. For example, "I need the incisal edges of the centrals 1.2 mm longer than on the model, and out labial .6 mm, please." Though admittedly quite crude, it surely is better than not even sending a study model and simply letting the technician do the best he can; which, incidentally, is exactly how most anterior crowns

and bridges are done–ask your technician!

Next–climbing the ladder of sophistication–would be to actually wax over the incisal edges, and perhaps even the labial surfaces of the maxillary anterior teeth, directly in the mouth with carding wax or something similar to create incisal length position and smile line. Simply take an impression of this directly waxed improvement, remove the wax from the impression if it comes off the teeth, pour it, and send it to the technician with the instructions that "This is about what we want– please finesse it to the ultimate."

Obviously, there are more sophisticated options like fabricating complete processed acrylic provisionals, which can be altered by trimming and/or adding compatible quick-cure resin while in the mouth until you create *exactly* what you want duplicated in the ceramo/metal final restoration. Custom incisal guide tables can then be made so that duplication of the essentials is ensured. In addition, a biscuit-baked trial for alteration is another possibility, although, candidly, I do not do this often.

My only comments on shades and staining are brief (*Vyronis,* 1980). First, learn open candid communication with your technician and don't be afraid to listen. Select shades together, where possible, and be understanding of the technician's problems in developing the aesthetics you want. Secondly, there is no way paint-on surface staining will take the place of proper basic shade selection in the body shade. Indeed, I feel the ultimate in vital shades and hues is achieved from the inside out, beginning with the proper opaque. Third, where multiple porcelain units are being done, be artistic and vary the shades and hues slightly from tooth to tooth. On elderly patients, do it with more gusto. Again, observe people and see if all their teeth are exactly the same color. It just makes sense to copy nature's irregularities.

Soft-tissue considerations are another aspect of optimum aesthetics. The technician seldom is afforded the luxury of seeing gingival papilla, especially on models! Be sure, therefore, that respect is paid to sufficient room for papilla by creating proper embrasures. As they say, for the technician and me, that inner proximal space is simply a place for the papilla, but for the papilla it is home! There are now techniques available to better simulate soft tissue on a final working model so that final contouring and staining can be accomplished in an atmosphere that better simulates the effects of soft tissue. Incidentally, if provisional bridges are to be used, as is often necessary with involved periodontal cases, proper provision for the interdental papilla is of paramount concern. We want the papilla maintained in a healthy state to enhance our ultimate restoration, but if it is impinged upon with the provisionals, finalizing the preparations and attaining an accurate final impression will become an unnecessarily difficult and bloody task. Once again, the single most important adjunct for achieving the ultimate in porcelain aesthetics is open communication between your technician and yourself. Remember, minds are much like parachutes; they function better when opened!

Occlusion

The other major factor mitigating against success in occlusal restoration in dental porcelain is the potential for adverse forces of occlusion, particularly in parafunction.

Candidly, in my judgment, providing for the proper criteria of optimum occlusion, both for function and parafunction, is the absolute key for successful reconstructive dentistry, regardless of the specific restorative materials used; but it is critical in porcelain. Assuming that the patient is doing his part to be healthy, most of the failures we see are either primarily or secondarily related to adverse forces brought to bear on either anatomic or prosthetic structures, that are ill-equipped to sustain such adverse loading. By primary etiology, the concern is direct fracture of either tooth structure or porcelain. By secondary causation, our concern is eventual periodontal breakdown, mobile teeth, and/or excessive wear. Although entire seminars and books are directed to this subject alone, let us reduce it to some essential basic concepts and begin with a little theory and then expand to the practical clinical applications. Briefly, for many years, most astute clinicians observed that although teeth may contact in both function (chewing, swallowing) and parafunction (perverted uses such as grinding and clenching), tissue damage to the dental structures (teeth, periodontium, TMJ articulation, and muscles) is infinitely more related to parafunction than it is to function. That observation is quite logical, since good scientific documentation in-

273

dicates that in functional uses, (chewing, speech, and swallowing) teeth only touch between 3–17 min./day (24 hours) probably at loads under 100 psi (*Gibbs,* 1981). They don't even touch in speech. The times they do touch are (a) during chewing, at the very end of the chewing stroke as they finally penetrate the bolus, the teeth meet in maximum intercuspation, and (b) in swallowing, as once again the teeth are brought into maximum intercuspation between 1,500 and 2,000 times a day, at very low loading. Conscious loading of the teeth and temporomandibular articulation in function, such as through hard meat, or carrots, or whatever, is still probably at low loading. These functional uses of the teeth somehow seem to be well protected by nature's stress-bearing governor, that is, our self-protective mechanism. I'm sure we agree that tissue damage from adverse forces–any tissue damage–is indeed a factor of intensity, duration, and frequency. Obviously, worn enamel, periodontal breakdown, and temporomandibular joint problems are hardly to be attributed to such light loads of such minimal frequency.

Parafunctional loading is another story, and to me a quite frightening one! If a patient can make occluding contacts in parafunction such as bruxing, it is possible he may be loading the teeth or prosthetic replacements, supporting periodontium, and temporomandibular mechanism with loads up to 1,000 psi for hours per day. Thus it seems clear that if damage is being done from adverse forces, it is from parafunctional uses rather than from functional uses.

Of courses, the difficult question still in need of additional scientific documentation remains: "Is the way a person uses his teeth in parafunction related to his occlusal scheme?" Or, asked another way: "Does lack of proper criteria of occlusion indeed cause or contribute to aberrant parafunctional activity?" I am aware of the research which seems to discount the effect of the occlusal scheme on parafunctional activity (*Rugh,* 1980). Even in this study, the introduction of an occlusal splint that provided a new occlusal program and presumably was constructed without occlusal discrepancies, had a dramatic effect in reducing parafunctional activity. Until we have more scientific documentation, I am forced to go along with the "state of the art" practiced by successful reconstructive dentists who nearly unanimously concur that proper criteria of occlusion seems to diminish abberrant parafunction. My experience finds me in concert with this position.

Surely, we are all aware that there is an increase in parafunctional patterns (bruxing) and, indeed, an increase in all the signs and symptoms of occlusal disease when the patient is under increased emotional stress. To assume, however, that headache, neck and shoulder pain, grinding and clenching, etc., are therefore simple stress problems, and that their solution lies only in stress reduction, is faulty. Perhaps an analogy will help. If we were to envision our brain as our master IBM computer, as long as the only stressful input into this computer were indeed the tooth-joint positional argument, our computer could probably handle the problem and figure out a way to get along without signs and/or symptoms. However, at the times when we add more stress into the computer–that is, the stresses of life to which we are all subjected–we simply overload the computer. It is as if the computer were saying, "Wait a minute, I could handle the tooth-joint problem relatively well for you but now that you are adding all this additional stress on me also, you are overloading my capacity to keep you comfortable; something has to go." Succinctly, this is precisely why so many of the signs and/or symptoms of occlusal disease are erroneously thought to be simply stress manifestations (muscle-tension headache). To put it more scientifically: as long as we don't exceed our physiological limits of tolerance, we cope. When we exceed these physiological limits, we come down with frank, clinical problems. Does stress then play a part? Of course it does, but, only in addition to a real tooth-joint problem. To treat just the stress is symptomatic care–though good–but treating the initiating cause might be efficacious also.

Let me say it simply. There is little question in my mind that occlusal discrepancies (tooth-joint positional disagreements) can surely be an etiological factor in parafunctional activity, especially in the presence of increased emotional stress. And, just as surely, the elimination of occlusal discrepancy by the establishment of proper criteria of occlusion will reduce or perhaps elminate the patient's parafunctional patterns.

The good news is that although, in the past, we were led to believe there was little or no agreement between the different philosophies in reconstructive dentistry, now I can assure you that there is substantial, near-unanimous, basic agreement on the essentials of the criteria of optimum occlusion. Sometimes, semantics get in the way and there are apparent disagreements, in the magnitude of the thickness of a few red blood cells (i.e., should anterior teeth just touch or just miss? Here we are talking of a few microns!). But agreement on basics is substantial.

Simply stated, the criteria of occlusion seem to be:

1. Good centric occlusion in harmony with centric relation. Or, simply said, ideal tooth position in harmony with ideal joint position. That is, maximum intercuspation of the posterior teeth while the joints are in their ideal position with the disc properly placed at an acceptable vertical dimension.
2. Eccentric touches are best placed on teeth farthest from the joint, that is, cuspids or anterior group disocclusion.
3. Posterior teeth should have sharp anatomy (within limits) both to reduce vertical loading and to provide for easy escape of posterior cusps through appropriately directed grooves without posterior cusp collision.
4. If there must be posterior tooth contact in eccentric movements, at least try to have it in a horizontal plane thus creating only a frictional force, rather than an immediate incline touch, which, if present, would be resolved

into an undesirable component of direct lateral force.

5. Provide for good anterior guidance in protrusive to immediately disocclude the posterior teeth in that excursive eccentric movement.

In a word, provide for both ideal vertical and horizontal considerations. Surely, techniques for the accomplishment of the above vary widely with philosophies, but basic agreement on the ideal occlusal scheme remains.

If achievement of this occlusal design with these criteria would assure, or at very least encourage that the teeth would only be used in function (chewing, speech, and swallowing, with mimimum time and force loading, i.e., 3–17 min./day, 100 pounds psi hrs./day), I think we could predict good success with our restorations, especially in porcelain. The work of *Williamson* (1978) at the Medical College of Georgia seems to support this. In synopsis, if we either have a bolus of food between posterior teeth, or have tooth-to-tooth contact posteriorly, the very strong masseter muscle continues to fire. Unload the teeth in eccentric movement so they can't touch and the masseter immediately stops firing. This is extremely significant for two reasons. First, it is this powerful masseter which has the potential for generating these very high loads, particularly in parafunction, where much of the force is a destructive nonaxial (lateral) vector. And, second, this work gives understanding and absolute scientific documentation to the mechanism by which the long-held theory of cuspid guidance laterally and anterior guidance

protrusively actually provides protection from the destructive parafunctional loading of the posterior teeth. Obviously, these same types of loads would be devastating to our porcelain reconstruction. But, you properly ask, how about the patient with wear on cuspids and anterior teeth? Think about that for a moment. *Ramfjord* (1971) and others indicate joints basically go to their "proper position" during reflex swallowing. If, while in their "proper position," only one posterior tooth is touching and thus taking all the load, it does not surprise me that nature's self-protective mechanism is invoked with a message from the tooth to the brain to assume an adaptive position—perhaps sitting on a front tooth or teeth, anteriors or cuspids. The only problem is that basic high school physiology tells us that the mandible positioning muscles cannot stay in this static contracted position (nor can any muscle) for more than a very few minutes. Lactic acid builds up in the static contracted muscles, causing pain, from which relief is accomplished by movement in the muscles, usually with the teeth still together. Thus anterior and cuspid wear faceting may be produced.

Show me anterior wear patterns on centrals, laterals, and cuspids, and I will show you posterior discrepancies between ideal tooth position and ideal joint position, commonly referred to as CO-CR discrepancies. In my judgment, anterior wear is clearly the *result* of an occlusal problem elsewhere. As *Peter K. Thomas* says, "The back teeth protect the front teeth; the front teeth protect the back teeth." A cliche? Certainly not! If the back teeth are arranged such that they meet in maximum intercuspation, in harmony with ideal joint position, the patient can comfortably get his teeth together at the end of a chewing stroke and during the 2,000 involuntary swallows per day and thus has no necessity to rest on his front teeth and grind them. Similarly, if proprioceptively the patient has good disoccluding anterior guidance and cuspid guidance for eccentric movements, that anterior disoccluding program keeps the patient from bruxing his posterior teeth.

Now, the ramifications of this become manifest in reconstructive procedures. If the posterior occlusion is built out of harmony with joints, muscles, tendons, and ligaments, that is, we build in posterior occlusal interferences in centric relation, we are inviting the patient to put horrendous forces on our ceramic-metal restorations (to say nothing of solder joints and weak frameworks), which have an excellent probability of porcelain fracture. Although it is convenient to blame our ceramic technician for this fracture, I am convinced that the vast majority of anterior porcelain fracture is a result of the patient's adaptive response to posterior disharmony. Further, most of the posterior porcelain fracture is not caused by the 100 psi loading on meat or carrots but rather due to the huge prolonged shearing lateral loads where the patient has eccentric contact (crown-to-crown or tooth-to-tooth), causing the powerful masseter to continue to contract. Providing proper criteria of occlusion then would greatly reduce these discouraging failures.

Porcelain or framework failure is, of course, the most dramatic problem that might be overcome by proper occlusal consideration. But, additionally, many other problems about the use of porcelain in reconstructive dentistry seem to evaporate with a proper understanding of occlusal forces and their cause. For example, the differences in the rate of wear of porcelain against natural tooth structure? If, indeed, the porcelain is only touching 3–17 min./day down the long axis and does not touch in parafunction, what is there to wear? The same goes for the controversy of glazed porcelain versus breaking the glaze. How about our concern about the strength inherent in the porcelain restoration? Can it withstand the horrendous potential forces of "function" in the mouth? Once again, be assured it can withstand *function*! The question is, can it withstand *parafunction*? Or better, by occlusal consideration, can we attenuate parafunction and render this a nonproblem? But, lest you think I'm making this all too simple, let there be no mistake–there is a real problem. Simply stated, even if I get all the criteria of occlusion properly accomplished at the time the case is seated, we all "know" it won't stay there, and as changes occur, we do have discrepancies with all the possible potentially destructive sequelae: parafunction with its inherent destructive forces. Obviously, I'd be less than astute to suggest that once occlusal harmony is established, it would never change. However, just as surely, most of the changes that are seen in the occlusion subsequent to cementation are seen because we "jumped into the restorative phase" too soon, before we resolved and stabilized the joints. This is perhaps the most important thing I can say to the young dentists learning reconstructive dentistry.

We are now assuming that we agree our restoration must have the criteria of occlusion, and the basis from which we begin is a treatment position where there is agreement between ideal tooth position and ideal joint position. Incidentally, with all the attention the joint and disc is getting today, skillful reconstructionists, I suspect, achieve a joint position within perhaps .05–.14 millimeter. Believe me, there is much more agreement than disagreement about treatment position. The problem is that the very patients in need of extensive rehabilitative dental procedures are, largely, the same ones who present with significant tooth-position, joint-position discrepancies. They generally lack the proper criteria of occlusion, and present with some or all of the classic signs and/or symptoms of occlusal disease–from headache, neck and shoulder pain, to frank TMJ dysfunction.

Unquestionably, success in rehabilitative dentistry will necessarily be predicated not only on first solving all the signs and symptoms of occlusal disease, but on following this therapy through to stability. It is important to note that a patient when treated may be asymptomatic but achieving ultimate stability is another matter.

Two important points must be made. First, the ability of the operator to solve occlusal disease signs and symptoms and achieve the proper criteria of occlusion–either with splints, provisional dentistry, direct equilibration, or with restorative dentistry itself–is absolutely dependent on learning skillful mandible manipulation (*Dawson,* 1973). Although acquiring this skill is far from easy, it is most certainly attainable and can be mastered with both competence and confidence.

Secondly, as tooth-joint discrepancies are resolved, the system is relieved of stress, joint positional changes will predictably occur over days, weeks, or sometimes months, observable as changes in the occlusion. This may be simply the relief of inflammation in the joint.

Alternatively, the joint position changes simply because our occlusal therapy has relieved the stress in the lateral pterygoid muscles, thus allowing the condylar head to seat more properly on the thin avascular articular portion of the disc. Indeed, changes can even result from true remodeling of the condyle itself (*Mongini,* 1977). But be assured, changes do occur. Then, too, if we envision the mandible as a beam, changes can just as surely occur remote from the condyle/disc/fossa, which also cause recurrent tooth-joint disharmonies. If teeth that have been held in abnormal position, either vertically or horizontally are relieved of stress, their position may also change slightly. The operator must be prepared, therefore, to continue to follow up minute refinements on either the "tops of the teeth" if direct prerestorative equilibration was the mode of therapy selected, or similarly to refine their plastic substitutes if splint therapy was the mode of choice.

Ten or fifteen years ago, the concept of joint changes following occlusal therapy was poorly understood. This is not a criticism, but simply a fact. I think it is safe to say that most dentists, at that time, doing occlusal therapy, regardless of mode (direct equilibration, splint therapy, or use of a deprogramming jig), generally agreed that occlusal therapy was a one-appointment procedure. Once the patient became comfortable, they were immediately ready for restorative dentistry. However, these conscientious dentists attempting to do occlusal therapy were universally perplexed to find at reexamination appointments that the patient did not stay in "centric" and that, indeed, significant changes in joint position were observed.

This is not to say that all these patients whose joints changed were again symptomatic. Indeed, the vast majority, though they had tooth-joint discrepancies, were totally symptom free, apparently because they were still well within their physiological limits of tolerance.

Some reconstructionists were more astute. They noted that changes occurred between the time of the "proper centric bite registration" until the time of cementation and thus realized the necessity for remount procedures. Interestingly, this was attributed much more to laboratory errors in the fabrication of the rehabilitative dentistry than to obvious resolution of joint problems.

Those who reported no change in their cases were categorically accused of not looking or not telling the truth. I think some whose cases did not change were just a bit smarter than the rest of us and had acquired the wisdom to go slowly and continue to refine the splints, existing occlusion, or provisionals (some even gold "provisionals") until these changes finally stopped. When the joints and teeth were well-stabilized prior to the final restorative phase, their reconstructions seemed to "stay" dramatically well.

We have learned much in this important area over the past few years. The *method* of solving occlusal disease signs and symptoms and attaining stability is unimportant: splint therapy, MORA's, direct equilibration on old existing restorations, or provisionals. What is important is that we must understand the necessity of subsequent refinement of the occlusion, natural or otherwise, over days, weeks, and even months until signs and symptoms stay resolved and the teeth and joints stay in a stable position. This stable tooth-joint relationship can be reached and then and only then should definitive restorative procedures be commenced.* To do so sooner is to court both frustration and case failure, regardless of the restorative material used.

Any discussion of changes that predictably occur in joint position during pre-restorative occlusal therapy, either utilizing splints, provisional dentistry, or equilibration procedures done directly on natural teeth (existing restorations), would be seriously inadequate and substantially flawed without specifically addressing three interrelated concepts:

1. The "un-ideal" dysfunctional joint position in patients presenting with signs and symptoms of occlusal disease.

* The assumption here is that we are not dealing with proven disc derangements (condyle off the disc) or frank systemic degenerative changes (degenerative arthritis and the like) nor permanent deformity of the structures due to traumatic injury.

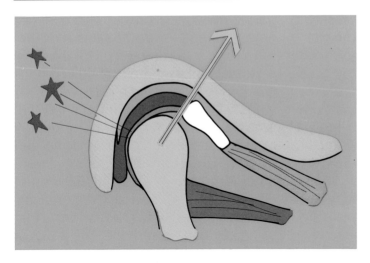

Fig. 7   Presentation of a condyle posteriorly displaced and impinging on the highly vascularized and innervated bilaminar zone of the posterior superior joint ligament.

2. What we consider to be ideal joint position.

3. Where is the unhealthy joint moving from and where do we feel it is actually going as these changes occur?

Candidly, this is quite controversial and indeed there are views that *seem* divergent or even appear contradictory. When astute and honest researchers and clinicians seem to report diametrically opposite findings, it is time to think and reason: there must be an explanation!

This apparent inconsistency about where the dysfunctional joint is, why it is painful, and what happens in successful occlusal therapy can be very simply explained in a most logical manner. At the outset, one qualification must be made. This discussion is *not* relevant to the truly anterior displaced disc (posterior displaced condyle), where the condyle is actually "off the disc." Unquestionably, a condyle may be truly off the disc. This, for example, could be manifested in an

extreme case with a marked "click" occurring late in the opening cycle and with a reciprocal click occurring just prior to maximum closure and may even be associated with restricted range of movement (Fig. 7). Currently TMJ dysfunction is receiving tremendous attention and discussions of "internal derangements of the joint" are very much in vogue. Indeed, we are even hearing that all joint noises (all clicks) are by definition diagnostic of the condyle being off the disc. It is my opinion that this is fallacious. The most practical way to verify a truly displaced disc would be by doing arthrograms in conjunction with either still radiographs (transcranial radiographs or preferably tomographs), or dynamic arthrograms done with fluoroscopic examination (*Mikhail* and *Rosen,* 1979). But this procedure has been classically ordered only on the more advanced, difficult pain patients, usually to verify the necessity of surgical intervention. Who orders arthrography for totally pain-free patients with slight nonreciprocating clicks occurring early in the opening cycle? Thus, when arthrograms consistently indicate disc displacement, it might be wise to reflect a moment on the severity of the problems manifested by the group for whom the procedure is being ordered, prior to jumping to the conclusion that all "clicks" equate with displaced discs.

The inference that all clicks are truly joint derangements (with the condyle off the disc) is a supposition to which I take exception and suggest rather that in many "early clicks" the condylar head is simply moving from one portion of the disc to another: from the thicker portion of the disc onto a more appropriate position on the thin avascular articular surface of the disc. This would explain why some arthrograms done in conjunction with fluoroscopic examinations on patients with classic joint noises show absolutely normal functioning condylar/disc assemblies. We have even seen this on patients where the arthrography is specifically being done to document a displaced disc and to confirm the subsequent "need" for surgery. So, though true "disc derangements" do occur, it is my judgment that they exist in nowhere near the numbers or percentages of the population that it is currently popular to indicate.

True disc derangement is not the subject of this discussion. Rather, let's address the many patients with varying degrees of discomfort in the TMJ elicited by history and palpation; more especially in palpation of the posterior joint space, done through the external auditory meatus, either with early noise or in the absence of joint sounds.

Let us look for a moment at this patient in historical perspective. For many years astute restorative dentists enjoyed good success in solving occlusal disease signs and symptoms, including joint pain and early clicks, by occlusal therapy predicated on skillful mandible manipulation, which was, in consensus, thought to be "back." Get the joints "back" was common terminology among occlusionists. The reason for this perception that skillful joint manipulation was to a "retruded position" or a "rearmost position" was quite simple. When the patient was guided to "proper joint position" or, said another way, "back to centric relation," a first prematurity was encountered, and as the patient squeezed his teeth into maximum intercuspation (habit bite), the mandible appeared to move in an anterior direction. Thus, the terminology of an "anterior skid" (Fig. 8). *Guichet* (1977) cogently explained that in an apparent large anterior skid, most of that distance was simply involved with the arc of closure and a very small portion was truly a linear displacement in an anterior direction (See Fig. 9). But the concept of guiding the mandible or condyles "back" persisted. Much credit must go to *Dawson* (1977) for describing proper joint position as being up and perhaps a little forward in the fossa. Or, said another way, on the posterior-superior portion of the eminentia with a properly positioned disc in place (Fig. 10). In this joint position, we note there is good approximation of compatible fibrocartilaginous tissue, that the microstructure in the bone is conducive to bearing stress, and that the direction of function of the masseteric

281

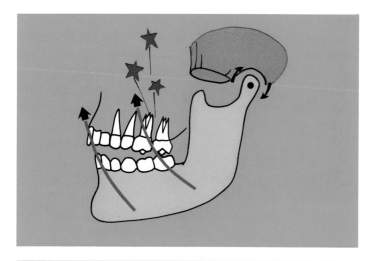

Fig. 8 Mandible manipulated to "proper" joint position, identifying the first prematurity commonly in the second molar region, ie–posterior fulcrumming.

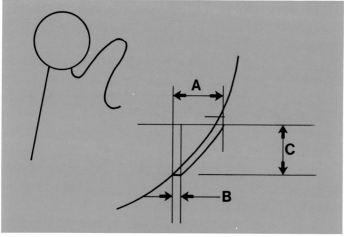

Fig. 9 Most of the anterior skid from the prematurity in guided CR closure to maximum intercuspation at CO (habit bite) is the natural arc of closure, not a linear anterior displacement.

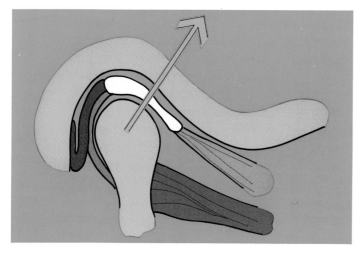

Fig. 10 Ideal joint position with the condyle centered in the fossa and articulating against the posterior superior portion of the eminencia. Note the condylar head is also seated against the articular surface of the disc and the direction of force is determined by the masseteric sling.

sling is compatible; all of which seem to lend credence to the logic of this assertion.

I am persuaded that regardless of mandible manipulation technique (chin-point guidance, thumb on the symphysis with forked fingers supporting the mandible, or bilateral mandibular manipulation), skillful occlusionists manipulate to a *very* similar position. And, although many still say "back", that is much more a semantic problem than a clinical one. In proper mandible manipulation, we all manipulate to a position up and a little bit forward. Unfortunately, however, some are still using the poor semantics of "getting their patients back."

Kantor and others did excellent studies on the replicability of joint position by various techniques and found that the differences between chin-point guidance, chin-point guidance with a deprogramming jig, and bilateral mandibular manipulation were small, indeed–the maximum being .09 mm (*Kantor,* 1972).

Chin-point guidance .14
Chin-point guidance with jig .07
Bilateral mandibular manipulation .05

Though there was actually much objective agreement among the "mandible manipulators," as to the position achieved by getting the condyles "back to proper joint position," the technique for achieving this was far from uncontroversial. Imagine, then, what happened when *Weinberg* (1972, 1976, 1978) reported his findings that pain patients with dysfunctional joints routinely exhibited condylar position too far back! He noted that transcranial radiographs taken on TMJ pain patients exhibited a striking correlation between pain and unequal joint space, with the condyles distally oriented in the fossa. The logical conclusion, therefore, was that to solve the pain, the condyles must be brought forward to a position of equal joint space (Fig. 11).

What may not have been actually stated, but was surely logically implied, was, "if the condyles are already too far back in the TMJ pain patient, with the condyle impinging into the highly vascularized and highly innervated bilaminar zone of the posterior superior joint ligament, surely any and all mandible manipulation techniques, or indeed philosophies of occlusal therapy, predicated on guiding mandible 'back' must be called into serious question. Proper therapy requires the opposite: that the condyle be brought forward."

Are these apparently diametrically opposed views contradictory? Certainly not! Succinctly, *Weinberg's* evidence is clearly correct. My pain patients have posteriorly displaced condyles. But this is critically important: I submit that proper occlusal therapy by skilled mandible manipulation, regardless of technique or mode of treatment, actually causes the condyle to come up and forward into its more ideal position.

When a patient is properly manipulated to joint position, his first premature contact is usually on a molar, which is, therefore, an obvious fulcrum. As the remaining teeth are brought into maximum intercuspation through the arc of closure, the anterior portion of the mandible and the anterior teeth rotate up about this

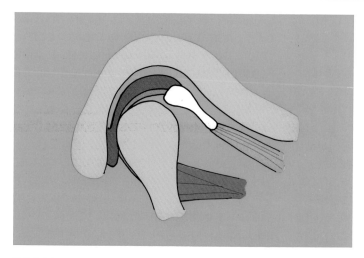

Fig. 11 Pain dysfunction patients commonly have posteriorly displaced condyles.

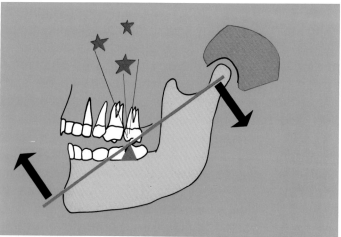

Figure 12

Figure 13

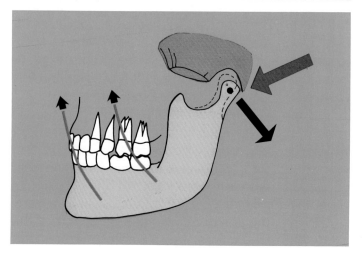

Fig. 12 and 13 If the patient has posterior fulcrumming in guided CR closure and can skid to a different CO (typical anterior skid), as THE INCISORS COME UP AND FORWARD, the condyle **must** go DOWN and BACK into the position typically found in pain dysfunction patients.

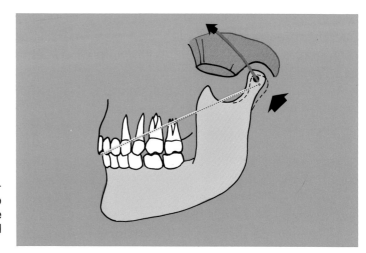

Fig. 14 Elimination of the posterior fulcrum causes the condyle to come up and forward to more equal joint space (proper occlusal equilibration to CR).

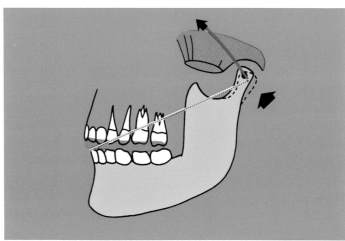

Fig. 15 Elimination of the fulcrum by proper occlusal appliance therapy.

fulcrum, while the other end of the bone, the condyles, just as obviously must rotate down and backward, particularly in cases where the gonial angle is largely obtuse (Figs. 12 and 13).

In its most basic form, any occlusal procedure that effectively eliminates this fulcrum (splints, jigs, MORA's, or equilibration) automatically causes the condyle to come up and forward, eliminating the posterior position of the condyle and bringing it instead to a position of more equal joint space. Will a pull-forward appliance do this? Surely! But, it will be just as surely affected by proper splint therapy or equilibration procedures if they are done so as to remove this fulcrum (Fig. 14 and 15).

Must this concept be accepted on faith alone? Certainly not! Even transcranial films (perhaps the least accurate joint films) (*Mikhail* and *Rosen,* 1979) taken first in maximum intercuspation in habit bite, and then with a jig in place (fulcrum removed) show the condyle has moved to better joint position up and forward. As noted earlier, however, this total change is not immediate and thus the necessity of subsequent refinement to stability. Finally, think of your own experience. The typical patient with CO–CR discrepancies has the incisal edges of his lower anterior teeth in close proximity to the lingual surfaces of the upper incisor in habit bite. Guided closure to the first prematurity indicates a fulcruming on the posterior teeth with a subsequent "anterior" skid to maximum intercuspation. Surely you have noticed that it is usual for these lower anterior teeth to contact the linguals of the upper anterior teeth *after* proper equilibration to CO–CR, in exactly (or nearly exactly) the same place they did in habit bite prior to occlusal therapy. You probably noticed this phenomenon when you equilibrated a Class I case tending toward Class III. In the "retruded position" (terrible semantics), there was a prematurity with an obvious anterior skid. You–like me–no doubt thought "Good! I'll pick up nice anterior guidance in this case," but you didn't. The anterior teeth ended exactly where they were in habit bite. This puzzled you and me. You no doubt noticed this phenomenon again, in a Class II with an anterior skid where you were sure occlusal therapy on this case would make the Class II worse. Perhaps you even worried that the case could not be equilibrated: that surely the lower incisors would end up off the lingual surfaces of the maxillary incisors and into the palate! But, once again, the anterior teeth

ended in the same place after therapy as before treatment.

How can this happen? If the distance between the lower central incisors and the condyle is a fixed value the only way the central incisors can possibly end in the same position after equilibration as they were prior to the procedure is for the condyles to move up and forward (Fig. 14). Fulcrum removal by whatever means (MORA's, splints, or direct equilibration procedures) predictably cause condyles to come up and forward from a posteriorly displaced position to a more properly centered one. The fulcrum in the occlusion caused the posterior aberrant condylar position: its removal causes proper positioning of the condyle in the fossa (Figs. 14 and 15).

Assuming the final restoration has been accomplished only after stability has been achieved, will there ever be the necessity of subsequent refinement? Realistically, yes, but it is my experience that it will be both seldom and very minor in magnitude.

Although there is broad agreement on the criteria of occlusion, I sense there is far less agreement about the importance of the need for minute specification in its achievement, nor is there much real agreement on how we test for it. *Guichet* speaks to this well when he suggests that the tops of the teeth (occlusal anatomy or scheme per se) in and of themselves are unimportant; they are important as they relate to muscles (*Guichet*, 1977). Thus, if, when the posterior teeth come together, there is perfectly even simultaneous contact, directed down the respective long axes, while the condyles are in their optimum functional position, there will be no need for adaptive protective muscle response to avoid the "hurt," i.e., muscle splinting.

But can we test for it? Assuredly, yes. The neuromuscular system can and will tell us when we have accomplished this specification within the patient's need: We will elicit what we call a neuromuscular release (Sometimes called a neuromuscular response–NMR). Specifically, the patient's neuromuscular system allows us to test for both his vertical and horizontal need for specification. When we have achieved even simultaneous vertical loading of the posterior teeth down their respective long axes, the patient will allow the operator to arc the mandible to forcible closure rhythmically or arrhythmically in arcs of 10–15mm (or much more) as measured in the incisor area without the induction of an inhibited self-protective response (*Guichet,* 1977). If discrepancies in the occlusion still exist, creating either uneven vertical loading or an adverse lateral vector force against a tooth or teeth in this vertical closure, the patient's self-protective mechanism will be invoked.

The problem is that there are different perceptions among well-intended dentists for the criteria of successfully finished occlusal therapy: skids gone, nice dot patterns, and good sound characteristic of all the teeth touching down their long axes simultaneously are all very helpful in determining a finished result, but when right is right, the teeth can and will tell you this by the attainment of this dramatic and immediate neuromuscular release. In my judgment, this NMR is the end-point for proper splints, provisionals, or equilibration procedures on natural teeth and just as surely must be the final test for the finished restoration in alloy, gold, or porcelain.

There is a similar NMR for eccentric movements that assures the achievement of proper eccentric criteria. When the patient has good eccentric criteria such that protrusive contacts are against the anterior teeth and lateral guidance is against cuspids (anterior group function and other compromises are surely viable), he will exhibit uninhibited free gliding excursive movements.

Once again, the operator's ability to achieve this specification as proved by the attainment of NMR is inescapably likened to his mastery of mandible manipulation.

So much for the theoretical aspects. The practical clinical applications that accrue to solving the patient's occlusal disease signs and symptoms and achieving stability prior to definitive care are many.

First and foremost, a totally relaxed musculature with stable joints allows the operator to more easily attain accurate, repeatable interocclusal centric jaw relation registration. As we know, the use of jigs in obtaining centric records is primarily to free the musculature and program joint position. Unfortunately, by definition, this recording will be at an increased vertical dimension that immediately prescribes the necessity of a precise hinge axis location for the face-bow transfer with its inherent difficulty and potential for introducing new error. But if a proper stable joint position has already been established prerestoratively by elimination of interferences, and it has been done to a neuromuscular release, i.e., a totally relaxed musculature (identical to that which can be attained with a deprogramming jig), we can now take centric registrations at the proper vertical dimension of occlusion. We need not open the bite with a jig to get muscle relaxation; we already have it on the natural teeth. Obviously, if it is your intention to open the bite, that is an entirely different story. I suspect the concern of most dentists is how to do effective porcelain rehabilitative procedures at the vertical dimension with which the patient presents, and this, therefore, is my thrust here.

Second, and an obvious extension of this, if harmony to a neuromuscular release is obtained prerestoratively in the existing dentition and/or old restorations, it allows the operator to sequence the reconstructive phase as the operator and the patient wish, always saving centric stops in the areas in which the operator is not working, thus maintaining the two most important guides: centric and vertical. Once we have a proper centric and vertical with patient comfort and stability, attained by our prerestorative occlusal therapy, why throw it away and try to regain it again later?

The dentist may wish to begin with anterior restoration. The centric stops are already on the posterior teeth for proper orientation of the working models in centric relation and at the proper vertical dimension. The dentist simply records the posterior condylar controls, either with pantography or check bites and works out ideal anterior guidance. If a centric bite registration is taken, it is taken only over the prepared anterior teeth at the proper vertical dimension with all posterior centric stops in contact tooth to tooth.

Alternately, the dentist may have a case that is simply a posterior reconstruction to be done in ceramo/metal, and may elect to do it in phases such as opposing quadrants; first on one side and then, at a later date, on the other side. Again, stability has been achieved by prerestorative therapy to a neuromuscular response and with a generous distribution of centric stops at the proper vertical dimension throughout the posterior on both sides.

Depending on your persuasion, you, like me, might even have a few microns clearance on the anterior. Here, we would simply do the preparations on the opposing quadrants and take the centric bite registration *only over the prepared teeth*. Once again, since we have a NMR, we can easily manipulate the mandible into the stops on the other sides where they remain and into the centric registration media on the prepared side with no inhibited muscle problems. Thus, we can get repeatable records at the proper vertical dimension and in centric relation. Once again, the posterior controls are recorded either by a pantograph or whatever means you elect, and the case is set up to be built.

Two further points are well in order. First, is it possible to do a porcelain reconstruction by single quadrants without a serious compromise in the final result? I think so. The obvious problem is that if we match the occlusion of the quadrant we are restoring to a less than ideal opposing quadrant, ultimately we will have perpetuated the un-idealness. The solution is simple. Once the quadrant of our choice has been prepared, take fifteen minutes and reshape the existing restoration and teeth in the opposing quadrant to more ideal anatomical form. It should be noted that we are going to cut them down later anyhow, so this is a perfect time to create more ideal anatomical form against which to match the quadrant being operated. Additionally, we might communicate to the laboratory technician that we want to plan ahead, and not "bastardize" our restoration for the sake of opposing anatomy, which eventually will also be changed. There are, of course, limits, but it's amazing what a little contouring and forethought can do to idealize the final restoration.

Even where I intend to do the entire mouth restoration as expeditiously as possible, I usually elect to do opposing posterior quadrants at an appointment rather than an entire maxillary or mandibular arch. My reasoning is quite straightforward. If I were to operate the entire maxillary posteriors, both sides, in one arch, I would be doing eight units. Similarly, if I were operating *opposing* posterior quadrants, I am also operating eight units. But, by doing my eight units in opposing arches, I need only capture four units perfectly in each impression, which is much easier than trying to get eight prepared teeth perfectly in one impression. The added bonus of doing the opposing quadrants is, again, preserving centric stops, which, of course, save vertical dimension and centric relation. And, of

course, this leaves the patient with a quadrant of uncut teeth upon which to function while half of the case is being fabricated at the laboratory.

With all this understood, let us finally address the old controversy of whether in fact it is possible to establish the proper criteria of occlusion with porcelain occlusion. Since many of the world's great dentists seem to have some pretty strong feelings that it is really impossible to do this in porcelain and, indeed, it can only be achieved in gold, it surely deserves some evaluation and comment. We must begin by putting this in historical perspective. When the original technology of actually fusing porcelain to precious metal became available in the late 1950s, and, therefore, porcelain occlusion became an option, much of the porcelain in use then shrank as much as 20 % in firing. Thus, the problem of porcelain occlusion was, "How can you overbuild the occlusion such that after slump and shrinkage of 20 % in the firing, it will be accurate?"

This is not easily achieved. Now, add to this the fact that most of these dentists were advocates of tripodized occlusion: that is, cusp tips did not go to stops on fossa but rather each cusp rested on three inclined planes, the resultant forces of which were directed down the long axis. Now, multiply this by four to five cusps per molar, and we need 12–15 even simultaneous loads on inclines whose cumulative resultant forces are down the long axis. It is safe to say that this was extremely taxing to accomplish in gold and was virtually impossible to accomplish after slump and shrinkage with the porcelain in use then. Therefore, the dentists practicing tripodized occlusion were absolutely right in indicating the impossibility of attaining their specifications in porcelain occlusion.

If, however, your specifications are simply even simultaneous stops of cusp tips on flat fossa areas, three to five per molar, as are mine, then it is possible to attain this, particularly today with porcelain that is approaching zero shrinkage. It should be noted that it is no easy task to simply get three to five touches down the long axis as I have described. Slump, however, may still be a problem. I think, there are some technicians who can come very close to accomplishing this specification with all porcelain occlusion. From a theoretical point of view, if your specifications are centric stops on cusp tips down the long axis on flat fossa, with immediate posterior disocclusion, and your technician can accomplish this so that either you have maintained those specifications upon cementation to a NMR or you can adjust the minute discrepancies on the porcelain after cementation to the same NMR, I'd say there is surely nothing wrong, per se, with porcelain occlusion. Candidly, I am attempting this on selected units, usually maxillary bicuspids and occasionally on maxillary molars, but I still feel it's extremely difficult to obtain proper specification of the criteria of occlusion in a total full-mouth posterior reconstruction in porcelain occlusals.

If, however, you advocate tripodized occlusion with the inherent necessity of a multiplication of stops, it would be very difficult to create a case to these specifications with full porcelain occlusion. I am confident, however, that the state of the art will eventually get us there. The issue, therefore, is not the material—porcelain—but rather whether you can utilize it properly to get your occlusal specification.

Conclusion

Restorative dentistry utilizing dental porcelain is both challenging and emotionally rewarding to the conscientious dentist committed to excellence, and its use fulfills the criteria of aesthetics, function, longevity, and practicality remarkably well.

When case failures are experienced with its use, they broadly fall into three categories: (1) The patient's expectations exceed our absolute ability to produce the result envisioned by them, often coupled with their unwillingness to accept responsibility for their state of health, (2) Objective aesthetic shortcomings, and (3) Fracture of the porcelain restoration itself or of the substructure framework.

The first problem can be resolved by realistic communication and perhaps the necessity of major reorientation in the understanding of our respective roles in the health services: theirs and ours. Problem two, aesthetic shortcomings, and, to a large degree, problem three, the propensity for fracture, can surely be minimized by the utilization of more intelligent preparation design. The third problem—fracture—seems to hold a special interest for me. The vast majority of failures due to porcelain fracture or framework fracture must surely be involved with potentially devastating forces of occlusion, particularly in parafunctional attitudes that present the biggest challenge to the restorative dentist. Solution of this problem clearly rests with the dentist's comprehensive understanding of occlusion the neuromuscular system, and of the etiological nature of stress as it relates to occlusal disease generally. Finally, the restorative dentist must come to terms with *his* or *her* expectations. We, too, must be realistic and recognize that even under the most advantageous circumstances, we are truly fallible human beings treating other humans loaded with variables. We must use vastly imperfect knowledge and inherently flawed technology. We will surely get better as improvement in scientific knowledge and technology become available, but there always will be some case failure. We must accept that as reality. We must cease looking upon this as our own very personal failure with the sense of guilt, stressful recrimination, and the negative self-image it engenders. Rather, let us remain secure, confident, and, yes, proud of our efforts and accomplishments in restorative dentistry with dental porcelain.

References

Dawson, Peter E. (1973): Temporomandibular joint pain dysfunction problems can be solved. J. Prosthet. Dent. 29:1 (Jan.). Read before the American Equilibration Society Meeting in Chicago, Illinois.

Gibbs, C. H. et al. (1981): Occlusal forces during chewing-influences of biting strength and food consistency. J. Prosthet. Dent. 46: 4 (Nov.)

Guichet, Niles (1977): Biologic laws governing functions of muscles that move the mandible. J. Prosthet. Dent. 38: 3 (Sept.). Paper read before the Academy of Dental Prosthetics, Washington, DC.

Guichet, N. (1977): Occlusion manual. Anaheim: Denar Corporation.

Guichet, N. (1977): Synopsis-occlusion in everyday dentistry, 3d ed. Anaheim: Denar Corporation.

Ingraham, R. et al. (1981): Rotary gingival curettage-technique for tooth preparation and management of the gingival sulcus for impression taking. International Journal of Periodontics and Restorative Dentistry 1: 4.

Kantor, M. E. et al. (1972): Centric-relation recording techniques–a comparative investigation. J. Prosthet. Dent. 28: 6 (Dec.).

Mikhail, M. G., and Rosen, H. (1979): The validity of temporomandibular joint radiographs using the head positioner J. Prosthet. Dent. 42: 4 (Oct.).

Mongini, Franco. (1977): Anatomic and clinical evaluation of the relationship between the temporomandibular joint and occlusion. J. Prosthet. Dent. 38: 5 (Nov.).

Pound, Earl. (1973): Personalized denture procedures. Anaheim: Denar Corporation.

Pound, Earl. (1973): Personalized denture procedures. Anaheim: Denar Corporation.

Ramfjord, S. P. and Ash, M. M. (1971): Occlusion, 2d ed. Philadelphia: W. B. Saunders Company.

Rugh, J. (1980): Paper read before the Society for Occlusal Studies Biannual Symposium, San Antonio, Texas, November.

Vyronis, P. (1980): Improving esthetics in porcelain-to-gold restorations. J. Prosthet. Dent. 44: 6 (Dec.).

Vyronis, P. (1979): Simplified approach to constructing porcelain margins. J. Prosthet. Dent. 42: 5 pp 592–593, (Nov.).

Weinberg, Lawrence A. (1972): Correlation of temporomandibular dysfunction with radiographic findings. J. Prosthet. Dent. 28: 5 (Nov.).

Weinberg, Lawrence A.: An evaluation of asymmetry in temporomandibular joint radiographs. J. Prosthet. Dent. 36: 4 (Oct.).

Weinberg, Lawrence A.: Posterior bilateral condylar displacement: its diagnosis and treatment. J. Prosthet. Dent. 40: 3 (Sept.).

Weiss, P. A. (1981): Toward reconcilling the esthetic potential of ceramco-metal restorations with established criteria for soft-tissue management. International Journal of Periodontics and Restorative Dentistry 1: 1.

Williamson, E. H. (1978): Laminographic study of mandibular condylar position when recording centric relation. J. Prosthet. Dent. 39: 5 (May).

A Clinician's View of Porcelain Reconstructions

Peter Schärer

Introduction

Several problems have arisen through the extensive use of porcelain crowns or porcelain-fused-to-metal reconstructions in oral rehabilitation. The great advantages of dental porcelain are its chemical durability and superior esthetic qualities, which are the main reasons why porcelain as a crown material has been so widely used during the last decades (Figs. 1a and b). Clinical problems, however, do arise from the use of this material:

1. Maintenance of periodontal health and the prognosis of fixed restorations constructed in porcelain-fused-to-metal.
2. The accuracy of the occlusion and articulation if the porcelain restorations are to meet specific gnathological standards.
3. The repair of fractured porcelain crowns.

This paper will discuss these three problems as seen by a clinician, using recent research data related to these topics.

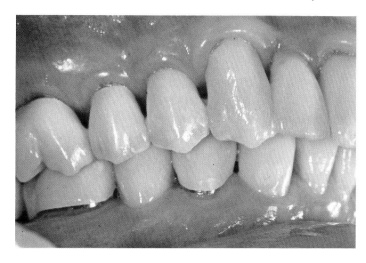

Fig.1a Porcelain-fused-to-metal reconstruction providing optimal esthetics and very good occlusal function. On posterior teeth, bevelled shoulder preparations, if possibly located supragingival, minimize gingival irritation in all areas where esthetics are not of primary consideration. Anterior crowns are full porcelain crowns or porcelain-fused-to-metal-crowns with facial shoulder baked in porcelain.

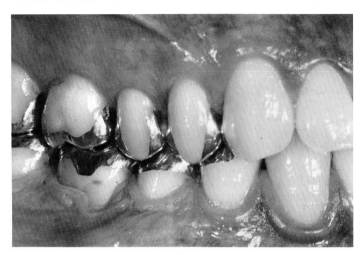

Fig. 1 b Overlay reconstruction on posterior teeth, with advantage of optimal control of the gold margin due to the possibility of burnishing during cementation and with minimal removal of natural tooth substance, especially for teeth that are not heavily destroyed.

Prognosis of Fixed Prosthodontics

An investigation by *Rüeger* (1979) on patients from the Dental School of the University of Zurich who wore fixed prosthodontics over periods of 10 to 30 years has shown that the long-term prognosis of fixed prosthodontics is far better than claims by certain groups, especially periodontists, who consider any kind of reconstructive work to be highly inferior to a natural healthy tooth (*Löe* 1968, *Waerhaug* 1968). This is true to some extent (*Valderhaug* and *Birkland*, 1976), but should not prevent the prosthodontist from attempting to improve the quality of reconstruction work so that it can be worn successfully by the patient for long periods of time–if possible, for a lifetime. These rather negative views towards reconstructive dentistry are not generally accepted in all countries, especially in the United States.

A study on the failure rate of fixed prosthodontics (*Schwartz* et al., 1970) considers the loss of any type of crown or bridge reconstruction before 10 to 15 years as a failure and indicates that fixed prosthodontics should normally last over a longer period of time. Our long-term controls (*Rüeger*, 1979) show that even after a period of 18 or more years, over 65% of the bridgework inserted at Zurich University still remains intact and functional (Fig. 2a). After a period of 10 to 13 years, only 13% of the crown and bridge work had to be removed or repaired. By extrapolating the life expectancy of fixed prosthodontics from this study, one can postulate that the "half-life time" of correctly constructed fixed prosthodontics should be within the range of 20 and 25 years. With our present knowledge in preventive dentistry and oral health, our increased awareness of the importance of periodontal considerations in fixed prosthodontics (influencing crown form, contour, and the positioning of the margin), and our greater understanding of occlusion and articulation, the hope is

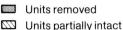

Units removed
Units partially intact
Units intact
A 10–13 years
B 14–17 years
C 18 or more years

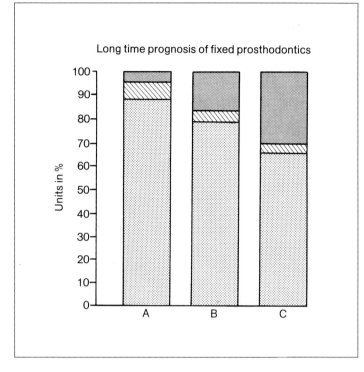

Long time prognosis of fixed prosthodontics

Units in %

Fig. 2 a Long-term prognosis of fixed prosthodontics.
After 18 or more years (Group C) almost 70% of the crown and bridge work is still intact and functioning correctly, showing that the long-term prognosis for fixed prosthodontics is rather good (*Rüeger*, 1979).

justified that reconstructive work (under the condition of proper oral hygiene and control) can last for a lifetime. Previous assumptions that over 10 to 20% of all crowned teeth become devital after cementation have not proven to be true (*Rüeger*, 1979), since the number of crowns that needed endodontic treatment during 18 or more years never reached the 5% level. With proper treatment and care during tooth preparation and cementation, the risk of pulp death is rather small. Through the use of new, more biologically compatible cements, the percentage of devitalized crowns can be kept even smaller (*Tobias* et al., 1978). Fixed prosthodontics is therefore still the best possible treatment in cases of destroyed or missing teeth.

Periodontal and Gingival Considerations in Porcelain Crowns

Examination by *Fankhauser* (1979) of 200 porcelain-fused-to metal crowns, worn by patients for at least three years, showed that certain gingival changes occurred in comparison with noncrowned teeth that were located on the opposite side of the patient's jaw (Fig. 2b). While the amount of plaque accumulation did not differ significantly from noncrowned teeth, there was a greater amount of gingival inflammation as determined by the papillary bleeding index (*Saxer* and *Mühlemann*, 1975). For this index, the amount of bleeding was measured while gently touching the gingival marging in at least two locations around the tooth. The

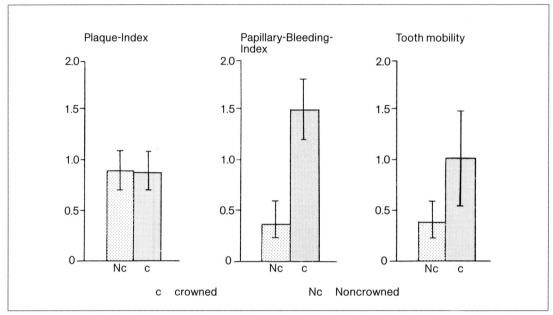

Fig. 2b Plaque index (*Silness* and *Löe*, 1964) and papillary bleeding index (*Saxer* and *Mühlemann*, 1975) in 255 porcelain-fused-to-metal-crowns.
Plaque accumulation on crowned teeth compared to natural teeth is no greater. However, a greater amount of gingival inflammation and also increased tooth mobility indicates that the crowning of a tooth creates a less favorable gingival situation in comparison to a healthy natural tooth (*Fankhauser*, 1979).

amount of plaque accumulation also was not different, probably due to the surfaces of the glazed porcelain or polished gold having similar roughness to a natural tooth. However, some additional gingival irritation develops through the insertion of a crown, and tooth mobility also is increased significantly. This again indicates some periodontal changes in crowned compared with healthy teeth. Various factors are responsible for the additional gingival inflammation observed in crowned teeth: By comparing the diameter of porcelain-metal crowns in an oral-facial direction (Fig. 3a), a very large amount of overcontouring can be observed. The mean value of overcontouring is about 0.5 mm; however, certain crowns are extensively overcontoured by up to 1.6mm. By relating the amount of overcontouring to the papillary bleeding index of the same teeth (Fig. 3b), we can see that a clear relationship exists, showing that even small amounts of overcontouring can markedly influence the degree of inflammation around the gingival margin.

Overcontouring is mostly due to insufficient removal of tooth substance during tooth preparation, thereby creating lack of space for the dental technician, who is then forced to overcontour the restoration in order to create an acceptable esthetic result. Other factors can add to increased gingival inflammation.

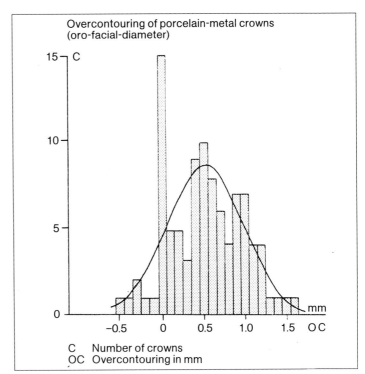

Fig. 3a Overcontouring of porcelain metal crowns in the orofacial diameter (255 crowns).
Most of the crowns are overcontoured, probably due to improper preparation, thereby not creating sufficient space for the laboratory technician to achieve an esthetic result without overcontouring (*Fankhauser*, 1979).

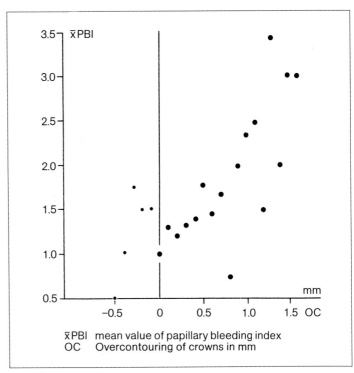

Fig. 3b The overcontouring of a crown usually occurs together with an increased bleeding tendency as indicator of a greater amount of gingival inflammation (*Fankhauser*, 1979).

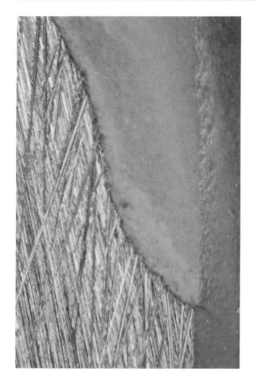

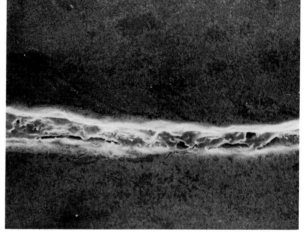

Fig. 4 a Improper porcelain build-up with the opaque layer reaching the porcelain surface. Opaque, because of its roughness, can add to the accumulation of plaque.

Fig. 4 b Marginal opening between porcelain crown and tooth (SEM, 110x magnification). Three factors are responsible for the inaccuracy of marginal fit: (1) preparation, (2) fitting of crown, (3) cementation and cement solubility. (Top: porcelain; bottom: enamel)

Improper Structuring of the Porcelain During Build-up

As first stressed by *Kuwata* (1980), due to improper build-up or finishing of the crown, an exposed opaque layer at the crown margin can increase the amount of plaque adherence in this very critical area, since the opaque will always produce a rough and unglazed surface to the crown (Fig. 4a).

Variations in the Marginal Opening of any Types of Porcelain Crown (Fig. 4b)

Theoretically, any kind of open margin will add to the possibility of plaque deposits in the gingival pocket and thereby increase the amount of inflammation. The width of the marginal opening between crown and tooth depends upon three factors:

1. Integrity of the tooth surface finishing line.

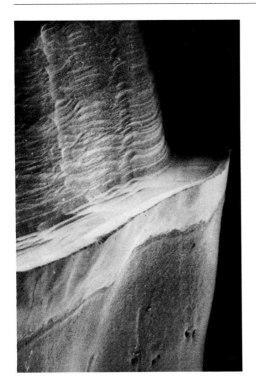
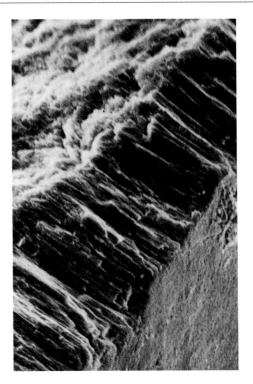

Fig. 5a Shoulder preparation (SEM, 17 x magnification).
The shoulder has been refined with a white Arkansas stone. Observe fractured enamel rods along the margin (*Zander* and *Lehner*).

Fig. 5b A preparation in which fracture has occurred along the edge of the shoulder is clearly related to the anatomical arrangement of the enamel (SEM, mag x 1710).

2. Improper handling of the margins during the construction of the crown by the technician.
3. Effect of cementation technique on accuracy and cement solubility.

Integrity of the Tooth Finishing Line

Regardless of the kind of tooth preparation used for the construction of a crown, either chamfer, bevel, shoulder, or bevelled shoulder, the preparation of the margin usually does not cut through only one structure around a tooth, but passes through dentin, areas of dentin covered with cement and areas of enamel. SEM pictures show (Figs. 5a and b), that no preparation can produce a perfectly smooth and sharp demarcation line when the preparation ends within enamel. Due to the anatomical alignment, the enamel rods tend to break off at an inclined angle if a right angle shoulder is prepared. Even carefully refined shoulder preparations, using superfine diamonds or stones,

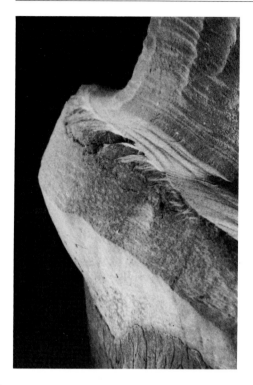 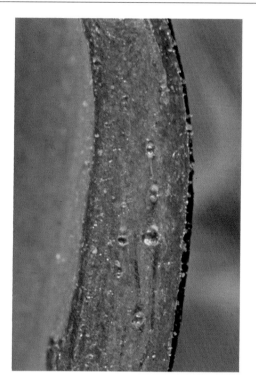

Fig. 6a Bevelled shoulder preparation. Due to the additional bevel, the finishing line is moved cervically away from ragged enamel rods at the shoulder joint (SEM, mag x 34).

Fig. 6b Marking of casting inaccuracies through the use of an indicator paste at the time of try-in of framework.

always display irregular and uneven fracture lines at their margin, particularly when passing through areas of thin enamel. Such fracture lines at the edge of the preparation can be observed equally in chamfer preparations, only the bevelled shoulder preparation removes the area of irregular enamel breakdown away from the preparatory margin, thereby creating a more even and smoother finishing line (Fig. 6a). Unfortunately, the bevelled shoulder preparation shows certain disadvantages in regard to esthetics and is therefore recommended mainly for posterior teeth. The accuracy

of the preparatory margin is therefore dependent not only upon the kind of diamond or stone used for the removal and the refining of tooth structure. Other studies have shown (*Baker* and *Curson*, 1974, *Barnes*, 1974) that the use of hand instruments to break off irregular enamel along the preparatory margin can also create uneven and irregular surfaces. One can therefore postulate that certain inaccuracies in our final crown margin are related to the original preparation, a problem that has not yet been solved clinically.

Incorrect Crown and Framework Construction

During waxing and especially during casting, certain irregularities in the framework structure can be frequently observed (Fig. 6b), and, if not eliminated, these can be the cause for an additional increase of the marginal opening between crown and tooth. These errors can be discovered clinically through the use of indicator pastes and then corrected either by the dentist or the technician, particularly with the aid of a stereomicroscope.

Effect of Cementation Technique on Accuracy

Only one method exists so far in restorative dentistry to achieve an optimal marginal fit between restoration and tooth: the burnishing of the gold margin during cementation in all those areas where access of burnishing instruments is possible (Fig. 7a). By the use of different types of burnishing stones or finishing burs (*Stiffler*, 1980), the marginal opening can be decreased from an average of 40 to 50 µm down to 15 to 20 µm. A 50% reduction of the opening was observed over the whole length of the controlled castings, but complete closure of the space between restoration and tooth seemed impossible (Fig. 8a), since under normal clinical conditions burnishing cannot be performed along the total length of the margin.

Measurements of the average opening of porcelain fused-to-metal-crowns (Fig. 7b) or of porcelain jacket crowns (Fig. 4b), constructed either on copper plated or stone dies, show rather encouraging results (*Schweizer*, 1979). Very little marginal defect was observed with both types of crowns, even though the possibility of burnishing does not exist and this applies particularly to nonprecious metals. The marginal fit of porcelain fused-to-metal crowns in comparison with the regular porcelain jacket crown is superior; however, the marginal deficiency of aluminous porcelain crowns ranging within 30 to 35 µm (Fig. 8b) is surprisingly small and well within the acceptable range as demanded by other authors (*Dreyer-Jörgensen*, 1965). The fact that porcelain, if properly handled can provide a marginal fit that is quite acceptable, leads to the increased use of labial porcelain shoulders on porcelain-fused-to-metal crowns. The advantages of this kind of crown are not only superior esthetics (Fig. 9a), but also the opportunity of using supragingival margins.

The use of supragingivally located crown margins without esthetic disadvantages can be of importance in maintaining gingival health, especially in cases with extensive periodontal pretreatment (Fig. 9b). Care has to be taken during crown construction that the porcelain shoulder is never larger than 0.3–0.5 mm, and that the metal shoulder of the framework is reduced labially only for the minimal amount necessary for esthetic reasons. By shaping the metal framework in such a way, the shrinkage of the porcelain shoulder during baking can be reduced to a minimum (Fig. 10a and b). Long-term studies show (*Fankhauser*, 1979) that already after 3½ years, most subgingivally

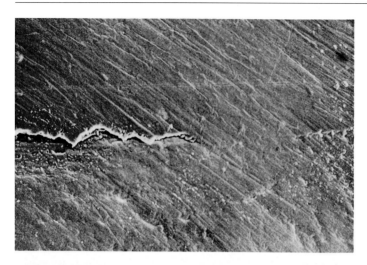

Fig. 7 a   The effect of burnishing of a cast gold filling. Marginal deficiencies can best be corrected by the use of a burnishable alloy (SEM, mag x 110).

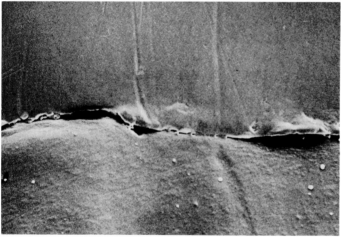

Fig. 7 b   Porcelain-fused-to-metal-crown. Burnishing is not possible in porcelain-fused-to-metal-crowns; however, the marginal deficiency is not very large provided careful crown adaption has been performed (SEM, mag x 100).

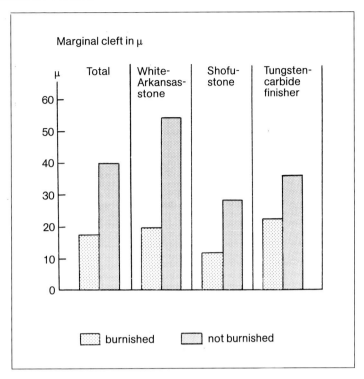

Fig. 8a Reduction of marginal deficiencies through burnishing of cast gold fillings using three different instruments (*Stiffler*, 1980).

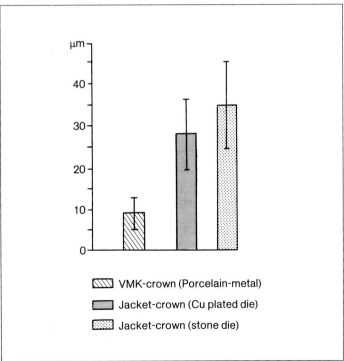

Fig. 8b Average marginal opening of VMK crowns and Vitadur aluminous porcelain jacket crowns built on copper plated or stone dies (*Schweizer*, 1980).

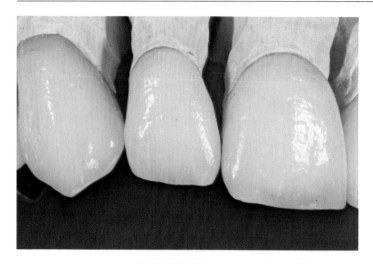

Fig. 9a   The advantage of a labial porcelain (shoulder) on porcelain-fused-to-metal-crowns is shown in the esthetic improvement.

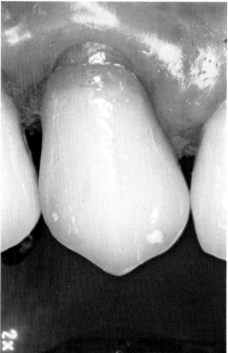

Fig. 9b   Esthetically acceptable, supragingival positioning of the crown margin for reasons of periodontal maintenance.

Fig. 10a and b   The metal frame-work should be cut minimally to reduce the amount of shrinkage of the porcelain shoulder during baking. The reduction of the metal framework should be done under the stereomicroscope.

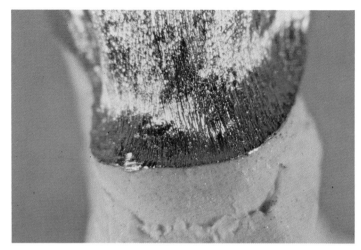

Figure 10a

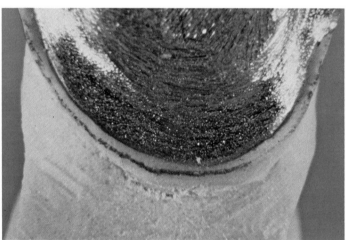

Figure 10b

placed crown margins are located very close to the gingival margin on the facial side. After a period of more than 10 years, the percentage of crown margins located either supragingivally or at the gingival level is markedly increased (Fig. 11). This occurs especially in patients who have to undergo extensive oral hygiene and homecare, since the length of attached gingiva, through excessive and often improper massage of the gums, becomes rapidly reduced and subgingivally placed crown margins are exposed. Porcelain shoulders with no metal margin in porcelain-fused-to-metal reconstructions are therefore indicated if long-term esthetics are of importance.

Successful cementation also depends on the cement used. Glass-ionomer cements, which have reached the market during the last years, have a much lower solubility in comparison to the traditional

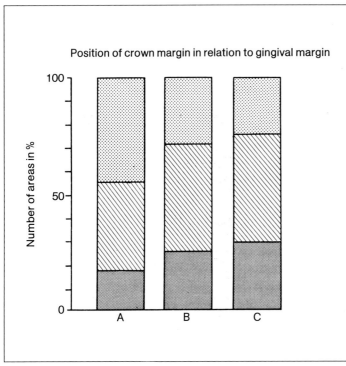

☒ subgingival
☒ on gingival level
☒ supragingival
A 10–13 years
B 14–17 years
C 18 or more years

Fig. 11 After long-term wear of fixed prosthodontics, an increasing number of crown margins become located supragingivally, indicating that even with good oral hygiene a tendency for gum recession exists, thereby exposing the previously subgingival crown margin (*Rüeger*, 1979).

Fig. 12a Cement solubility in vivo (14 months) (*Sidler*, 1982).

Fig. 12b Force required to remove crowns cemented with three luting cements applied on dentinal surfaces with different roughness (*Zumstein*, 1982).

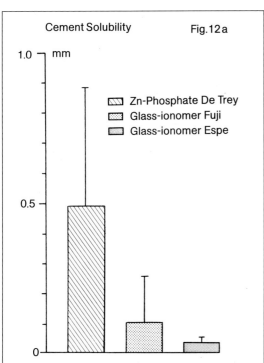

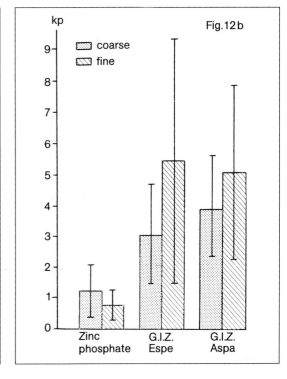

zinc-phosphate cements (*Sidler*, 1982). They give a better chance that marginal deficiencies are at least filled out by the cement substance and not washed out after a short time. The improvements in regard to solubility still continue in the area of glass-ionomer cements (Fig.12a). Care has to be taken that when using glass-ionomer cements, the tooth surface is not finished with coarse diamonds advocated for zinc-phosphate cements. On the contrary, the retention with glass-ionomer cement (possibly mechanical and chemical) is greatly improved if the tooth is refined to a very smooth and polished surface (Fig. 12a) (*Zumstein*, 1982).

Occlusion

Any discussion of porcelain occlusion and its disadvantages in comparison to gold seems to be greatly exaggerated. There are suffcent qualified laboratory technicians worldwide who can show that a porcelain occlusion can be built up to exactly the same accurate gnathological standards as gold occlusions, regardless of the fact that during the baking of porcelain, the shrinkage factor has to be considered. Problems related to occlusion can also be reduced if one attempts to use occlusal concepts, which create minimal horizontal shearing forces during functional movements, but provide a straight loading of the porcelain in centric occlusion.

If one considers the three dominant occlusal concepts mainly used today in dentistry,

- bilaterally balanced occlusion (balanced occlusion)
- unilaterally balanced occlusion (group function occlusion)
- mutually protected occlusion (*Hobo*, 1971),

of all the occlusal concepts used, the mutually protected occlusion concept provides the safest basis for posterior teeth for axial loading and for the reduction of shearing forces during function. *Kuwata* (1980) has discussed the proper framework design and even-thickness porcelain build-up (Fig. 13a), which are especially necessary for reconstructions built according to the group function concept. Very difficult problems arise in these cases with regard to the control of occlusal forces on posterior porcelain teeth of the working side. By using a cuspid disclusion on the working side (Fig.12b) and complete disclusion on the idling side, no shearing forces occur on the posterior teeth and much less clinical and technical efforts are necessary to achieve an optimal result. However, diagnostic wax-up procedures prior to extensive reconstructive work according to the methods originally developed for gold occlusions (*Lundeen*,1969), seem to be even more necessary for the successful build-up of porcelain (Figs.14a and b). The technician can thereby achieve an optimal functional relationship with no shearing forces on posterior teeth (Figs. 15a and b). The mutually protected

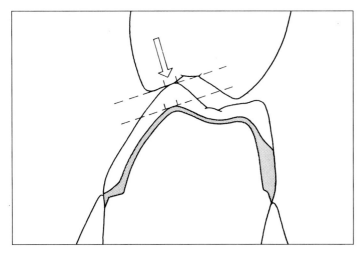

Fig.13a Diagram of porcelain stress during function according to *Kuwata* (1980). This diagram is based on the group function concept.

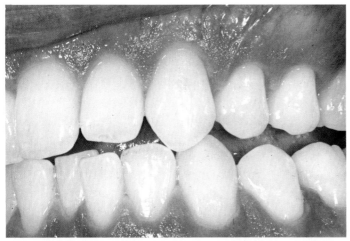

Fig.13b The mutually protected occlusion concept, with cuspid rise anterior disclusion and no horizontal or lateral shearing forces on posterior teeth, reduces occlusal stress on posterior porcelain crowns.

Fig.14a and b Gnathologically constructed porcelain crown using the diagnostic wax-up method prior to the build-up of porcelain (from *Rinn*, in *Schärer, Rinn, Kopp*, 1982).

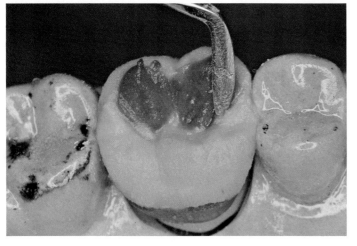

Figure 14a

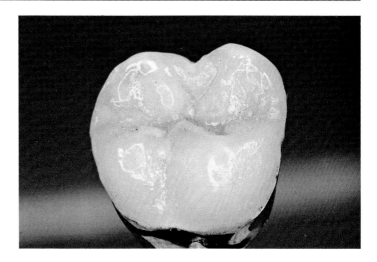

Figure 14 b

Fig. 15 a Build-up of a porcelain occlusion against an occlusal model of a previous diagnostic wax-up. Through the diagnostic wax-up procedure (*Kuwata*, 1980) porcelain occlusions can be created, step by step, to a high degree of accuracy.

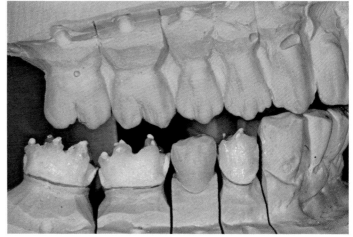

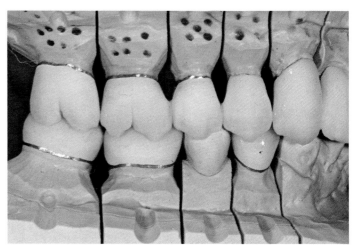

Fig. 15 b The same finished porcelain occlusion case in the biscuit-bake stage.

309

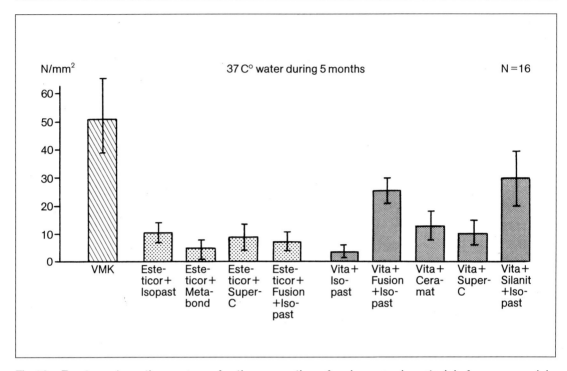

Fig.16 Fracture strength necessary for the separation of various repair materials from a porcelain specimen. None of the tested material has the same retentive values recorded between porcelain and metal in a VMK porcelain metal crown (*Notter* and *Belser,* 1982).

occlusion concept creates the least amount of potential occlusal problems in porcelain reconstructive work if built according to a diagnostic wax-up.

Porcelain Repair

Porcelain repairs due to fractured porcelain crowns in porcelain-fused-to-metal-crowns can be greatly reduced through:

1. Proper framework design (*Kuwata,* 1980),

2. Proper occlusal design (disclusion according to the mutually protected occlusion concept).

Several repair materials have been recommended during the last years, if fracture of porcelain should occur. Through the use of such materials, high quality porcelain is replaced by lower quality composite material. The patient should therefore always be informed that the longevity of the reconstruction has been reduced. After a five-month period, *Notter* and *Belser* (1982) observed that the forces required to tear off such repair material from porcelain test specimens was always lower compared to the force necessary to fracture porcelain from its framework (Fig. 16). Because the best repair materials provide only about 60% cohesive strength compared with the normal retentive strength between porcelain and metal, adequate repair of fractured crowns is not yet possible and in most cases professional ethics demand the remake of a fractured crown.

Summary

From a clinician's point of view, the esthetic advantages of porcelain veneers in present day reconstructive dentistry have solved some of the problems, but have also created new ones. The long-term prognosis of fixed prosthodontics is much better than is often stated in the literature. However, a greater degree of gingival inflammation can be observed on all teeth filled with porcelain crowns, even though the amount of plaque deposition is not different from natural teeth. The main reasons for such gingival alterations are either overcontouring of porcelain-fused-to-metal crowns due to improper preparation or incorrect porcelain build-up. In addition, the marginal opening between crown and tooth adds to plaque accumulation. Poor marginal fit is due to inherent problems in tooth preparation, incorrect framework construction, and partly due to the fact that porcelain-fused-to-metal-crowns cannot be burnished during cementation. Facial porcelain margins on porcelain-fused-to-metal-crowns are of increasing importance because of esthetics and periodontal reasons (supragingival crown margins).

Occlusal problems in porcelain crowns can be solved through correct framework design and porcelain build-up on the basis of a diagnostic wax-up and by providing anterior disclusion to the posterior teeth as postulated by the "mutually protected occlusion" concept. All these factors can minimize the amount of repair necessary due to fracture. No repair material equals in retentive strength the bonding between metal and porcelain of a normal porcelain-fused-to-metal-crown or the cohesive strength of dental porcelain.

References

Baker, D. L., and Curson, I. (1974): A high speed method for finishing cavity margins. Brit. Dent. J. 137: 391.

Barnes, I. E. (1974): The production of inlay cavity bevels. Brit. Dent. J. 137: 379.

Dreyer-Jørgensen, K. (1958): Prüfungsergebnisse zahnärztlicher Gußverfahren. Dtsch. Zahnärztl. Z. 13: 461.

Fankhauser, G. (1979): Clinical investigation of metallo-ceramic crowns. (German) Thesis, Univ. of Zurich.

Hobo, S. (1971): Atlas of occlusion. Los Angeles: University of California.

Kuwata, M. (1980): Theory and practice for ceramo metal restorations. Chicago: Quintessence Publishing Co., Inc.

Löe, H. (1968): Reactions of marginal periodontal tissues to restorative procedures. Int. Dent. J. 18: 759.

Notter, O. R., and Belser, U. C. (1982): Porzellanreparaturmaterialien – experimentelle Untersuchungen der Haftfestigkeit verschiedener Produkte. Schweiz. Mschr. Zahnheilk. 92: 33.

Rüeger, K. (1979): Investigation on long-term prognosis of fixed prosthodontics. (German) Thesis, University of Zurich.

Saxer, U. P., and Mühlemann, H. R. (1975): Motivation und Aufklärung. Schweiz. Mschr. Zahnheilk. 85: 905.

Schärer, P., Rinn, L. A., and Kopp, F. R. (1982): Esthetic Guidelines in Reconstructive Dentistry. Chicago: Quintessence Publishing Co., Inc.

Schwartz, N. L., Whitsett, L. D., Berry, T. G., and Stewart, J. L. (1970): Unserviceable crowns and fixed partial dentures: Life-span and causes for loss of serviceability. JADA 81: 1395.

Schweizer, J. (1979): SEM investigation of the marginal fit of two ceramic crown systems. (German) Thesis, Univ. of Zurich.

Sidler, P. (1982): In vivo investigation of the solubility of three luting cements. (German) Thesis, Univ. of Zurich.

Silness, J., and Löe, H. (1964): Periodontal disease in pregnancy. Acta Odont Scand. 22: 121.

Stiffler, H. P. (1980): Burnishing effect of three different burnishing instruments for cast gold fillings. (German) Thesis, Univ. of Zurich.

Tobias, R. S., Brown, R. M., Plant, C. G., and Ingram, D. V. (1978): Pulpal response to glass ionomer cement. Brit. Dent. J. 144: 345.

Valderhaug, J., and Birkeland, J. M. (1976): Periodontal conditions in patients 5 years following insertion of fixed prosthesis (Pocket depth and loss of attachment). J. Oral Rehabil. 3: 237.

Waerhaug, J. (1968): Periodontology and partial prostheses. Int. Dent. J. 18: 101.

Zander, A., Lehner, Ch. Influence of crown preparation on hard tooth structure (in preparation).

Zumstein, T. A. (1982): Retentive strength of three luting cements on teeth with different dentin surface roughness. (German) Thesis, Univ. of Zurich.

Accuracy of Porcelain Occlusals

Sumiya Hobo

Ceramo-metal restorations have been used in fixed prosthodontics for over two decades and are now the most frequently used restoration in complete veneer crown work. The ceramo-metal restorations combine both aesthetics and strength, and generally satisfy the patient's demand for optimum appearance without showing metal on the facial and occlusal surfaces.

In the first decade of the ceramo-metal restoration, the porcelain veneer was used rather conservatively, being applied only on the facial and part of the proximal aspects. During the second decade, however, the veneering surface of porcelain has been extended, so that today the porcelain may cover the entire surface of the coping and include both facial, lingual, and occlusal surfaces.

It has been stated that a full porcelain veneer ceramo-metal restoration has better strength characteristics than a partial porcelain veneer ceramo-metal restoration because stresses are more evenly balanced between porcelain and metal (*McLean*, 1979). For this reason, the full porcelain veneer has superior physi-

cal characteristics combined with better aesthetics.

Development of base-metal alloy may be one of the other reasons that the full porcelain veneers have become popular. Base-metal alloys have superior sag resistance and maintain their dimensions better after firing the porcelain. In addition, they can be used for longer span fixed partial dentures.

Some brands of base-metal alloy may discolour at the ceramo-metal junctions and full porcelain veneers can reduce this by preventing excessive oxidation on exposed metal. Base-metal alloys are also not suitable for use on occlusal surfaces because of their hardness, difficulty in working, colour, and texture, when compared with the noble metal alloys.

Although full porcelain veneers are now very popular, much controversy exists over their use. Factors such as accuracy of reproduction, physiological acceptance, and fragility are but a few of the questions raised (*Monasky* and *Taylor*, 1971).

Porcelain occlusals, once adjusted intraorally, must be glazed. Glazing will minimize the abrasiveness, or wear potential, against opposing teeth and reduce the number of surface microcracks, which can cause stress concentrations and subsequent fractures (McLean, 1979). On the other hand, if porcelain occlusals distort severely during the glazing procedure, precise occlusion will not be obtained.

It is generally believed that accuracy of gold occlusals is better than that of porcelain occlusals (Johnston et.al., 1967, Hobo and Shillingburg, 1973, McLean, 1979). However, the patient's demands for optimum aesthetics is one that a dentist cannot ignore. The dentist must ensure the accuracy of porcelain occlusals if he is to satisfy the requirements of physiological compatability as well as aesthetics.

In this paper, techniques for fabricating porcelain occlusals of posterior ceramo-metal restorations were investigated, and the accurary of porcelain occlusals produced from these techniques is discussed.

Methods and Results

Distortion of Porcelain Occlusals

It is a well-known phenomenon that porcelain slumps while firing to high temperature, resulting in a rounded configuration of porcelain. The following test was made so that the amount of distortion occurring on the cusps and fossae during the glazing cycle could be determined (Hobo, 1982).

A maxillary bicuspid epoxy die was prepared with a full shoulder preparation.

This die was mounted on, and perpendicular to, a flat plastic base. A standard metal coping for a full porcelain veneer ceramo-metal crown was fabricated on this die. With the coping seated on the die, ten metal models of duplicates were fabricated, using Degudent gold alloy in one piece.[1] The base of each metal model was trimmed as flat as possible (Fig. 1).

Two brands of porcelain, Ceramco[2] and Vita VMK 68[3], were employed for veneering the copings. An opaque layer 0.3 mm thick was applied and fired prior to applying the body porcelain. After firing the body porcelain to a biscuit bake, total porcelain height of a cusp was adjusted to 1.5 mm, and that of a fossa to 1.0 mm (Fig. 2).

Height of the cusps and depth of the fossae were measured in relation to the flat base using a micrometer with an accuracy of $\pm$ 1.0 µm (Fig. 3). Measurements were made at the stage of the biscuit bake, at the first glazing, and after the second glazing. Between the first and the second glazings, the surface was ground to simulate occlusal adjustment.

The following observations were made during the investigation:

1. Every cusp and fossa measured decreased in dimension after the firings.
2. Cusps distorted more than fossae in dimension.
3. The amount of distortion of porcelain occlusals during the second glazing was less than during the first glazing (Table 1).

[1] Degussa, Frankfurt, W. Germany.
[2] Ceramco, Inc., East Windsor, N.J.
[3] Vita Zahnfabrik, Säckingen, W. Germany.

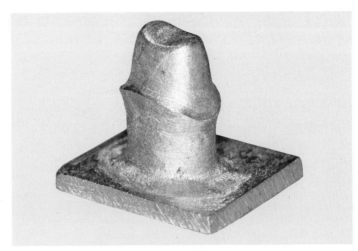

Fig. 1   Solid gold test model for full porcelain veneer.

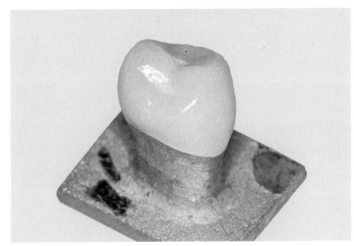

Fig. 2   Glazed test sample.

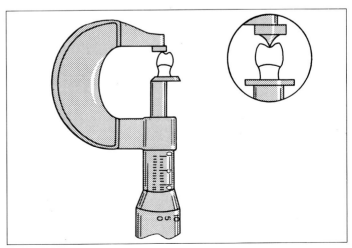

Fig. 3   Measurement of cusp height and fossa depth.

Table 1   Distortion of Occlusal Porcelain Without Cone (Microns)

	1st Glaze (S.D.)		2nd Glaze (S.D.)	
	Cusp	Fossa	Cusp	Fossa
Ceramco	− 22.7 (8.90)	− 7.6 (2.55)	− 13.9 (2.85)	− 5.2 (2.66)
Vita	− 24.2 (6.29)	− 10.9 (8.60)	− 10.5 (2.99)	− 3.5 (2.68)

(From Hobo S., J. Prosthet. Dent. 47: 154, 1982)

Table 2   Distortion of Occlusal Porcelain With Cone (Microns)

	1st Glaze (S.D.)		2nd Glaze (S.D.)	
	Cusp	Fossa	Cusp	Fossa
Ceramco	− 24.0 (4.76)	− 7.6 (1.94)	− 8.1 (2.33)	− 4.5 (1.78)
Vita	− 23.5 (4.30)	− 6.0 (1.94)	− 6.3 (2.58)	− 3.4 (1.78)

(From Hobo S., J. Prosthet. Dent. 41: 154, 1982)

Techniques for Obtaining Accurate Porcelain Occlusals

How can distortion of porcelain occlusals during firing be minimized? There are two popular techniques for fabricating porcelain occlusals. One is the technique using opaque cusp cone (Hobo, 1982), and another is the technique advocated by McLean (1980).

1. Opaque Cone Technique

The amount of distortion or shrinkage of porcelain during the firing process is approximately in proportion to the thickness (or bulk) of porcelain applied. Since the thickness of porcelain on the cusp portion is approximately 1.5 mm, the amount of distortion on the cusp is greater than that of the fossa, where thickness of porcelain is approximately 1.0 mm. To minimize distortion of the porcelain cusps due to slumping during firing, use

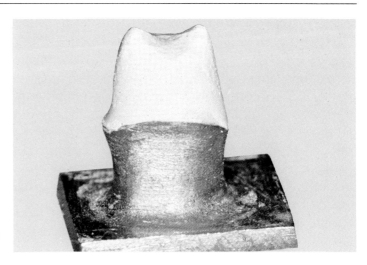

Fig. 4 Elevated opaque cones on the locations of cusps.

of the cusp cone with opaque porcelain is advocated.

The same ten dies used in the previous investigation were employed to examine the accuracy of porcelain occlusals fabricated by means of the opaque cone technique. Opaque porcelain was applied and shaped to form elevated cones at the location sites of cusps (Fig. 4). These cusp cones were 0.8 mm above the original opaque layer in height. After the opaque porcelain was fired, body porcelain was applied over the opaque layer and fired. After the biscuit bake, adjustment was made so that total porcelain height of the cusp was 1.5 mm and that of the fossa was 1.0 mm from the flat table. By means of a micrometer, measurements were made after occlusal contouring of the biscuit bake, after the first glaze, and after the second glaze (Table 2).

After the glazing cycle, every cusp and fossa decreased in height. The amount of distortion during the second glaze was less than that during the first glaze. The opaque cone technique provided better dimensional accuracy than the standard technique without opaque cones, when related to the distortion of porcelain during the second glaze. There was also no significant difference between the two brands of porcelain employed in these tests.

When using cusp cones with Vita VMK opaque porcelain, a dimensional change in height of 6.3 µm and 4.3 µm was found on cusp and fossa portions respectively, after the second glazing cycle. If occlusal adjustment was completed before the second glazing, then any occlusal discrepancy found subsequently was so small that it would be tolerated by present clinical standards of accuracy.

According to the results obtained, it was proved that occlusal adjustment after the first glaze could provide better dimensional accuracy than that at the biscuit bake stage, and the superiority of the opaque cone technique was verified.

2. Technique Advocated by *McLean* (1980)

An occlusal linear shrinkage of approximately 20% occurs when porcelain is fired, and the amount of distortion is generally in proportion to the thickness (or bulk) of porcelain applied. In essence, the thicker the layer of porcelain applied, the greater the amount of distortion; conversely, the thinner the layer applied, the less the amount of distortion. In order to compensate for the high shrinkage of porcelain, *McLean* (1980) introduced a technique for building accurate porcelain occlusal surfaces. Briefly the technique is as follows: after the opaque porcelain is fired, body porcelain is applied so that full contours are developed. Prior to firing, the articulated casts are occluded in intercuspal occlusal position to determine the proper occlusal relationship. After firing, an occlusal linear shrinkage of 20% occurs. Since the thickness of porcelain is about 1.5 mm on the occlusal surface, a space of about 300 μm is left between the porcelain and the antagonist after the first biscuit bake. This space of 300 μm is filled with body porcelain at a second application. The articulation instrument is then closed, bringing the opposing cast into its intercuspal occlusal position. After the second biscuit bake, a space of 60 μm (300 μm x 20%) is left. The third application of body porcelain is made in the same manner, and fired, consequently, 12 μm (60 μm x 20%) of occlusal discrepancy is left (Table 3). This amount of occlusal discrepancy may be accepted by current gnathological standards (*Thomas* and *Tateno,* 1979).

McLean's technique provides the superior surface characteristic of occlusal porcelain since thinner layers of porcelain develop a dense ceramic body with minimum porosity, and gases or entrapped air can escape more easily via the porcelain grain boundaries. This effect can be independent of the vacuum applied.

Opaque Cone Technique versus *McLean* Technique

The following investigation was made to compare dimensional accuracy of porcelain occlusals fabricated by means of the opaque cone technique and the *McLean* technique. A mandibular first molar epoxy die was prepared for a full porcelain veneer ceramo-metal crown. A mandibular epoxy cast including the prepared die was duplicated with stone material, and six identical mandibular stone casts were fabricated. Six sets of maxillary epoxy casts and mandibular stone casts were mounted on the Denar centric relator, respectively. The Denar centric relator can only perform pure hinge movements and therefore has excellent accuracy.

Ten metal copings for posterior ceramo-metal crown were fabricated with Degudent gold alloy for each of six dies. Six technicians participated in the test, and each of them made ten full porcelain veneers as specimens, five of the specimens being made by the opaque cone technique and the remaining five by *McLean's* technique. A total of 60 specimens were fabricated. Two out of six technicians participating were consid-

Table 3   Estimated Occlusal Discrepancy Due to Shrinkage of Porcelain by McLean's Technique

Discrepancy	
1st Bake	300 μm (1.5 mm x 0.2 = 0.3 mm)
2nd Bake	60 μm (0.3 mm x 0.2 = 0.06 mm)
3rd Bake	12 μm (0.06 mm x 0.2 = 0.012 mm)

ered to be highly experienced, two of them were average, and two of them were beginners.

Every full porcelain veneer crown was fitted on the dies, and occlusal contacts against the antagonist were examined with silicone impression material. The set impression material was removed from the casts, and the number of perforations made by the occlusal contacts was counted on an X-ray viewer.

As the control, a full gold crown with ideal occlusion was fabricated on the die. The number of perforations in the silicone impressions made by occlusal contacts was counted by means of the same procedure and the number of occlusal contacts was determined as eight.

To simplify the results, the numbers of occlusal contacts made by porcelain occlusals was calculated on a percentage basis where the average number of occlusal contacts made by gold occlusals represent 100%.

Average occlusal contacts reproduced on the porcelain occlusals by six technicians was 82.8% for the opaque cone technique and 81.7% for the *McLean* technique. There was no significant difference between these two techniques (Table 4).

Of the six technicians, 63.3% could reproduce 100% of the occlusal contacts by the *McLean* technique, while 36.6% could achieve it by the opaque cone technique. When considering a success rate of less than 100%, in the case of the opaque cone technique, 40.0% of the technicians could reproduce 85% of the occlusal contacts. However, 10.0% of the technicians reproduced less than 60% of the occlusal contacts by either the *McLean* technique or the opaque cone technique (Table 5).

This investigation also revealed that about 65% of technicians could reproduce more than 85% of the occlusal contacts by the *McLean* technique, and about 75% of technicians could reproduce more than 85% of the occlusal contacts by opaque cone technique.

Table 4   Accuracy of Reproduction of Occlusal Contact Between Two Techniques

Operator	McLean (%)	Cone (%)
A	71.4	81.4
B	81.4	85.7
C	75.7	85.7
D	75.7	81.4
E	85.7	67.1
F	100.0	95.7
Mean (%)	81.7	82.8

Table 5   Reproduction of Occlusal Contact Between Two Techniques

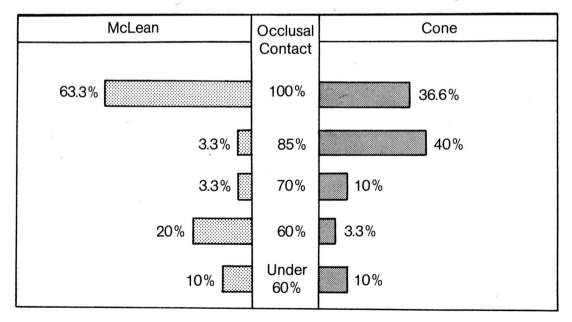

McLean	Occlusal Contact	Cone
63.3%	100%	36.6%
3.3%	85%	40%
3.3%	70%	10%
20%	60%	3.3%
10%	Under 60%	10%

Clinical Procedure for the Opaque Cone Technique

The following clinical procedures are suggested to fabricate accurate porcelain occlusals.

Fabrication of the Coping

Sheet wax is applied to the die, and wax is removed 1 mm above the margin of the coping (Fig. 5). Inlay wax is added to make the marginal collar (Fig. 6). Excess inlay wax is trimmed and a 1 mm wax collar is made in the facial surface extending to a height of 3 mm on the lingual.

Miller (1980) recommends a coping to have cuspal contour on the occlusal surface, permitting definite porcelain sculpturing of cusps, which are supported by the metal substructure. This technique, however, may not be appropriate, due to stress concentrations on the tips of sharp cusp cones, where fracture occurs.

After the correct wax-up is established, the wax coping is invested and cast. The metal collar of the facial aspect is adjusted so that 0.3 mm height of metal band is left. It is easier to make the wax collar rather thick, and subsequently to trim the metal. This method preserves marginal fit of the coping. The ceramo-metal junctions of the metal supporting structure should be formed in shoulder or heavy chamfer shape so that porcelain and metal meet at right angles.

It is the author's recommendation to remount the finished metal copings prior to the porcelain application (Fig. 7). There are two major causes of occlusal discrepancy. One is the distortion of the porcelain itself, this being an inherent problem, and the other is the misfit of the metal coping. Occlusal discrepancy caused by the latter problem can be minimized by means of the remount procedure where the metal coping is seated in the mouth to check the fit and then transferred to the remount cast. Porcelain is then applied to the metal coping seated on the remount cast which eliminates the difference in seating of the coping between the die and the prepared tooth and prevents undue occlusal discrepancy.

Application of Opaque Porcelain

A layer of opaque porcelain 0.3 mm thick is applied to the metal substructure after the recommended treatment such as cleaning and oxidation of the metal is finished (Fig. 8). After the first opaque firing, the coping is seated on the remount working cast and the location of the cusps is determined. When applying the second layer of opaque, the opaque cusp cone is placed on the location of the cusp (Fig. 9). At this stage, the tip of the opaque cone should be in contact with the antagonist (Fig. 10). After the second bake of opaque porcelain, the tip of the opaque cone is ground to a dome shape with ceramic stones and adjusted to a height of 0.8 mm (Fig. 11). Consequently, a distance of approximately 0.3 mm to 0.4 mm is left between the tips of the cusp cones and the antagonist (Fig. 12).

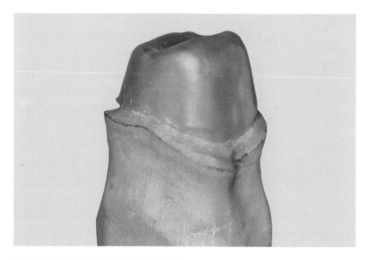

Fig. 5   Sheet wax applied on the die, wax coping 1 mm above the margin being eliminated.

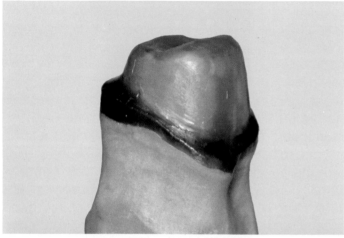

Fig. 6   Inlay wax is added around the margin to form wax collar.

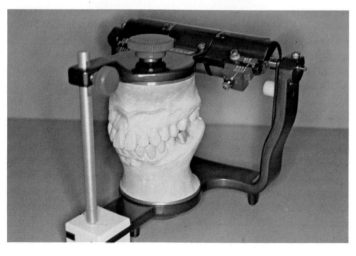

Fig. 7   Metal coping prior to porcelain application.

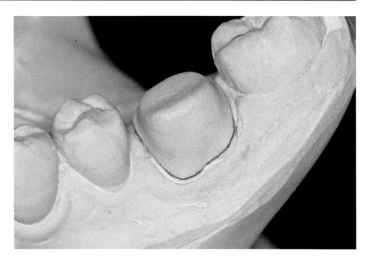

Fig. 8 Opaque porcelain applied 0.3 mm thick on the metal substructure.

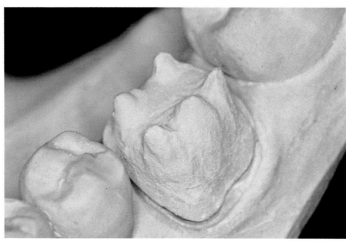

Fig. 9 Opaque cusp cones placed on the remount working cast.

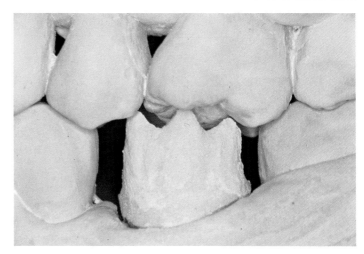

Fig. 10 Tips of the cusp cones make contact with the surface of the opposing tooth.

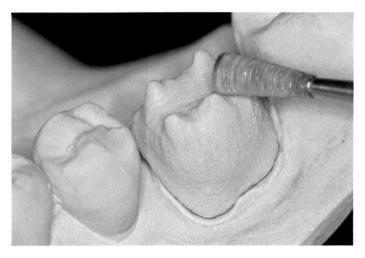

Fig. 11 Tips of the cusp cones rounded after the second bake of opaque porcelain.

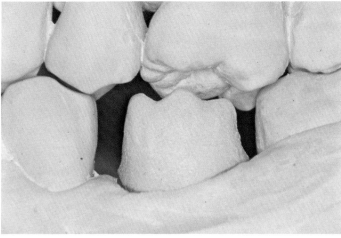

Fig. 12 0.3 mm to 0.4 mm space left between the tips of the cusps and the opposing tooth.

Application of Body Porcelain

The full contours are developed in the dentine powder, and then the dentine powder is cut back to allow for overlay of enamel and incisal powders (Fig. 13). Once the crown contours, including occlusal aspects, are formed, the articulated casts are occluded in intercuspal occlusal position to determine the proper configuration and occlusal relationship (Fig. 14). At this stage, the occlusal surface of the porcelain should have morphologically correct occlusion (Fig. 15). Excess porcelain is then removed and the anatomy of the occlusal surface is refired (Fig. 16).

After the first bake of body porcelain (Fig. 17), proximal contacts are adjusted and the crown is seated on the working cast. A distance of about 0.3 mm will be left between the occlusal surfaces of porcelain

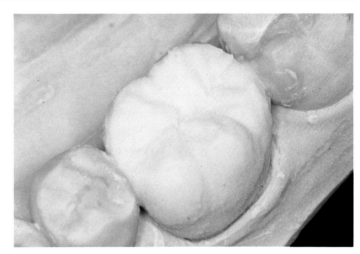

Fig.13 Full contours developed in body porcelain.

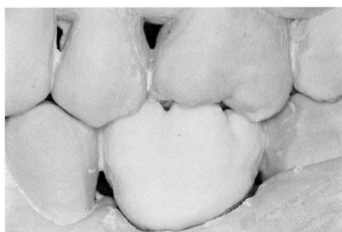

Fig.14 Articulator closed and the casts are in occlusion.

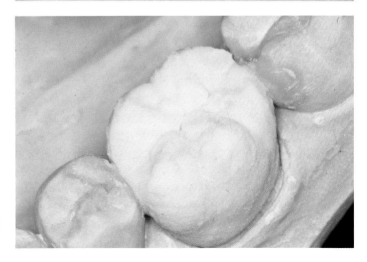

Fig.15 Morphologically correct configuration on the occlusal of porcelain.

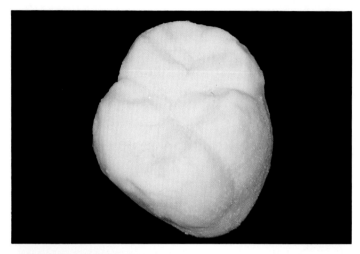

Fig.16 Porcelain crown after trimming.

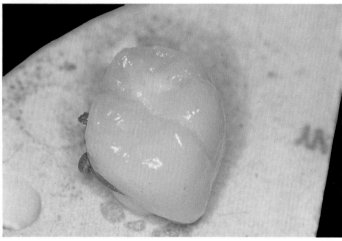

Fig.17 First biscuit bake of the crown.

and the antagonist due to the shrinkage of the porcelain during firing (Fig.18). This space is filled with incisal porcelain and the occlusal anatomy is corrected so that the porcelain occlusals and antagonist are in contact (Figs. 19 and 20).

After the second bake of body porcelain, the crown is seated on the working cast where it will be found that a distance of about 0.06 mm is left between the occlusals (Fig. 21). This space is filled with inci-sal porcelain, and abnormal occlusal configurations such as irregularity and small cracks are corrected (Fig. 22).

After the third bake, the crown is seated on the working cast, where a distance of only about 0.012 mm (12 μm) is left between the occlusals. Occlusal discrepancy may be checked with occlusal registration strip (Fig. 23). This space is filled with incisal porcelain (Fig. 24), and fired so that occlusal discrepancy is minimal.

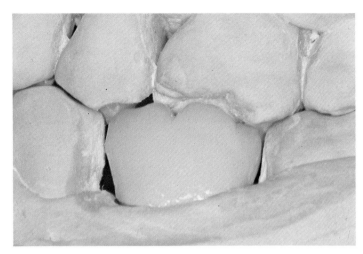

Fig. 18   300 micron space left between the occlusals due to shrinkage of porcelain.

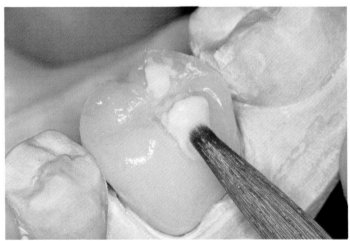

Fig. 19   Incisal porcelain added to fill the space.

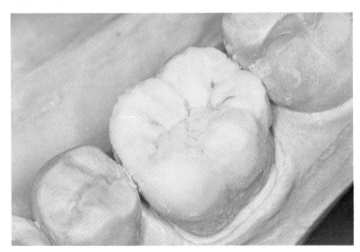

Fig. 20   Crown finished after application of porcelain.

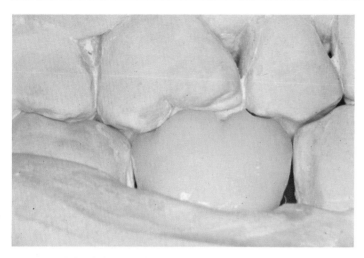

Fig. 21   60 micron space left between the occlusals due to shrinkage of porcelain.

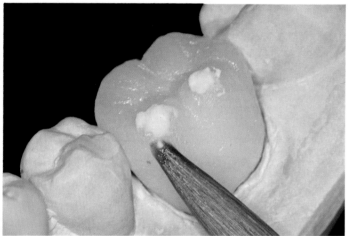

Fig. 22   Incisal porcelain added to fill the space.

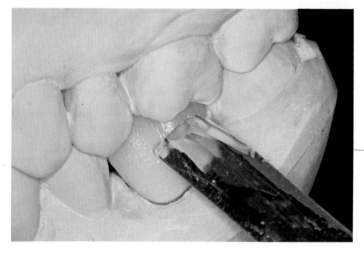

Fig. 23   12 micron space left between the occlusals. Occlusal registration strips are employed to examine occlusal discrepancy.

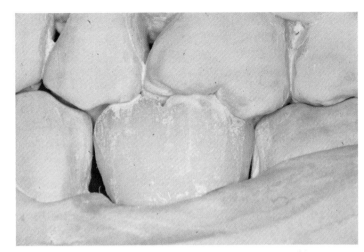

Fig. 24 Incisal porcelain is added, and the casts are occluded.

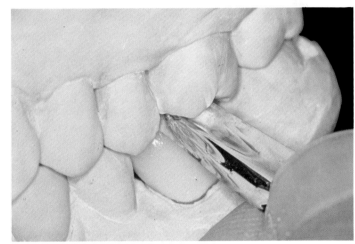

Fig. 25 Occlusion checked by occlusal registration strips after the third biscuit bake.

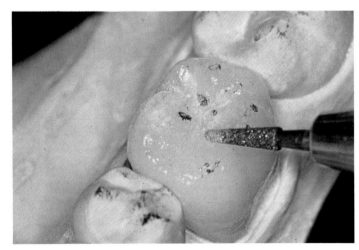

Fig. 26 Occlusal anatomy improved without eliminating occlusal contacts marked.

It will be seen that the occlusion is developed to an acceptable degree at each of three biscuit stages (Fig. 25). Occlusal contacts may be marked with articulating paper and, if necessary, the crown contours should be improved in final shape so that proper anatomical contours are provided prior to glazing. Occlusal surfaces, however, need not be entirely completed since slight distortion may occur during the glazing cycle and further adjustment may be needed (Fig. 26).

Glazing

Since cusps decrease in dimension (height) by 20 μm to 25 μm and fossae decrease in dimension by 6 μm to 10 μm during the first glazing cycle, it may be better to have occlusal contacts slightly greater in height and area at the biscuit bake stage. When the first glazing is made (Fig. 27), the crown is seated on the working cast and occlusion is checked. It may not be advisable to carry out further occlusal adjustment on the articulated remount cast unless severe occlusal discrepancy exists. It is believed that the working cast mounted on the articulator has a dimensional discrepancy of more than 12 μm and for this reason, it should be appreciated that the occlusal surface of the crown after the first glaze has increased in dimension.

The final adjustment of the occlusion is made in the mouth, the crown being completely seated on the prepared tooth (Fig. 28). The occlusion is checked with articulating strip (Fig. 29) and necessary occlusal adjustment made (Fig. 30). The maximum degree of accuracy of occlusion should be provided at this stage (Fig. 31). After the final adjustment, the remaining glazed surface of the crown is removed with a white rubber wheel (Fig. 32). This prevents the surface from becoming too glassy after the second glazing cycle. Occlusal contacts should be maintained during removal of the glaze.

The crown is now subjected to the second glazing cycle (Fig. 33). Since the amount of distortion occurring on the occlusal surface during the second glazing cycle is less than 10 μm, the occlusion is subjected to very little change in dimensions through this process (Fig. 34).

Intraoral Adjustment

The occlusion is checked again before the cementation and any adjustment by spot grinding made with a Shofu white point.[1] Grinding should be strictly limited to the areas of occlusal interference, and care should be taken to avoid unnecessary removal of the glazed surface. The ground surface is polished with a Shofu polishing wheel.[2]

The surface of porcelain finished with a Shofu polishing wheel is so smooth that the possibility of wear of the antagonist is very little.

When three consecutive applications of porcelain are applied in thin layers, the occlusal surface of the porcelain is very dense and the ceramic body has minimal porosity. For this reason the internal structure of porcelain allows grinding to a depth of about 10 μm.

[1] Shōfu Inc., Kyoto, Japan.
[2] Shōfu Inc., Kyoto, Japan.

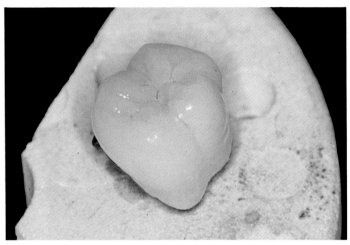

Fig. 27   The first glaze.

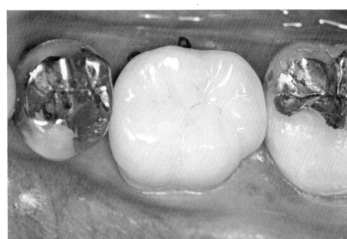

Fig. 28   Crown inserted in the mouth.

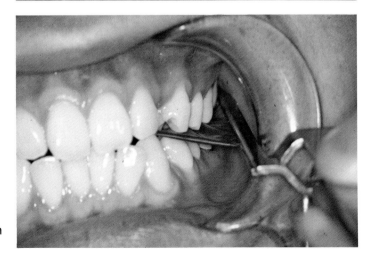

Fig. 29   Occlusion examined with articulating strip.

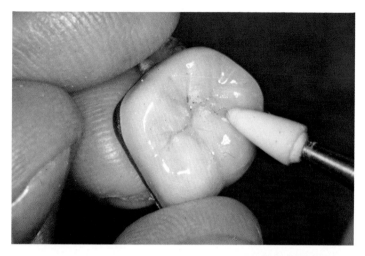

Fig. 30 Occlusion is adjusted with white point.

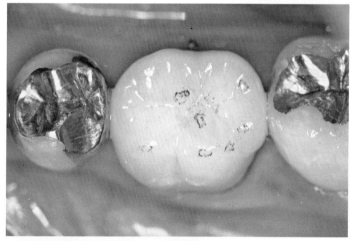

Fig. 31 Crown properly adjusted.

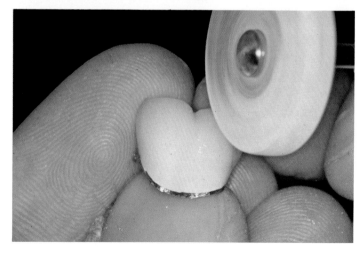

Fig. 32 Glazed surface is removed prior to the second glazing.

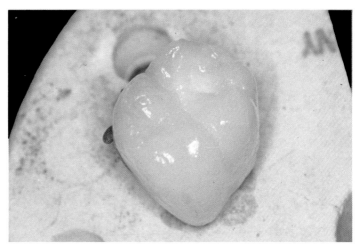

Fig. 33   Crown after the second glazing.

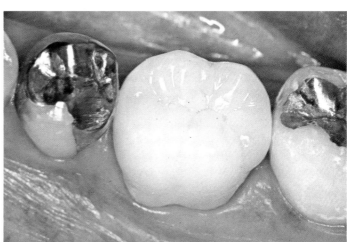

Fig. 34   Crown seated in the mouth. Amount of distortion on the occlusal surface is less than 10 μm.

Summary and Conclusions

The use of complete porcelain occlusal surfaces is becoming popular not only to meet the patient's aesthetic demands but also to avoid exposing metal in the mouth, particularly where base-metal alloys are used.

Since the dimensions of the cusps and fossae of the porcelain decrease during firing, thicker layers of porcelain will result in greater distortion. To improve dimensional accurarcy of porcelain occlusals, application of opaque cusp cones of 0.8 mm high is suggested (*Hobo,* 1982).

The volume shrinkage of porcelain is in approximate proportion to the amount of thickness of porcelain applied. *McLean* (1980) advocates the technique of applying and firing body porcelain in three consecutive stages so that dimensional accuracy of porcelain occlusions is improved. According to the *McLean* technique, occlusal discrepancies found after the biscuit bake, the first glazing, and the second glazing were approximately 300 μm, 60 μm, and 12 μm, respectively.

Porcelain shows rather large distortion during the first glazing cycle, while less than 10 μm distortion occurs during the second glazing cycle. Based on this fact, it may be advisable that occlusal adjustment is made after the first glazing, and ground surfaces are glazed again so that the least dimensional change of occlusal surface occurs.

A technique for fabrication of accurate porcelain occlusals was introduced based on the findings in these tests. By means of this technique, approximately 75% of the dental technicians engaged in this study could reproduce occlusal contacts with an accuracy greater than 85% when compared with an ideal gold occlusal surface. Furthermore, less than 10 μm of occlusal discrepancy was found after the glazing cycles, using the opaque cone technique.

References

Hobo, S. and *Shillingburg, H. T.* (1973): Porcelain fused to metal: tooth preparation and coping design. J. Prosthet. Dent. 30: 28.

Hobo, S. (1982): Distortion of occlusal porcelain during glazing. J. Prosthet. Dent. 47: 154.

Johnston, J. R., Mumford, G., and *Dykema, R. W.* (1967): Modern Practice in Dental Ceramics. Philadelphia: W. B. Saunders & Co.

McLean, J. W. (1979): The science and art of dental ceramics. Volume I: The nature of dental ceramics and their clinical use. Berlin: Quintessence Publishing Co., Inc.

McLean, J. W. (1980): The Science and Art of Dental Ceramics. Volume II: Bridge design and laboratory procedures in dental ceramics. Berlin: Quintessence Publishing Co., Inc.

Miller, L. L. (1977): Framework Design in Ceramo-Metal Restorations. Dent. Clin. N. Am. Oct.

Monasky, G. E., and *Taylor, D. F.* (1971): Studies on the wear of porcelain, enamel, and gold. J. Prosthet. Dent. 25: 299.

Thomas, P. K. and *Tateno, G.* (1979): Gnathological occlusion. Tokyo: The Shortin Ltd.

Saturday Morning, April 24, 1982

Panel of Experts: Dr. *William L. Comcowich,* Prof. *Sumiya Hobo,* Prof. *Peter Schärer,* Dr. *David Koth*

Chairman: Dr. *J. W. McLean*

Participant

Prof. *Schärer,* do you find adverse pulpal reaction to the polyacrylic acid in glass-ionomer cements?

Prof. Schärer

Not that I know of, but I must say that there is some controversial literature about the toxicity of glass-ionomer cements. Some recent German papers show that they may not be as bland as we expect. However, some of the data relating to toxicity are practically related only to tissue cultures. We do not know of any reactions *in vivo.* Personally I believe that there is more scientific experimental evidence that is favorable, but I am not entirely sure.

Prof. McLean—written question

Dr. *Comcowich,* how do you determine that a stable joint exists before neuromuscular release?

Dr. Comcowich

I would like to have my patient be able to return at successive appointments, perhaps over a period of at least a month, and detect no changes in the occlusion as I guide to a joint position. At the time we finish our first prerestorative occlusal therapy, we should be at the point where we feel a neuromuscular release in which the teeth touch so evenly that the muscles tell us that we are there. Routinely at a subsequent visit, perhaps after a week, we find changes. We would refine that again. I would not be happy to continue with the reconstructive dentistry until at least a month later and we see that the patient is exactly as the previous appointment. Maybe there are no changes, or very few between the first appointment and the second one. If changes continue, we sort them out until after at least a month there are no further changes. Then rehabilitative procedures begin. I find that the stability remains relatively well. Of course it will not stay that way forever. However, I find that subsequent refinements two, three, or four years later are minute and very readily corrected.

Prof. McLean—written question

Are your procedures for this determination different between symptomatic and asymptomatic joints?

Dr. Comcowich

If the patient is symptomatic, meaning that the patient has either discomfort in the joint, headache, neck, shoulder pain, or anything to report or we notice something, it is my experience that those patients need more refinement. If the patient's joints are not involved, they usually need less subsequent refinement. If the joints are symptomatic, that is an indication to me that we will need much more refinement from our initial occlusal therapy. If the joints are relatively stable as shown by absence of discomfort, less subsequent refinement is necessary.

Prof. McLean—written question

Dr. *Hobo,* what purpose do computers have in your school?

Prof. Hobo

What you saw was not a computer, it is a porcelain furnace. But, in fact, we have three computers in my school. One of them has special purpose for measuring mandibular movement. It exactly measures the six degree freedoms of the movement of the mandibile to an accuracy of 0.06 mm.

Prof. McLean—written question

Dr. *Jones,* do you use vibration to seat crowns during cementation?

Dr. Jones

Our studies show that the glass-ionomer cements have a much higher film thickness, and the polycarboxylate cements have the lowest film thickness if used in relation to their correct working time. Vibration significantly reduces the film thickness of all types of cements. This has a greater effect than stress or even $\pm10\%$ in the powder: liquid ratio.

Prof. McLean

I assume, Dr. *Jones,* that you refer here to the current glass-ionomer cements using polyacrylic acid liquid in the bottle, not the new water-hardening variety like Ketac-cem. As you know, there are two types of systems available now. There is the water-hardening glass ionomer, in which the polyacrylic acid powder is mixed in the glass powder and water plus a little tartaric is added. By contrast, the current materials on the American and European market dispense the liquid as a solution of polyacrylic acid. Professor Schärer uses the new water-hardening type.

Prof. Schärer

I think basically Dr. *Jones* is right. The beauty of the old zinc phosphate cement was that you could put it in your refrigerator and you could modify the working time to allow burnishing of the inlay margins. We were measuring the margin in our *in vivo* study, and we obtained larger margins on those cemented with the glass-ionomer cement than with the zinc phosphate cement. It's too bad, we have a material that is much more acceptable and which has a lower solubility, but it's more difficult to handle, and we haven't controlled it yet.

We have not used vibration yet because there has been one study on vibration that showed that most of the cement leaks out again because of vibration. Perhaps by combining vibration with the glass-ionomer cement, we can overcome this problem. However, we still are not so sure how we can lengthen the working time for burnishing with glass-ionomer cement. That is the biggest handicap that I see.

Ketac-Cem can be refrigerated, too, but with the zinc phosphate cement, working time can be extended by up to 20 minutes. Cooling a glass-ionomer cement may increase it 3–10 minutes, which still is not enough. Here I still see a problem.

Prof. McLean

Work we did on the water-hardening glass-ionomer cement (Ketac-Cem) showed that it had the lowest film thickness and best rheological properties of any cement on the market. We were at 20 µm using the B.S.I. test for film thickness. I don't agree that you should have a very long working time with cement because you run the risk of increasing solubility and with low powder-to-liquid ratios, mechanical weakness. The essence is to develop cements with 6–7 minutes working time, with a snap set and then the aluminum ions are extracted to crosslink and make the whole body water resistant. That is the cement we have developed at the Laboratory of the Government Chemist.

339

Prof. Schärer

I have to teach undergraduate students how to cement gold cast restorations, and this is a very particular problem. Personally, I am completely satisfied with up to 10 minutes, but maybe I am looking at this primarily from the viewpoint of a teacher.

Participant

How does changing from a rearmost, uppermost position of the condyle as the ideal position change your technical treatment to accomplish a forward, upward position predictable? Is the risk of bruising the angle of the ramus the same as the risk of bruising the chin?

Dr. Comcowich

First of all, I think the chin-point guidance has gotten an undeserved bad reputation. Chin-point guidance is a manipulative procedure that was popularized by Niles Guichet, and if you study his writings as recently as 10 years ago, you will find that he does not advocate forcing condyles back. His information is that your thumb is simply a stethoscope on the symphysis of the chin, by which you feel the condyles seating to proper position.

I know that I am accused of that, as I happen to use a lot of chin-point guidance as a teaching aid. Let me say clearly that the thumb should be simply like a stethoscope on the symphysis, to feel condyles seating. The condyles are seated by the musculature.

The question still arises whether the position we are treating really is not rearmost nor uppermost, but rather is in the posterior superior portion of the eminentia and how can we get that position by chin-point guidance? The answer to that is very difficult, but I will simply say to you that published research indicates that replication of that position is within 0.14 mm without a jig in place and as much as 0.07 mm with a deprogramming jig. The research indicates clearly that the patient can reproduce that position, which is virtually the same within 0.02 mm of the guided position done by bilateral manipulation. Bilateral manipulation certainly is more accurate, but only to the extent of about 0.02 mm. We must think of the clinical significance in teaching skilled dentists about mandible manipulation technique. Often in their initial foray into mandible manipulation, they miss this position by millimeters sometimes, and yet we discuss a difference of 0.02 mm. In summary, we are neither bruising rami of mandibles at the angle nor are we bruising chins by doing manipulative procedures.

Participant

Do you think it is possible that we dentists are fortunate that the resistance of the host allows successful results even when experts change the direction of arrows on their graphics?

Dr. Comcowich

When Dr. *Frank Celenza* says that the precision of that position is more important than the position itself, it is a valid comment. Perhaps that indicates why the Myomonitor of Dr. *Jankelson* seems to work, and the skillful manipulation by various techniques seems to work relatively well. I think by skillful mandible manipulation we arrive at the same place. There is much more agreement than disagreement here.

Participant

If canine disclusion is accepted as being best to protect the porcelain posterior occlusion – and porcelain cusps are relatively susceptible to fracture – why is it necessary to restore all occlusions with such highly cuspated forms? All cases shown today seem to be built to achieve maximally steep posterior occlusions.

Dr. Koth

It's a matter of creating efficiency and therefore reducing the vertical forces on the tooth – which maybe are the least important forces. A mutually protected occlusion is no doubt the easiest to reproduce. I think that is why we favor it.

Prof. Schärer

I think so, too. I think occlusion, like centric relation and the mutually protected occlusion concept, is easier for us. We really should not make a religious faith of this. We have to accept it as one physiologically acceptable way of making life easier for us. There is nothing wrong with this if your patients accept it. As to the steep canine, maybe it's just conforming with what some lab technicians consider an ideal cuspid. The amount of tip length does not determine the guidance; it depends on anatomic acceptability, and on the age of the patient. For a patient 30–40 years old, I would not make the canines too flat. If the patient is 50–60, I would flatten them.

Dr. Comcowich

If we accept Dr. *Williamson's* work, which indicates the desirability of immediate unloading of posterior teeth, then it would seem that the way to unload posterior teeth – and prevent these horrendous loads on the teeth – would be to have sharp occlusion directed through properly directed grooves to avoid posterior cusp collision. If big, rounded cusps move down into a *fossa*, obviously it is harder to get a big round cusp to escape immediately. Sharp occlusion permits more immediate disclusion more readily than flatter teeth. That is the reason why I would like to have sharp occlusion: to have immediate posterior disclusion.

Participant

Do the glass-ionomer cements have the same adhesive qualities as zinc phosphate to bond mechanically to sandblasted internal metal surfaces of crowns?

Prof. McLean

The glass-ionomers probably have more adhesion to tooth structure than zinc phosphate because of the carboxyl group and ionic bonding. They are similar to zinc carboxylate. If you want to attach the glass-ionomers to gold inlays of the Type III alloy, which are really not highly oxidized surfaces, then I suggest that you tin-plate them with about 2µm of tin to provide an oxidized surface that could bond to the glass-ionomer. If you are using alloys such as the high gold alloys for ceramic bonding, they already are made as oxidizable alloys, and you will have no problem in bonding to the glass-ionomer. The glass-ionomer needs only an oxide surface for bonding.

Participant

Please explain how the condyle can be forced down on the same side of the interference if one places the insertion of the muscles of closure as shown in Dr. *Comcowich's* slide. The insertion of these muscles appears to be posterior to the interfering tooth and would have the opposite effect.

Prof. McLean

I assume that what is being said, in fact, is that you have not turned the jaw into a Class I lever; it is still a Class III.

Dr. Comcowich

When we place splints or manipulate to a position, we certainly see classic posterior fulcrum action. To support the thesis that in habitual position the condyle is indeed cocked downward and backward, I suggest preparation of some transcranial radiographs, or preferably tomographs would show it better. When the patient has the teeth in maximum intercuspation, you will find either equal or unequal joint space. In poor posterior fulcrum function, routinely we see that the transcranial film taken in habitual bite has unequal joint space with the joint downward and backward, as *Weinberg* points out. How do we make a transcranial radiograph in proper joint position? We make a deprogramming jig and remove the interference so that the teeth are not in the wrong position with the deprogramming jig in place. A film prepared now shows the condyle more centrically related, or concentricity in the *fossa.*

Participant

As a clinical dentist, I don't have research facilities, but I see that the condyles are distally displaced in habitual bite and by placing a deprogramming jig, which separates the occlusion and effectively removes the fulcrum, I see a repositioning of the condyle. This is not total definitive repositioning, but the condyle comes to a more centric position in the *fossa*. How can that happen with the muscles closing the mandible? According to the literature, cadaver anatomy is much distorted relative to the swelling of tissue. Do you think it is dangerous to draw conclusions about condyle-fossa relationships from cadavers?

Dr. Comcowich

Yes, and I think it is dynamic. There is much more to be learned and I want to caution all of us. There is a lot we do not know about the temporomandibular joint and I am sure that my position will be altered somewhat in the light of future research.

Participant

Dr. *Hobo* went through an intricate technique of opaque buildup of cusps to reduce porcelain shrinkage. Why not just cast the metal framework to the proper dimensions to provide proper porcelain support and eliminate these additional procedures?

Prof. Hobo

Dr. *Miller* recommends the technique you mentioned. I don't like it because you may create sharp metal cusp points. There will be a concentration of the porcelain stress in that particular region, and a significant fracture of the porcelain may occur.

Prof. McLean

The biggest factor in preventing cusp breakage is the width of the occlusal table. The stress analysis done by Jorgenson showed quite clearly that fractures are more likely to occur when preparations are out of parallel and the occlusal table is not sufficient to support the porcelain. This was in relation, of course, to crown preparation, not fused porcelain to gold, but the analysis is relevant to gold copings. Our technicians find that building too much metal into the cusp areas leads to poor esthetics. Thus, there is a limit to the amount of metal you can use. If the cusp developed is too sharp, re-entrant angles may be created. Porcelain will not easily wet and sinter in re-entrant angles or concavities.

343

Participant

What do you do for patients who subluxate consistently and chronically? In those patients who need full-arch splints in full-mouth reconstruction and have a history of bruxing with the classic signs and symptoms of occlusal traumatism, would you use ceramic occlusions on posterior teeth?

Dr. Comcowich

A patient who chronically subluxates has really sick joints. In the truly displaced disc—and there are some, as you know—there are condyles that are off the discs in an unstable situation. In such patients, surgery may be the answer. Perhaps fewer than 5% of TMJ patients are in that category. Patients with truly unstable disc-joint-fossa relationships should be referred for the procedure in which a little wedge section is taken from the posterior superior joint ligament, the disc is tied down, and stability is achieved before any reconstructive procedures. Would I be happy with porcelain occlusion in such a patient? Once a stable position is possible, the material used is not important. Rather getting the criteria of occlusion is important. Then I have no strong feelings at all about whether porcelain or gold is used. With modern ceramic technology, it can be done, as Professor *Hobo* has very well shown. Many good dentists have said that there is no place for porcelain on the tops of the teeth. But by and large, these dentists were advocating tripodization and, historically porcelain was shrinking 20% at the time of their work.

It would be very difficult to create tripodization with porcelain. My criteria for good occlusion does not require tripod support. I would like to have three to five stops down the long axis of a posterior tooth. That can be done in gold—and, incidentally, it is difficult—and it can be done in porcelain.

Prof. Hobo

My feeling is a little different. The patient who has chronic subluxation may requires occlusal readjustment after cementation. This patient requires long-term temporary cementation. Porcelain occlusal restorations are not good for such a case, because porcelain is not easy to adjust in the mouth. Therefore, it is safer to use gold, if patients' T.M.J. is not healthy.

Dr. Comcowich

Normally the buccal surfaces and buccal cusp tips on my mandibulars, are in porcelain and the central fossa of both the maxillary and the mandibular teeth, and the maxillary lingual cusps are in gold. Thus, three of four sites are adjustable in gold if need be.

Prof. Schärer

I don't think I would rehabilitate the patient who consistently and chronically subluxates. Here, I disagree completely. The patient really must be brought to a stable situation with a cessation of subluxation. Otherwise, I will not rehabilitate. Just to make sure, I keep the patient on bite-plates or whatever is needed, but I would not put anything permanent into the patient's mouth. These are the worst patients; they usually wear down their own teeth. Our rule is very simple—don't have different materials working against each other in those patients.

The worst situation is porcelain against natural teeth, because then you have to build in a bite-plate to protect such patients from their own china, these patients must be counselled.

Participant

We use the same technique and conception as Dr. Comcowich for occlusion therapy with *Bruhl's* anatomical research. Can you explain how you determine the vertical dimension of occlusion in your full reconstructions? The vertical dimension is very important when we think that the condyle must come into its own position.

Dr. Comcowich

Many of the problems that have been laid at the doorstep of vertical dimension are much more criteria of occlusion problems than vertical dimension problems. Vertical dimension ought to be determined by establishing the position of the anterior teeth according to function and esthetics. If we establish the anterior teeth in the position—which is not arbitrary—to get the *f* and *s* sounds properly, and then align the mandibular teeth in the *s* sounds almost to approximate the maxillary teeth, then skeletally the patient is either a Class I, II, or III. If the patent tends to be Class III when the anterior teeth are in their proper position, the patient needs virtually no freeway space to speak and function. Class III patients need 0–2 mm freeway space, so we can build the case virtually at that vertical dimension. Conversely, patients who need the greatest amount of freeway space are in Class II. If a Class II person says an *s* sound, the mandible moves forward and upward, and hence it is not uncommon for a Class II subject to need as much as 3–8 mm of space between the posterior teeth. Therefore, it is essential that the vertical dimension of occlusion be based on anterior guidance and the anterior determinants of occlusion. There is an acceptable range. As Professor *Schärer* has shown, vertical dimension, working in the front portion of the mouth and the back portion, are interrelated.

345

Prof. McLean

I would like to respond to a question directed to me. Are the new glass-ionomer cements recommended for gold or porcelain surfaces or both? There is no reason why they should not be used against pure porcelain, because the glass-ionomers have a very high modulus and are very stiff materials. They are mechanically strong but, like zinc phosphate, they do not bond chemically to porcelain.

Participant

Why do you say the mandible is displaced anteriorly if the first premature contact is on the second molar? If the fulcrum is on the second molar, the force of the masseter muscles would displace the mandible up toward the condyle.

Dr. Comcowich

It is an apparent anterior skid. To speak of anteriorposterior discrepancies is basically a misnomer. Most of that is simply the arc of closure and there is very little anterior displacement of the mandible in that situation.

The Evolution of Porcelain-Fused-to-Metal (PFM) Alloy Systems

Joseph J. Tuccillo and Paul J. Cascone

Introduction

Eighty-one percent of all the fixed bridge-work placed today in the United States is porcelain-fused-to-metal (*Rand survey,* 1981). This would come as no surprise to Dr. *Abraham Weinstein,* who is generally credited with developing the first commercially successful dental gold alloy and porcelain composite.

But, the alloy developed and marketed by Dr. *Weinstein* in the 1950s contained 84% gold, whereas the majority of PFM restorations today are fabricated from dental casting alloys with no gold content.

Two recent survey findings (*Rand survey,* 1981) emphasize the amazing technological change that has occurred in the United States in materials for fixed PFM prostheses. The changes wrought in the past 20–25 years were not brought about by accident. Rather, they were the direct result of research efforts of the major dental gold alloy and porcelain manufacturers in response to pressures from the dental profession. Some of the developments were prescient, however, in that the research and development efforts were begun before the need arose. The development of the palladium-silver system is one example. When this system was introduced in 1974, it created hardly a stir in the marketplace, yet, when the price of gold reached $850/oz early in 1980, the system was there, ready, and waiting. The survey previously referred to suggests that palladium-silver is today the most widely used precious PFM alloy system in the Unites States.

The purpose of this paper is to trace the evolution of casting alloys for PFM restorations from their inception in the 1950s. Generally speaking, each new alloy development or improvement came about as a solution to a problem. Some of the problems found by alloy developers are listed as follows together with their solutions:

Problem	Solution
Low physical properties in the Au-Pt-Pd System	Addition of Fe
"Hot tears" in castings	Fine grain alloys
U.S. Government "frees" gold price from $ 35/oz support.	Au-Pd-Ag System
Rise in price of gold to over $ 800/oz	Pd-Ag System and nonprecious alloys
Discoloration caused by silver content of Pd-Ag System	Au-Pd System

These and others will be discussed in detail to show how they wove the fabric of evolutionary change in PFM casting alloys.

Before tracing the why and how of this evolution, let us consider how an alloy is developed or an existing one improved. What properties and characteristics must be built into an alloy so that it meets the requirements of a demanding technology as well as solves a specific problem?

Basic Characteristics of Dental Alloys

All crown and bridge alloys, PFM or other, must possess certain basic characteristics:

A. The physical properties must meet the minimum standards for a particular type of restoration. Generally, the physical properties cited by ADA Specification No. 5 are used as a guide.

B. Resiliency or the capacity to absorb mechanical energy in the elastic region on repeated flexure. Flexing in a PFM alloy is particularly serious because of the brittle porcelain veneer.

C. Tarnish resistance–a fundamental requirement of all dental alloys. Precious metal alloys should not lose their metallic appearance nor dissolve in the mouth fluids. In the case of nonprecious metals, passivation must take place so that the metal becomes inert and remains so in the mouth.

D. Toughness or the ability to absorb occlusal stresses.

E. Fatigue resistance or the ability to withstand the repeated flexure occurring in a bridge during mastication.

348

Working Characteristics of Dental Alloys

In addition to basic strength characteristics, dental alloys must possess acceptable working characteristics:

A. Ease of casting: The alloy must be easily melted, using today's technology, and must faithfully reproduce the mold cavity and produce a casting that fits the original model acceptably.

B. Ease of soldering: This characteristic is especially important in long-span bridgework where fit is sometimes a problem. Good fit and good solderability are hallmarks of precious metal alloys; whereas nonprecious metals, by comparison, are inferior in both respects.

C. Burnishability: This is an important requirement of alloys used primarily for inlays and crowns. Here again, gold alloys are superior by far in this property.

Environmental Characteristics of PFM Alloys

Besides the basic strength and working characteristics required of all crown and bridge alloys, PFM alloys must possess functional characteristics peculiar to their particular environment:

A. Thermal stability and sag resistance (*Tuccillo* and *Nielsen,* 1967). The castings must be capable of supporting their own weight during the normal porcelain firing cycle. Marginal integrity of the copings must be maintained, and there must be no lateral movement of bridgework due to relief of casting stresses. PFM alloys must withstand the thermal cycling that takes place during porcelain application without any phase changes occurring that would affect the size, shape, or functional characteristics of the restoration. The problem of movement, especially in margins during porcelain firing, is not uncommon. Who has not had the experience of a bridge that fitted well prior to porcelain application but not at all after firing! PFM alloys have also been known to undergo phase changes during porcelain firing with a concomitant change in coefficient of expansion producing delayed porcelain failure (*Rowe* and *Asgar,* 1976).

B. Fine-Grained: A PFM alloy that is not fine-grained will produce coarse-grain (larger than 50 microns) castings, which are susceptible to "hot tearing" or "rock candy" fractures (Fig. 1). Grain refinement began a new era in precious metal alloys. Reducing the grain size of castings from approximately 150 microns to 50 microns by the addition of grain refiners such as iridium or ruthenium to dental alloys resulted in superior physical properties. Besides eliminating "hot tearing" in PFM alloys, it raised the yield strength and elongation and also produced a more homogeneous casting that had better tarnish resistance. An important aspect during manufacture was that the properties of the alloy varied less from melt to melt.

C. Free of possibly toxic elements: Although this was a major consideration in

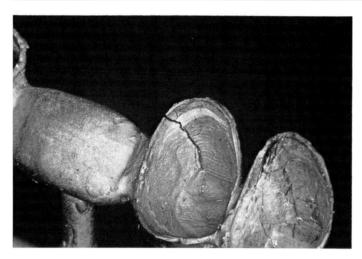

Fig. 1 Hot tear in casting.

1968 when beryllium-containing nickel alloys first appeared, apparently this does not appear to be so much a cause for concern today, at least in the United States, for reasons related to the price of gold. However, there are still some countries; Germany, Japan, Scandinavia, that continue restrictions on elements such as nickel and beryllium.

D.   Compatibility with porcelain: Traditionally, porcelain-metal compatibility has meant that both the alloy and the porcelain have the same thermal expansion coefficient at the set point of the porcelain. The set point of the porcelain is the temperature at which the porcelain becomes rigid upon cooling. Once the porcelain is rigid, stresses begin to build up which may eventually result in porcelain fracture. In order to prevent a high stress level from occurring in the porcelain, *the alloy and porcelain must contract together, as closely as possible, from the set point of the porcelain to room temperature.*

The above statement defines compatibility in its strictest sense.

In the past, it was assumed that the closer the thermal expansion coefficients of the materials, the more compatible was the porcelain-metal pair. Clinical experience did not confirm this theory, however; so other factors that affect the expansion coefficients were investigated.

Compatibility Range

Empirically, it is found that, for any given alloy, the thermal expansion of the porcelain must be within an acceptable range (Fig. 2). Outside this range, the porcelain will fracture.

It should be noted that this is only a casual relationship; there are no scientific principles that define the allowable extent of the porcelain's expansion deviations (plus or minus) from the expansion of the alloy. Also, for any porcelain-metal pair, the range is found to be relative; that is,

350

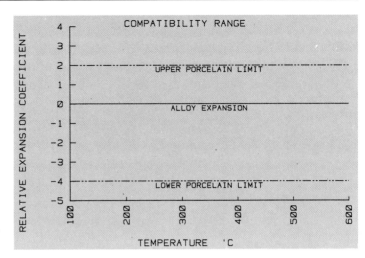

Fig. 2 Alloy-porcelain compatibility range.

for different alloys (different expansions), there will be different acceptable limits for the porcelain.

Although the "compatibility range" idea has no basic scientific foundation, the concept is useful in understanding other factors that affect porcelain-metal compatibility.

Heating/Cooling Rate

Dental porcelain is basically glass and, therefore, very sensitive to thermal processing. The thermal expansion (contraction) and the set point of the porcelain will change as the heating (cooling) rate changes. This is probably the main reason for the poor correlation between thermal expansion tests and˙ clinical tests. Typically, thermal expansion tests are conducted at a heat rate of 5° F/ minute. In use, however, the porcelain is heated at a rate of 100° F/minute and cooled at a rate of 500° F/minute. The

thermal behavior of the porcelain will change significantly due to the different rates. Unfortunately, direct measurement of the porcelain's expansion/contraction behavior at the high rates is not possible presently (which is why actual numbers are not shown in Fig. 2).

The thermal expansion and contraction of the porcelain are therefore constantly changing throughout the normal firing procedure.

Despite the fact that the actual expansion coefficients are not known, the porcelain can be designed to work within a particular heating and cooling cycle. Any deviation from the recommended cycle (underfiring, overfiring, slow cooling) may move the expansion behavior outside the acceptable limits and cause the porcelain to fracture.

Note: Slow cooling refers to the temperature drop in the restoration within the first ten seconds after firing. Most porcelain-metal pairs cannot tolerate a cooling rate slower than 300° F/minute. Some automatic porcelain ovens cool the restoration at a slower rate than this, producing a thermal check.

E. Capacity for bonding with porcelain: The theory of bonding for dental porcelain-fused-to-metal systems is analogous to that for glass-to-metal seals and enameled metals.

The principles involved with glass-to-metal bonding have been described in a series of experiments performed in the Ceramic Laboratory at the University of California (*Zackay* et al., 1953) and at the Battelle Memorial Institute (*King* et al., 1959). These principles have been applied to particular dental porcelain-alloy pairs by one of the authors (*Cascone,* et al., 1977 and 1978).

The formation of a chemical bond is crucial for adherence. The basic requirement, as discussed by *Pask* (1964), for the formation and maintenance of a chemical bond is that a continuity of atomic and electronic structure exists across the interface. This requires a transition zone that is compatible with both the alloy and the glass (porcelain). A metal oxide serves the purpose if the glass at the interface is saturated with the metal oxide. The problem is then one of developing and maintaining saturation of the glass at the interface with a suitable metal oxide.

The processes involved in developing saturation are twofold: First, the glass must wet the metal surface. This generally requires the presence of a metal oxide on the alloy surface. Secondly, the glass must dissolve the metal oxide until the glass at the interface is saturated with the lowest-valence oxide of the metal.

In order for these processes to occur, the following factors are important:

1. The dental porcelain must produce a sufficient amount of glass during the first opaque firing. This is a function of the porcelain's composition and firing cycle.

2. For precious dental alloys, the base metals have to diffuse to the surface of the alloy and oxidize.
   For nonprecious dental alloys, the oxide present on the alloy surface must be adherent and must be partially soluble in the glass.

3. The metal oxide that is dissolved by the glass must readily saturate it within the short time available during the opaque firing cycle. This is a function of the oxide and glass compositions.

Maintenance of a chemical bond requires that the glass at the interface remain saturated with the lowest-valence oxide of the metal throughout further porcelain firings. The precious dental alloys are relatively simple systems since they contain one or two easily oxidizable elements that take part in the bonding process.

For the case of a single metal oxide, saturation is maintained if the diffusion rate of the oxide in the glass is less than the dissolution rate of oxide in the glass. In other words, the oxide at the interface is being replenished at a faster rate than the diffusion rate of the oxide away from the interface.

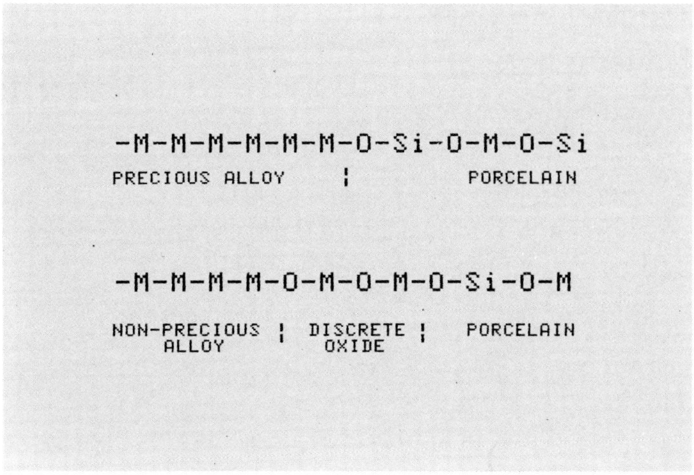

```
-M-M-M-M-M-M-O-Si-O-M-O-Si
PRECIOUS ALLOY          ¦          PORCELAIN


-M-M-M-M-O-M-O-M-O-Si-O-M
NON-PRECIOUS ¦  DISCRETE  ¦   PORCELAIN
   ALLOY         OXIDE
```

Fig. 3 Schematic representation of transition zones for precious and nonprecious alloys.

If two metals are involved, redox reactions occur that maintain saturation of one of the oxides at the interface.

Due to the nature of the base elements used in precious alloys (e.g., indium, tin), these processes occur readily. The glass is able to dissolve almost all of the oxide off the metal surface, with the result that only a few molecular layers of oxide remain between the alloy and the porcelain.

The nonprecious dental alloys undergo very complex oxidation processes because all of the elements present are able to be oxidized. Generally, the glass is not able to dissolve the entire oxide off the metal surface, resulting in a discrete oxide layer between the alloy and the porcelain. Further heating increases this layer and may also alter the nature of the oxide adjacent to the metal surface. A chemical bond may be maintained between the oxide layer and the porcelain, but adherence may be lost between the oxide layer and the alloy.

Figure 3 illustrates, schematically, the final chemical bond for precious and nonprecious alloys at an atomic level. Note that the lack of a discrete oxide layer in the precious systems decreases the possible modes of failure thereby producing a more reliable system.

The possible modes of failure for the precious metal systems are:

1. Failure in the porcelain
2. Failure between the porcelain and the alloy

The failure modes for the nonprecious alloy systems are:

1. Failure in the porcelain
2. Failure between the oxide and the porcelain
3. Failure in the metal oxide
4. Failure between the oxide and the metal

Terminology for PFM Alloys

From the preceding discussion of environmental characteristics, it is obvious that PFM alloys are different from crown and bridge alloys. They differ also in composition; thus the usual terminology is not applicable. Generally, the nomenclature for crown and bridge alloys is based on ADA Specification No. 5, which classifies alloys by function (Type I, II, III, IV) none of which was intended for PFM alloys. Recently, the ADA set up an *Acceptance Program* that includes PFM alloys and that classifies them as follows:

	Au + Pt Group
High Noble Metal	Greater than or equal to 90 %
Medium Noble Metal	Less than 90 %; greater than or equal to 70 %
Low Noble Metal	Less than 70%
Base Metal (Nonprecious)	0%

This classification falls short, however, in describing the PFM alloy systems available today; therefore, for purposes of this paper, the following terminology and nomenclature will be used:

A.   When one element in the alloy is greater than 50%, the alloy will be designated by the element name and may be modified by color.

Examples:

1. Composition −Gold 88%, platinum 6%, palladium 5%

   Designation −Gold alloy or yellow gold alloy

2. Composition −Gold 53%, palladium 30%

   Designation −Gold alloy or white gold alloy

3. Composition −Nickel 70%, chromium 20%

   Designation −Nickel alloy

4. Composition −Palladium 60%, silver 28%

   Designation −Palladium alloy

B.   Where no one element constitutes at least 50% of the total composition, then the two major elements will be used to designate the alloy.

Examples:

1. Composition −Gold 45%, palladium 30%, silver 10%

   Designation −Gold-palladium alloy

2. Composition −Palladium 45%, silver 40%

   Designation −Palladium-silver alloy

C.   A second or third element may be used in the alloy designation if it is considered important for the functional use of the alloy and provided it follows the alloy designation with the modifying participle "containing" or the preposition "with."

Examples:

1. Composition −Nickel 70% chromium 20%, beryllium 2%

Designation   −Nickel alloy containing beryllium

2. Composition   −Gold 45%, palladium 30%, silver 16%

Designation   Gold-palladium alloy with silver

D.   When designating an alloy system, as many elements may be used as deemed neccessary for an adequate metallurgical description of the system.

Examples:

1. Composition   −Gold 88%, platinum 6%, palladium 5%

Designation   −Gold-platinum-palladium system

2. Composition   Gold 51%, palladium 28%, silver 10%

Designation   −Gold-palladium-silver system

Major Developments in the Evolution of PFM Alloys

Now, with the terminology and chief requirements of PFM alloys in mind, let us consider the major PFM alloys systems, why they evolved, and how.

No alloy system available today satisfies completely all the needs of the dentist, technician, and patient. Each improvement within an alloy system or evolution to a different alloy system was an attempt to solve a problem or fulfill a need. Viewed in this perspective, the changes we have seen since the 1950s seem straightforward and logical. In effect, they demonstrate a cooperative relationship between the profession and craft on one hand and the industry on the other. The dentists and technicians tell the manufacturers what they need; the manufacturers develop and deliver the products; and the field responds with acceptance or rejection.

The first commercially successful porcelain-metal combination was the work of Dr. *Abraham Weinstein,* who patented specific alloy and porcelain compositions (*Weinstein, Katz,* and *Weinstein,* 1962) and started a company, "Permadent," to produce both products. Several other systems developed earlier had serious problems that precluded their commercial success. Besides composition of metal and porcelain, Dr. *Weinstein's* patents specified precise coefficients for each material as well as the relationship of one to the other. He also described the construction technique and the use of palladium in the alloy to adjust expansion coefficient. The Permadent materials solved three basic problems of previous composites. First, the coefficient of expansion of both porcelain and metal was "compatible", i.e., the porcelain did not crack when applied to the metal and cooled to room temperature. Second, the porcelain did not "pop off" the metal. There was, apparently, a tenacious bond of one material to the other. Third, the technique was acceptable to the technician, and the esthetics were acceptable to the dentist and the patient.

The Problem

However, there were problems with the alloy that may be explained as follows. The original gold-platinum-palladium alloy had the following composition:

Au	84.10%
Pt	10.00%
Pd	2.00%
Ag	3.00%
Sn	0.40%
In	0.50%

The physical properties were as follows:

UTS (psi)	41,700
YS (psi)	16,500
Elongation	8%
Hardness	90

The melting point of the alloy was 2130° F.

The main problem with the alloy was its low strength and hardness. The strength was equivalent to that of a Type II crown and bridge alloy, barely acceptable for full crowns, let alone fixed partial dentures. A secondary problem related to the higher melting range and casting temperature as compared with those of conventional gold-copper-silver crown and bridge alloys. The gold-platinum-palladium system could not be melted with a gas-air torch, and the investments available at that time used a gypsum binder that dissociated at the higher casting temperature of the PFM alloy (*O'Brien* and *Nielsen,* 1959).

The Solution

Solutions to these problems were not long in coming. Researchers found that by adding as little as 0.5% iron to the original alloy, strength levels were raised significantly. Whereas the gold-platinum-palladium system without iron had a Brinell hardness of approximately 110, the 0.5% iron addition raised this to 165. The hardening mechanism is due to fine-particle strengthening caused by the precipitation of an ordered iron/platinum-type compound dispersed as a submicron second phase. This phase forms upon cooling from above 900° C and, once formed, is thermally stable beyond 1000° C, (*O'Brien* et al., 1964; *Smith* et al., 1970; *Leinfelder* et al., 1969; *Leinfelder* et al., 1966; *German,* 1980; *Tuccillo* and *Cascone,* unpublished).

Meanwhile, investment manufacturers developed phosphate-bonded investments as substitutes for the gypsum-bonded crown and bridge investments. However, as is often the case, solutions create new problems, and the stronger phosphate investments caused "hot tearing" of the coarse-grain alloys common at that time.

The answer was found in grain refining, and so began the era of fine-grained dental casting alloys. Today, most, but not all, alloys are fine-grained. The first publication on the benefits of fine-grained dental alloys appeared in 1966 (*Nielsen* and *Tuccillo*) and showed that iridium and ruthenium are potent grain refiners of gold alloys with only 50 to 250 parts per million necessary to reduce the as-cast grain size from about 300 microns to 50

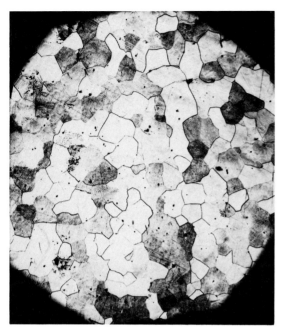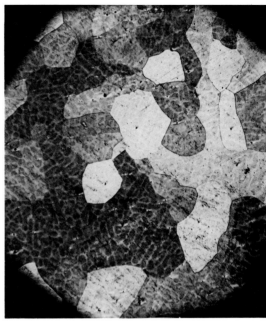

Fig. 4   Photomicrographs of alloys with large and fine grain size (original magnification 125x).

microns (Fig. 4). Reducing the grain size improves the tensile strength and elongation of as-cast alloys by providing additional grain boundaries that act as obstructions to the passage of dislocations. Figure 5 shows this increase for Type III and Type IV gold crown and bridge alloys. The function of indium and tin in the alloy was shown to be crucial to the development of a chemical bond between the metal and porcelain (*Shell* and *Nielsen*, 1962). In a classic paper, *Shell* and *Nielsen* described a bond test indicating not only that the bond was chemical in nature, but that a "smooth" metal surface would bond as well as a "roughened" surface. They theorized that the tin and indium formed surface oxides that were the ba-

sis of the chemical bond. Their findings were confirmed in later microprobe studies (*Lautenschlager* et al., 1969, and *Nally, Monnier, Meyer,* 1968).

One important offshoot of this work was in the area of design considerations. With the knowledge acquired from the *Shell–Nielsen* study, prosthodontists were freed from the need to "anchor" the porcelain to the metal as must be done with acrylic facings, and the functional design of bridgework began evolving to its present form.

The importance of "wetting" of the metal surface by the porcelain was another critically significant offshoot of this study. Bond failures often could be traced to the improper firing of opaque porcelain on

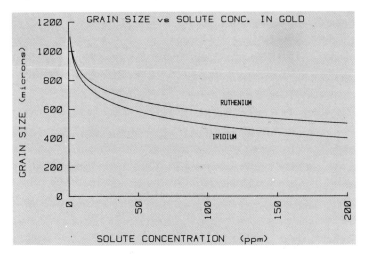

Fig. 5 Effect of grain refiner concentration on grain-size of gold.

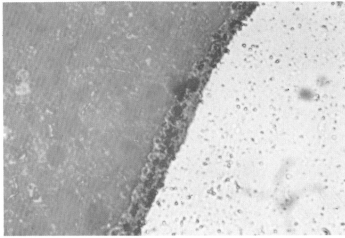

Fig. 6 Photomicrograph of interfacial zone between a nonprecious alloy (white) and porcelain, illustrating a thick oxide layer (original magnification 750x).

the metal. If the opaque were not fired high enough to thoroughly "wet" the metal surface, then the bond would be less than complete. The importance of wetting was pointed out in a study by *O'Brien* and *Ryge* (1965).

The question of wetting of the metal surface by the porcelain was also to be a determining factor in the bonding of porcelain to nonprecious metals. Whereas the oxides found on precious metals are thin, tenacious, and easily "absorbed" by the porcelain, the oxides formed on nonprecious metals are none of these but, in fact, are thick and brittle (Fig. 6); for this reason metal bonding agents were developed to reduce or change the oxides or force the formation of more favorable ones. The use of special glasses in the opaque porcelain to promote wetting was also an additional help.

Following the introduction of PFM alloys

and up to 1968, researchers were engaged in improving the original gold-platinum-palladium alloy and ancillary products to solve the problems that had surfaced. However, not all the problems were solved. Reports from the field indicated that the modulus of elasticity of the alloy was too low for long-span bridges and the homologous temperature of the alloy was also too low, which meant that its thermal stability needed improvement. There were indications that dimensional changes occurred due to casting stress annealing at the porcelain firing temperatures.

The solution to these problems of the gold-platinum-palladium system was known at that time. The answer was the substitution of palladium for gold. Such a substitution would improve the thermal stability and the modulus of elasticity. However, it would also produce a white gold, not a yellow gold, alloy. Was the profession ready for this? It may seem strange today to ask such a question, but it was a real concern in 1968.

The Revolution Begins with the Gold-Palladium-Silver System

If one can pinpoint a specific time, 1968 was the starting point for the development of the gold-palladium-silver system. The decision of the U.S. Government to "free" gold accelerated the work in dental alloy research. No longer was gold "pegged" at $35 per ounce, and it was not difficult to see over the horizon. The price of gold would rise, and the profession would demand casting alloys of lower in-

trinsic cost. The stage was set to substitute palladium for gold.

The solution was the development of the gold-palladium-silver system in which the gold content was reduced, platinum eliminated, and palladium and silver increased (*Katz* patent, 1974; *Tuccillo* patents, 1976).

This alternative was immediately successful, both functionally and economically. The physical properties were superior to those of the gold-platinum-palladium system; thermal stability was improved; the handling characteristics were better; density was 25% lower; and the intrinsic cost was reduced.

The general composition of this system is as follows:

Au	50%
Pd	30%
Ag	12%
In and Sn	8%

The hardening mechanism for this system is solid-solution strengthening. Generally, the elements added to the gold-palladium-silver system form substitutional solid solutions. In other words, the tin or indium atoms enter into the face-centered-cubic lattice in place of the gold, palladium, or silver atoms. Hardening results from interactions between dislocations and solute atoms (e.g., indium, tin).

There are many types of interactions that can occur (*Flinn*, 1962); however, the two of most interest are elastic and electrical.

Elastic interactions occur between the stress field of a dislocation and the stress

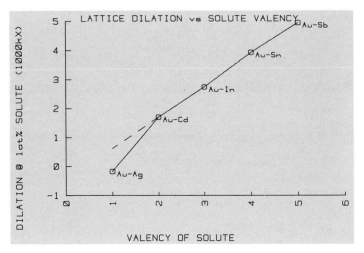

Fig. 7 Lattice dilation of gold with various solute additions.

field around the solute atom. Substitutional solute atoms either expand or contract the lattice, causing some degree of lattice distortion. Generally, the greater the difference in size of the solvent and solute atoms, the greater will be the stress field. This size factor is directly related to the solubility of the solute in the solvent.

Electrical interactions occur between the screened charge of the solute atom and the altered electron density around a dislocation. These interactions produce the same general effects as the elastic interactions.

Figure 7 (redrawn from *Owen and Roberts*, 1945), relates the increase in lattice parameter of gold due to the addition of 1 atom % solute to the valence of the solute. For the polyvalent solutes, the lattice dilation is directly proportional to the valence, demonstrating that the elastic and electrical interactions are related.

Figure 8 relates the accompanying increase in hardness with the addition of 5 atom % solute to the solute valence. The rapid hardening due to the inclusion of tin is evidence that the elastic and electrical interactions can be compounded.

The higher palladium content results in a melting range that is approximately 100° F higher than that of the gold-platinum-palladium system. Thus, there is less chance of thermal distortion during the porcelain firing cycle.

Since the gold-palladium-silver system has such high nobility, technical manipulation is not a problem and casting fit is very satisfactory. Soldering is at least as uncomplicated as with the gold-platinum-palladium system, and the techniques are the same.

In this instance, the higher gold price worked to the advantage of technology, forcing the introduction of a technically superior metal. The fact that the alloy was white ceased to be a negative consideration, for as the price of gold increased, the demand for a gold-colored alloy decreased.

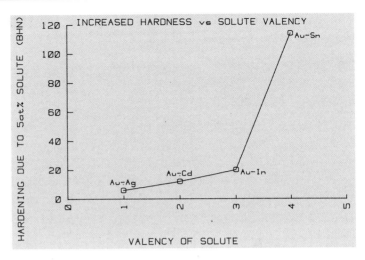

Fig. 8 Hardening response of solute on gold.

The nickel-chromium-beryllium system of nonprecious alloys was also introduced after 1968. Its initial penetration of the market was nil. In 1976, when gold was about $130 per ounce, an NADL survey suggested a 25% penetration. By 1980, when gold was $800 per ounce, it was estimated at about 50%. In 1968, however, the gold price was around $38 per ounce, and there was little incentive to switch to an alloy system that was more difficult to cast, fit, grind, polish; impossible to solder; and that had a proclivity to reject porcelain.

About that time, environmentalist groups became quite concerned about the use of beryllium in dental alloys and forced some of them off the market. This aspect will be considered later.

The Palladium-Silver System

The Era of "Goldless" PFM Alloys

Although the alloys of the gold-palladium-silver system were quite satisfactory, research continued on the development of precious alloys of even lower intrinsic value. A concentrated effort was made to eliminate gold completely by substituting palladium and silver. The choice of substitutional elements considered at that time was restricted to the noble/precious metal group, i.e., ruthenium, rhodium, palladium, osmium, iridium, platinum, and silver. On the basis of physical and chemical characteristics, palladium and silver were the two elements of choice, but a careful metallurgical balance was necessary. Whereas substituting palladium for gold in an alloy raises the melting range and lowers the coefficient of expansion, silver has the reverse effect. Indium and tin for hardening and bonding completed the system. Thus was born the palladium-silver system of PFM alloys in 1974.

361

The general composition of the palladium-silver system is as follows:

Pd   55–60%
Ag   25–30%
In and Sn   10–20%

The high noble and precious metal content (80–90%) of this system assured its acceptance by the dental profession and craft. It literally worked like the gold-palladium-silver system.

The palladium-silver system undergoes solid-solution hardening in much the same way as the gold-palladium-silver system except that it is perhaps more straightforward since size effects are not a factor and valence effects dominate.

The palladium-silver alloys have a density of 10.8 gms/CM^3, and this, in conjunction with their low intrinsic cost, means a substantial decrease in total metal cost as compared with the gold-containing alloy system. A further advantage is their handling characteristics and also their physical properties are comparable.

However, the palladium-silver system is not without problems. First of all, the technique for handling this system successfully is somewhat more complicated and time-consuming because of the high silver content. Silver is a colorant for porcelains and sometimes imparts a yellow-green hue to the porcelain at the porcelain-metal interface. The mechanism is not understood completely, but we can speculate on the possibilities.

The green-yellow discoloration of porcelain is due to the precipitation of minute silver particles in porcelain. The color of stain varies from green to yellow to orange as the amount of silver absorbed in porcelain increases and as the size of the silver particles increases (*Doremus*, 1965). These two factors are dependent upon the composition of the porcelain and the firing cycle. Silver is absorbed by the porcelain at elevated temperatures while the precipitation of the particles, and therefore the discoloration, occurs during the cooling cycle.

How the silver is transported from the alloy to the porcelain is still not completely understood, but one mechanism has been defined. At the firing temperature of porcelain, silver has a high vapor pressure resulting in the alloy releasing silver from its surface as a gas. This gaseous silver produces two effects:

1. Silver gas travels throughout the porcelain furnace and condenses in the cooler regions. During the normal heating and cooling cycles, the silver revaporizes and condenses upon anything cooler in the furnace, including the restoration.
2. The silver gas is very active near the surface of the alloy and is therefore readily absorbed onto the surface of the porcelain.

The first effect is seen after prolonged use of silver-bearing alloys. If the porcelain furnace is not properly decontaminated at regular intervals, alloys containing no silver can be found to be discolored. The second effect seems to explain why the discoloration generally appears only near the juncture of porcelain and metal.

There are ways of reducing the occurrence of discoloration. The two most suc-

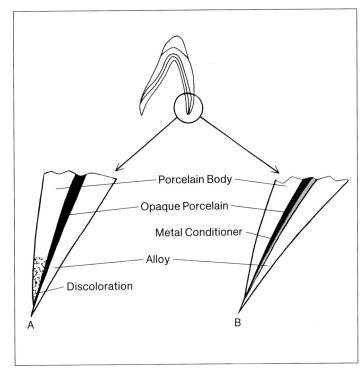

Porcelain Body

Opaque Porcelain

Metal Conditioner

Alloy

Discoloration

A

B

Fig.9a   Silver discoloration occurs when body porcelain flows onto metal surface.

Fig.9b   A ceramic metal conditioner acts as a barrier layer preventing the body porcelain from flowing onto the alloy.

cessful methods are the use of a gold metal conditioner or a ceramic metal conditioner. Each works in a different way to impede staining.

1. Gold Metal Conditioners: The 24-Karat gold metal conditioners reduce the apparent silver content on the surface of the alloy when properly fired. In other words, as the gold metal conditioner is fired, the surface of the alloy becomes rich in gold. If the alloy originally contained 25% silver, theory predicts that the silver content at the surface drops dramatically to about 15% due to the addition of the gold. As the percentage of silver decreases, so does the probability of discoloration.

2. Ceramic Metal Conditioners: These materials act as a barrier layer between the metal and porcelain, preventing the porcelain from coming in contact with the metal surface.

So long as the furnace is not contaminated, discoloration occurs only when the body porcelain (or superglaze) touches the metal surface (Fig.9a). Ceramic metal conditioners can be applied thinly and, when properly fired, form a thin glass coating. By slightly overextending the opaque line with the metal conditioner, a barrier is established between the body porcelain and the alloy (Fig.9b).

Many other ways of preventing discoloration have been suggested. The success

363

of the different techniques varies depending upon the shade and type of porcelain, as well as on the technician; but two are definitely not recommended. They are: (1) Underfiring the opaque or gold metal conditioner, which will prevent proper porcelain adherence; and (2) Acid treatments. The palladium-silver alloys are more susceptible to acid attack than the gold-bearing alloys. Acids such as nitric or hydrochloric will seriously weaken the alloy.

There are no magic products that can eliminate discoloration, but there are ways of controlling it, the most effective being the ceramic metal conditioners.

A second problem with the palladium-silver system has to do with its use with porcelains manufactured in Europe. The system was developed to work with U.S.-manufactured porcelains, which generally have higher coefficients of expansion.

Figures 10 and 11 illustrate the relationship of porcelain and PFM alloys manufactured in the United States and Europe. The U.S. systems have a broader range of thermal expansion. There is a significant difference between the palladium-silver and the gold-palladium-silver systems of U.S. manufacturers and the European porcelains.

It became obvious in laboratory use that the European porcelains were not always workable with the two systems, the porcelain cracking under certain laboratory techniques that exacerbated the mismatch between the materials.

The solution to both problems–discoloration and coefficient of expansion too high for European porcelains–was not long in coming. In 1977, the gold-palladium system was introduced, and a patent has since been issued covering developments in this area (*Cascone, 1978*).

This system became an immediate anomaly in the marketplace. Just when the industry was swinging toward alloys of lower intrinsic value, it reversed course to an alloy system of higher intrinsic value. In fact, in the period between 1977 and 1980, the gold-palladium system became by far the most used PFM alloy system, displacing the gold-palladium-silver system. This attests to the working characteristics and properties of this system. Although higher in cost than the gold-palladium-silver system, the higher cost was offset by the superior working characteristics of the gold-palladium system, which resulted in labor savings.

The composition covered in the gold-palladium patent is as follows:

Au	52	%
Pd	38	%
Ag	0	%
In	8.5	%
Ga	1.5	%

The removal of silver accomplished two purposes: it eliminated the discoloration problem and, by substituting palladium for the silver, the coefficient of expansion was lowered. However, although the gold-palladium system was sufficiently low for the European porcelains, it was, alas, too low for some of the U.S. porcelains with their higher coefficient. Here again, a solution to one problem created another.

The industry adapted by learning which combinations of porcelain and metal to use. Unfortunately, this sometimes becomes a trial-and-error experience since there are so many variations of technique that can affect the successful combining of porcelain and metal. For example, there are vacuum porcelain furnaces that utilize a slow furnace cool from the porcelain firing temperature. Whereas this may work successfully in some cases, there are combinations of porcelain and metal which, when slow-cooled, develop overwhelming interfacial stresses, especially when pontics are involved. Of course, rapid cooling can also be detrimental and cause cracking through the porcelain. In general, the safest procedure is to remove the restoration from the furnace once the firing cycle is complete and allow it to cool naturally to room temperature. The reason for this becomes clear when considering the heat dissipation patterns of a pontic and a coping.

Thermal Gradients and Design

The two basic designs employed in porcelain-metal restorations are the coping and the pontic. Upon cooling from the porcelain firing temperature, the temperature gradient within the coping is very different from that within the pontic. By simplifying the designs, the effect of the gradients can be studied.

The pontic can be considered to be a sphere of metal surrounded by porcelain. In order for the alloy to lose any heat, the heat must be conducted through the porcelain. Because porcelain conducts heat about 1,000 times more slowly than the metal, the metal stays hot for a long time, as does the porcelain-metal interface. The surface of the porcelain, then, is the coolest area. The porcelain will set first at the surface and last at the porcelain-metal interface. The coping is simply a layer of porcelain on top of a layer of metal. Since the metal has one surface open to the air, it can lose heat rapidly. The porcelain-metal interface is found to be cooler than the surface of the porcelain. The porcelain sets first at the porcelain-metal interface and last at its surface.

As previously mentioned, any difference in the contraction behavior between the porcelain and the alloy will produce stresses in the porcelain.

In the case of the coping, most of these stresses can be relieved, since the surface of the porcelain sets last. However, for the pontic, because the surface sets first, the stresses are allowed to build up and may even be accentuated (This may result in a time-delay fracture).

Due to this difference in thermal gradients, thermal checking of porcelain is seen more on pontics than on copings. In fact, some porcelain-metal pairs can be used successfully on copings but not on pontics or long-span bridges (*Cascone, 1979*).

The stage was now set for the dramatic increase in the gold bullion price between the fall of 1979 and early 1980. The alloys available to dentists and technicians were gold alloys, palladium-silver alloys, and nonprecious metals.

When gold began its meteoric price climb in 1979, use of the palladium-silver system started to increase dramatically. By now, technicians had learned how to handle the problems associated with the palladium-silver system by making the necessary technical adjustments. Most notably, the use of ceramic surface coatings alleviated the problem of discoloration. Technicians also learned to purge their vacuum porcelain furnaces periodically and to make whatever adjustments were needed in their spruing and casting techniques to offset the gas absorption proclivity of the system.

As the price of gold increased, it became economically feasible to take the extra technical steps that were called for by the palladium-silver system.

Nonprecious Alloy Systems

Concurrently with the above developments, technicians were also learning how to handle the nonprecious alloys. Although the nickel-chromium-beryllium system had been available for many years, its use was limited because of the technical difficulties associated with nonprecious alloys. It was also the general opinion that nonprecious alloys produced inferior PFM restorations from the standpoints of casting fit (*Nitkin* and *Asgar,* 1976) and porcelain bonding (*McLean* and *Sced,* 1976), as well as other functional characteristics (*Duncan,* 1980). Today, there are at least four nonprecious systems in use: nickel-chromium, nickel-chromium with beryllium, cobalt-chromium, and cobalt-chromium

with ruthenium. Some typical compositions are as follows:

Nickel-Chromium	77 Ni	13 Cr	4 Mo	6 Al	
Nickel-Chromium-Beryllium	79 Ni	13 Cr	4 Mo	2 Al	2 Be
Cobalt-Chromium	67 Co	21 Cr	8 Mo	4 Al	
Cobalt-Chromium-Ruthenium	53 Co	27 Cr	10 W	3 Ga	3 Ru

Of the four systems, the nickel-chromium-beryllium is considered the best to work with.

However, all nonprecious alloys are considered technique-sensitive and more difficult to handle than precious metals. They require special waxing and investing procedures to help compensate for their greater solidification shrinkage, and still the quality of fit is often questionable. Nonprecious alloys are very difficult to solder and to finish because of their high hardness, and nonprecious restorations are difficult to remove from teeth.

Another serious disadvantage of nonprecious metals is inconsistency in bonding to dental porcelains. Oxide formation during heating and cooling as required in porcelain application is not always controllable. The use of beryllium in nickel-chromium alloys helps considerably in preventing the formation of a brittle nickel-chromium spinel. Without beryllium, bonding agents must be used. In addition, to reduce oxide formation, most manufacturers of nonprecious alloys specify special surface treatments such as sandblasting techniques or steam-cleaning, or both. Short firing cycles and special opaques are sometimes recommended. A minimum number of porcelain firing cycles is also suggested by some.

As *McLean* states (1979):

"In the case of the base metal alloys, more work has yet to be done on casting accuracy and development of new investments…Even assuming the casting problem is overcome, no solution has yet been found to controlling oxide production at the interface of a nickel-chromium/porcelain interface. Use of these materials should therefore be confined to the specialist and research laboratory."

The message is clear. When using nonprecious metals, one must expect to spend more time, utilize more skilled labor, follow more precisely the prescribed techniques, and be prepared for more failures than when using precious metals.

However, the fact remains that perhaps 40% of all PFM restorations made in the United States today are nonprecious, solely on the basis of two advantages that are perceived by much of the dental profession to more than offset the many disadvantages. These advantages are:

1. A modulus of elasticity 2.5 times higher than that of precious metals and a higher strength, which permits the fabrication of light, thin copings.
2. Low cost.

Undoubtedly, that last advantage is the primary reason for using nonprecious metals, yet, the metal cost of a PFM unit cast from a palladium-silver alloy is probably less than $ 5.00, or only about 2% of the patient's total fee. In addition, the accuracy of the claim that nonprecious alloys can be used in significantly thinner section than precious metal alloys will be challenged by *Dr. Jones* in this symposium.

Another factor to be considered with nonprecious usage is the cloud of controversy about the allergenic and carcinogenic potentials of nickel. Nickel alloys have been used in fixed prostheses for a limited time, and little research has been done to determine their biological safety. It is known, however, that nickel produces more allergic reactions than all other metals (*Fisher*, 1967). It has also been shown that nickel-sensitive patients exhibit adverse reactions to intraoral dental alloys containing nickel and that reactions can occur in parts of the body far removed from the mouth (*Bergman, Berman,* and *Soremark,* 1980).

The technician, too, should be concerned personally with the health factor since inhalation of grinding dust and vapors from these alloys, as well as skin contact, may be a hazard. Inhalation of nickel dust has proven carcinogenic in animal studies, and nickel is a well-established carcinogen among nickel workers (NIOSH, 1977).

If a nonprecious alloy is to be used, one solution to the nickel and beryllium problem would be the cobalt-chromium system. These alloys, however, are more difficult to melt and cast than the nickel-chromium alloys with beryllium. Also, unless ruthenium is used to lower the coefficient of expansion of the straight cobalt-chromium system, these alloys are not recommended for the lower thermal expansion European porcelains. Whichever alloy is used, very strict adherence to the recommended technique is mandatory.

Economic considerations are an important aspect of any decision involving the use of nonprecious alloys. At the present time, with the cost of palladium-silver alloys averaging less than $ 5.00 per unit for metal and with the advantages that precious metals have over nonprecious alloys, it is questionable whether there is an economic advantage in using a nickel-chromium or cobalt-chromium alloy.

Conclusion

The alternative alloy systems available to the dentist and technician for PFM restorations have evolved since the 1950s in response to specific needs. So will it be in the future.

What may we expect in the years ahead?

1. Although, in the United States, about 70 % of all restorations are made from alloys that do not contain gold, this is not the case in the rest of the world. Europe is just beginning to lower the gold content of acceptable alloys in order to lower the cost. South America and Asia have just begun to swing over to the palladium-silver and nonprecious systems. Although gold-containing alloys will always be the systems of choice for PFM restorations, it would appear that their share of the market will continue to give way to alternative systems.

2. The problem of discoloration with palladium-silver alloys will be solved metallurgically by developing diffusion barriers within the alloy structure. Therefore, we can expect to see "goldless" alloys of even lower palladium content and intrinsic cost.

3. Alloy development will continue to be directed toward non-nickel, nonprecious alloy systems, and systems will soon evolve that are significantly different from any available today.

4. Castable ceramics are a definite probability. Materials for single units have already been introduced. Whether the problem of fit can be solved remains to be seen, but, certainly to some degree, the technique is prominent in the future development of veneer porcelain restorations.

5. Gold alloys will continue to be an important and preferred choice, but the gold content will be even further reduced.

6. If the price of gold remains in the $ 400–$ 450 per ounce range or drops even lower, the market share of gold alloys will stabilize. But it is questionable that it will ever increase.

References

Bergman, M., Berman, B., and Soremark, R. (1980): Tissue accumulation of nickel released due to electrochemical corrosion of non-precious dental alloys. J. Oral Rehab. 7: 325.

Cascone, P. J. (1978): U.S. Patent 4,123,262.

Cascone, P. J. (1979): Effect of thermal properties on porcelain-to-metal compatibility. IADR Abstract 683, 57th General Session.

Cascone, P. J., Massimo, M., and Tuccillo, J. J. (1978): Theoretical interfacial reactions responsible for bonding in porcelain-to-metal systems. Part II: Oxidation of alloys. IADR Abstract 872, 56th General Session.

Cascone, P. J., and Tuccillo, J. J. (1977): Theoretical interfacial reactions responsible for bonding in porcelain-to-metal systems. Part I—Palladium-base alloys. AADR Abstract 640, Annual General Session.

Doremus, R. H. (1965): Optical properties of small silver particles. J. Chem. Physics 42: 414.

Duncan, J. D. (1980): Casting accuracy of chromium alloys: marginal discrepancies. J. Dent. Res. 59: 1164.

Fisher, A. A. (1967): Contact Dermatitis. Philadelphia: Lea & Febiger.

Flinn, P. A. (1962): Solid solution strengthening. In: Strengthening Mechanisms in Solids, Chap. 2, ASM.

German, R. M. (1980): Hardening reactions in a high-gold content ceramo-metal alloy. J. Dent. Res. 59: 1960.

Katz, M. (1974): U.S. Patent 3,819,366.

King, B. W., et al (1959): J. Am. Ceram. Soc. 11: 504.

Lautenschlager, E. P., et al (1969): Microprobe analysis of gold-porcelain bonding. J. Dent. Res. 48: 1206.

Leinfelder, K. F., O'Brien, W. J., Ryge, G., and Fairhurst, C. W. (1966): Hardening of high-fusing gold alloys. J. Dent. Res. 45: 392.

Leinfelder, K. F., Servais, W. J., and O'Brien, W. J. (1969): Mechanical properties of high-fusing gold alloys. J. Prosthet. Dent. 21: 523.

McLean, J. W. (1979): The Science and Art of Dental Ceramics, Vol.I, Chicago: Quintessence Publishing Co., Inc.

McLean, J. W., and Sced, I. R. (1976): The base-metal alloy/porcelain bond. Trans. Brit. Ceram. Soc. 5: 235.

Nally, J. H., Monnier, D., and Meyer, J. M. (1968): Distribution topographic de certains éléments de l'alliage et de la porcelaine au niveau de la liaison ceramo-métallique. Schweizerische Monatsschrift für Zahnheilkunde, 78.

Nielsen, J. P., and Tuccillo, J. J. (1966): Grain size in cast gold alloys. J. Dent. Res. 45: 964.

NIOSH (May 1977): Criteria for a Recommended Standard ... Occupational Exposure to Inorganic Nickel. U.S. Government Printing Office, Washington.

Nitkin, D. A., and Asgar, K. (1976): Evaluation of alternative alloys to Type III gold for use in fixed prosthodontics. JADA 93: 622.

O'Brien, W.J., Kring, J.E., and Ryge, G. (1964): Heat treatment of alloys to be used for the fused porcelain technique. J. Prosthet. Dent. 14: 955.

O'Brien, W. J., and Nielsen, J. P. (1959): Decomposition of gypsum investment in the presence of carbon. J. Dent. Res. 38: 541.

O'Brien, W. J., and Ryge, G. (1965): Contact angles of drops of enamels on metals. J. Prosthet. Dent. 15: 1094.

Owen, E. A., and O'Donnell, R. (1945): The solubility of certain metals in gold. J. Inst. Metals. 71:213.

Pask, J. A. (1964): Modern Aspects of the Vitreous State. Vol. 3. J. D. Mackenzie, d. London: Butterworth.

Rand Research, Inc. (1981): Alloy direct mail research report. Chicago.

Rowe, A., and Asgar, K. (1976): Thermal study of porcelain substrate metals. IADR Abstract 505, 54th General Session.

Shell, J. S., and Nielsen, J. P. (1962): Study of the bond between gold alloys and porcelain. J. Dent. Res. 41:1424.

Smith, D. L., Burnett, A. P., Brooks, M. S., and Anthony, D. H. (1979): Iron-platinum hardening in casting golds for use with porcelain. J. Dent. Res. 49:283.

Tuccillo, J. J. (1976): U.S. Patens 3,961,420 and 3,981,723.

Tuccillo, J. J., and Cascone, P. J.: Unpublished work, J. F. Jelenko & Co., Armonk.

Tuccillo, J. J., and Nielsen, J. P. (1967): Creep and sag properties of a porcelain-gold alloy. J. Dent. Res. 46:579.

Weinstein, M., Katz, S., and Weinstein, A. B. (1962): U.S. Patents 3,052,982 and 3,052,983.

Screening Tests for Metal-Ceramic Systems

Kenneth J. Anusavice

Introduction

Laboratory evaluation of new materials and devices is a prerequisite for ensuring the safety, efficacy, and economy of these products for intraoral use. The porcelain-fused-to-metal (PFM) prosthesis is a multicomponent structure typically consisting of metal substrate, interaction zone, opaque porcelain, body (dentine) porcelain, incisal (enamel) porcelain, and a glaze layer. The clinical success of PFM restorations is dependent on alloy castability, alloy sag resistance, porcelain-metal adherence, porcelain-metal compatibility, porcelain-porcelain compatibility, physical properties of the individual components, design of the prosthesis, quality of the solder joints (if present), resistance to intraoral degradation, and esthetic characteristics.

Because of the great complexity of discussing each of these variables in depth, this chapter will consider the four variables which have a major effect on the clinical success of PFM prostheses, namely, bond strength, compatibility of alloys and porcelain, alloy castability, and alloy sag resistance. Although other variables are also important, the test methods and resulting data are fairly well established and some of these tests have been used to predict clinical performance with a reasonable level of success.

Screening Tests for Metal-Ceramic Adherence

Considerable efforts have been made during the past thirty years to develop test methods that could quantitatively discriminate between excellent metal-ceramic adherence and poor or clinically unacceptable adherence. The search for an "ideal bond test" still continues because of the uncertainty that exists in the interpretation of existing bond test data. Certain metal-porcelain systems, which have demonstrated relatively high bond strength values, may fail in vivo more frequently than other systems exhibiting comparable levels of adherence. Conversely, predictions of low levels of adherence for certain base metal alloy-porcelain combinations have not generally been realized in subsequent clinical practice.

Test methods may be classified according to the principal stresses induced in the test specimens. Tensile, shear, flexure, tensile-shear, and torsion test designs have been employed. Most of these tests have been conducted using a single stress cycle. Although clinical prostheses are subjected to many cycles of stress before failure occurs, few data are available to evaluate metal-ceramic bond strength under cyclic loading conditions. Impact loading methods, such as the free-falling sphere test employed in the ceramics industry and the "hammer test" used by dental alloy manufacturers, provide a means of qualitatively characterizing the appearance of the fracture surfaces.

Perhaps the chief difficulty associated with interpretation of bond test data is the lack of information on the stress distribution and the types of stress generated within each test specimen. For the shear-type tests, it is usually assumed that the stress distribution is uniform along the entire interfacial region and the failure load is divided by the interfacial area to calculate the failure stress or bond strength.

Secondly, assumptions are made that the lateral stress distribution is uniform and that stress concentration effects are neglible; thus the conclusion is frequently made that fractures occurring in porcelain away from the interfacial region are an indication that the bond strength is either equivalent to or exceeds the cohesive strength of porcelain. Obviously, if higher stresses occur away from the interface due to the test design or because of stress concentration factors, this conclusion would be erroneous. One would not be measuring the interfacial bond strength but merely the strength of the porcelain alone.

The rate of loading and type of stress distribution produced could markedly affect the fracture path within a bond test specimen. Other variables such as metal-ceramic thickness ratio and length and width of the interfacial zone could affect not only the magnitude of bond strength but also the location of the point of fracture initiation and the path of crack propagation. DeHoff et al (1980) reported that the metal-to-porcelain thickness ratio in a four point flexure test could markedly affect the point of peak tensile stress and possibly the point of fracture initiation. Koji (1976) reported that, in the pull-through shear test, a 10 mm long interfacial zone results in a threefold increase in bond strength compared to specimens with a 5 mm interface length.

One should exercise caution, therefore, when assessing the fracture origin based solely on the appearance of a fracture surface with a mixed mode fracture pattern. Furthermore, one should consider these effects when comparing bond strength values obtained from test designs of different specimen dimensions. Bond strength testing of alloy specimens veneered with different porcelain products may also yield differences due to variations in residual stress and in the tensile strength values of the porcelain selected. This factor is important in most

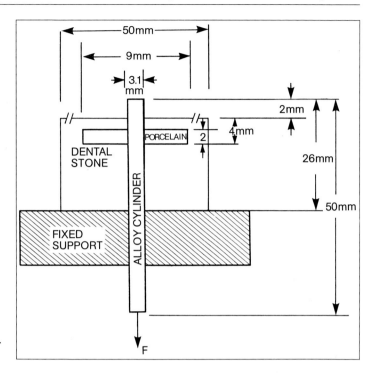

Fig.1 Pull-shear bond test design.

of the test designs since a higher probability of tensile failure than shear stress failure exists with many of the tests commonly used in dental research applications (*Anusavice*, 1980). Stress analyses performed in this study on a variety of test configurations revealed significant stress concentrations in ten of the eleven test designs evaluated.

Pull-Shear and Push-Shear Tests

Perhaps the most widely accepted bond test designs are the push-shear test and the pull-shear test (Fig.1). A finite element stress analysis (*Anusavice*, 1980) of these specimens (Fig. 2) reveals that maximum shear stress develops at the interfacial region closest to the applied force and decreases to less than one-half of this value at the interfacial region farthest from the applied force. A slightly more uniform stress distribution results in the pull-shear mode.

Shell and *Nielsen* (1962) reported that pull-shear testing resulted in a sizable scatter of data points due to Griffith flaw effects. As stated by *Kingery* (1960), "An important consequence of the theory that brittle fracture is initiated at *Griffith* flaws is that the fracture strength of a brittle solid is statistical in nature, depending upon the probability that a flaw capable of initiating fracture at a specific applied stress is present. This is the main explanation of the scatter of results normally found for the strength of ceramic materials." *Shell* and *Nielsen* (1962)

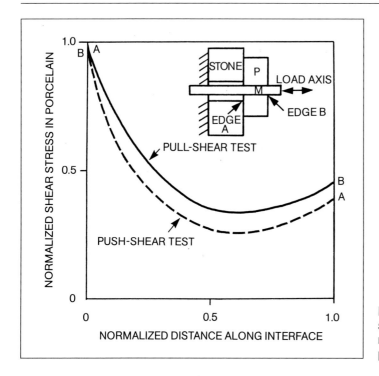

Fig. 2 Normalized porcelain shear stress along porcelain-metal interface in pull-shear and push-shear bond test specimens.

reported that roughening of a platinum alloy surface had no effect on bond strength. However, the addition of trace metal elements to a gold alloy resulted in significantly higher bond strengths. These tests were performed using 14 gauge alloy wire with a maximum interface length of 2.5 mm to avoid plastic deformation of the wire.

One of the first studies of base metal alloy-porcelain bond strength was reported by *Moffa* et al (1973). Pull-shear bond strength values were 95.8 MPa (13,900 psi) for a Ni–Cr–Be alloy and 73.1 MPa (10,600 psi) for a high gold content alloy veneered with Ceramco porcelain (Ceramco, Inc.).

Koji (1976) reported a pull-shear bond strength of approximately 31.3 MPa (4,538 psi) for a Ni–Cr alloy (Wiron S) and Ceramco porcelain with an interfacial zone 10 mm in length. For specimens having a 2.5 mm interfacial zone length (along a 3 mm dia. rod), the bond strength varied from about 7.4 MPa (1,067 psi) to 19.6 MPa (2,845 psi).

Koji (1977) also determined the effect of alloying additions on the bond strength of an 80 wt.% Ni–20 wt.% Cr alloy. The bond strength of the binary alloy veneered with Ceramco porcelain was 17.9±1.4 MPa (2,589±199 psi). The addition of 6 wt.% Ti increased the bond strength by 75% to 31.3±0.8 MPa (4,537±114 psi). The addition of 6 wt.% Sn caused an increase of 34% in the measured bond strength. A 2% Ta addition increased the bond strength by 20% while a 6% Ta addition

Table 1 Pull-Shear Bond Strength Data of Lubovich et al. (1977)

Alloy	Alloy Type	Shear Strength (MPa)	
		Ceramco Porcelain	Vita Porcelain
SMG–3 (J. M. Ney Co.)	Au–Pt–Pd	89.9 ± 10.2	110.9 ± 9.5
SMG-W (J. M. Ney Co.)	Au–Pd–Ag	118.3 ± 11.2	118.3 ± 4.3
Nobil-Ceram (Nobillium Corp.)	Ni–Cr–Be	59.2 ± 12.3	52.3 ± 19.3
Permabond (Permadent, Inc.)	Ni–Cr–Be	119.5 ± 14.7	105.1 ± 13.7
Victory (Unitek Corp.)	Ni–Cr	99.1 ± 5.5	79.0 ± 15.9

resulted in a 2% decrease in bond strength.

Using alloy rods approximately 2mm in diameter veneered with a porcelain disc 2mm in height, *Lubovich* et al. (1977) coated the specimen surfaces above and below the porcelain disc with silicone grease prior to surrounding them with dental stone cylinders 38mm in diameter and 32mm in height. A summary of these test data using the pull-shear test is given in Table 1.

From this study it was concluded that there was no significant difference in bond strength between the Ceramco and Vita porcelains despite the presence of checking in 7 of the 46 Vita porcelain specimens. The alloys demonstrated significantly different bond strengths, and base metal alloys performed better with Ceramco porcelain (Ceramco, Inc.) than with Vita porcelain (Vita Zahnfabrik AG). The surface preparation and resulting surface roughness may have played a significant role in the resulting bond strength differences between the Nobil-Ceram and Permabond specimens. The Nobil-Ceram alloys were ground with heatless stones and preoxidized while the Permabond specimens were preoxidized and then sandblasted with 50 μm Al_2O_3 abrasive.

Carpenter and *Goodkind* (1979) further evaluated the effect of roughened and highly polished alloy surfaces on pull-shear and four point flexure test results. No change in four-point flexure strength was detected for either alloy-porcelain

Table 2   Pull-Shear Bond Strength Data for Ni–Cr–Be Alloys (Moffa, 1977)

Alloy	Manufacturer	Shear Strength (MPa)
Ultratek	Metals for Modern Dentistry	97.9± 9.0
Nobil-Ceram	Nobillium Corp.	88.9± 9.6
Microbond 2000	Howmedica Inc.	51.0± 7.6
Gemini II	Kerr Mfg. Co.	51.7± 6.9
Permabond	Permabond Co.	48.3± 8.3
Vera Bond	Albadent, Inc.	87.6±20.7

Table 3   Pull-Shear Bond Strength Data for Beryllium-Free Ni–Cr Alloys (Moffa, 1977)

Alloy	Manufacturer	Shear Strength (MPa)
Wiron S	Williams Gold Co.	88.2±10.3
Victory	Unitek Corp.	70.3± 5.5
Omega VK	Omega Dental Products, Inc.	97.9±13.8
Alpha MS	Omega Dental Products, Inc.	74.5±10.3
Microbond N/P	Howmedica, Inc.	85.5±12.4
Microbond N/P^2	Howmedica, Inc.	80.7±11.0
Jelbon	J.F. Jelenko & Co.	64.8± 4.8
Neydium	J.M. Ney Co.	106.2±25.5
Ceramalloy	Ceramco, Inc.	88.9±10.3

Table 4   Bond Strength Data for Gold-Base Alloys (Moffa, 1977)

Alloy	Alloy Type	Manufacturer	Shear Strength (MPa)
Ceramco "O"	Au–Pt–Pd	J.F. Jelenko & Co.	73.1± 6.9
Jelenko "O"	Au–Pt–Pd	J.F. Jelenko & Co.	88.9±11.7
Degudent U	Au–Pt–Pd	Degussa	111.0± 8.3
Cameogold	Au–Pd–Ag	J.F. Jelenko & Co.	103.4±18.0
Will-Ceram W	Au–Pd–Ag	Williams Gold	86.9± 8.3
PG	Pd–Ag–Au	Nobillium Corp.	69.0± 4.1.

system as a function of surface roughness. The pull-shear test design employed a layer of platinum foil above and below the porcelain attachment area and a felt pad for load distribution.

Some claims have been made that base metal alloys containing beryllium are associated with greater bond strength than beryllium-free alloys. *Moffa* (1977) summarized an extensive study of the bond strength of Ceramco porcelain to numerous beryllium-containing and beryllium-free alloys using the pull-shear test design. For these measurements he employed the silicone grease lubricant and dental stone embedding technique. He found no generalized difference in bond strength between the two types of alloy nor between base metal alloys and gold base alloys. A summary of these data is given in Tables 2, 3, and 4. Note that the bond strength value in Table 2 for Nobil-Ceram is 30 MPa higher than the values given by *Lubovich* (Table 1) and the value for Permabond is about 71 MPa lower than the values reported by *Lubovich*.

Asgar and *Giday* (1978) reported lower coefficients of variation for the push-shear test (25–41%) compared to the pull-shear test (12–21%). Ceramco porcelain was used on all specimens. In this study, the porcelain-metal specimens were coated with wax prior to embedding them in dental stone. A summary of these bond strength measurements is given in Table 5. This study revealed lower bond strength values for Wiron S, Ultratek, Cameogold, and Jelenko "O" compared to the Moffa study (Tables 2–4).

Malhotra and *Maickel* (1980) evaluated the effect of the pull-shear versus push-shear test on bond strength data for four gold-base and one palladium-base alloy veneered with three commercial products. They also reported higher bond strength values with the push-shear test. Based on this study, bond strength values were higher for Biobond porcelain (Dentsply International, Inc.) than for

Table 5   Comparison of Push-Shear and Pull-Shear Bond Test Data of Asgar et al. (1978)

Alloy	Alloy Type	Push-Shear Bond Strength (MPa)	Pull-Shear Bond Strength (MPa)
Wiron S	Ni–Cr	58.5±14.3	70.0± 9.9
Gemini II	Ni–Cr–Be	65.2±21.6	64.9± 7.8
Ultratek	Ni–Cr–Be	68.4±19.0	68.8± 9.7
SMG-W	Au–Pd–Ag	93.6±38.1	71.7± 9.1
Cameogold	Au–Pd–Ag	117.4±25.9	71.1±15.0
Jelenko "O"	Au–Pt–Pd	89.8±32.2	76.1± 9.6

Table 6   Push-Shear Versus Pull-Shear Test Data of Malhotra et al. (1980)

| Alloy* | Alloy Type | Shear Bond Strength (MPa) | | | | | |
| | | Biobond | | Ceramco | | Vita | |
		Push	Pull	Push	Pull	Push	Pull
Ceramco Gold	Au–Pd–Pt	118 (13.2)	83.7 (6.8)	82.5 (10.7)	66.8 (6.3)	88.8 (7.0)	68.2 (4.7)
Ceramco "L"	Au–Pd–Pt–Ag	93.5 (8.4)	83.8 (9.2)	74.3 (9.2)	61.2 (3.4)	78.9 (8.2)	66.1 (6.0)
Cer-Mate	Au–Pd	123.4 (15.2)	94.8 (18.6)	88.3 (11.4)	75.3 (9.0)	100.5 (6.4)	72.9 (8.4)
Ceramco White	Au–Pd–Ag	99.8 (5.0)	82.7 (8.8)	81.7 (4.3)	65.2 (5.2)	97.4 (9.5)	83.1 (7.0)
Pors-On	Pd–Ag	98.7 (10.8)	63.9 (6.8)	69.8 (4.2)	60.0 (5.5)	69.2 (3.9)	60.6 (4.3)

* All alloys supplied by J. Aderer, Inc., Long Island, N.Y.

Ceramco or Vita porcelain. The Au–Pd alloy showed relatively higher push-shear bond strengths for all three porcelains. A summary of these test data is given in Table 6.

Kawasaki (1980) investigated the pull-shear bond strength of Ni alloys containing between 0 to 10 wt.% Co and 0–25 wt.% Cr. It was found that bond strength increased with increasing Co content in all alloys. Bond strengths were lowest at compositions of 15 wt.% Cr in the Ni–5 wt.% Co–Cr system and at 20 wt.% Cr in the Ni–10 wt.% Co–Cr system.

Three-point and four-point loading designs have been used for bond strength evaluation. Finite element stress analysis of these test configurations has revealed extremely high stress concentrations at the porcelain end points (*Anusavice,* 1980). The shear stress distribution in porcelain along the porcelain-metal interface is shown in Figures 3 and 4 for the three-point and four-point loading test specimens, respectively. In each case, the shear stress drops off sharply from the porcelain end points (A and B) and is essentially negligible along the rest of the interface. For most test designs, the shear stresses are lower than the tensile stresses. This implies that the probability of tensile failure is greater than the probability of shear failure. This effect is shown in Figure 5, which is a plot of the area under the shear stress curves versus the ratio of maximum tensile stress to maximum shear stress. The area index is inversely proportional to the relative stress concentration effects within each bond test specimen. An ideal bond test would have an area index of 1.0 (no stress concentration effects) and a 100% probability of shear failure (σ max/τ max = 0).

It should be pointed out that there are two tensile stress components that are generated under flexure conditions: one of these is a direct tensile stress, which develops perpendicular to the interface, and the other is the tensile component of bending stress, which acts parallel to the interface. It is not clear which of these stresses is the primary cause of failure.

Caputo, Dunn, and *Reisbick* (1977) proposed a four-point flexure test design that was selected to overcome the porcelain tensile failures experienced by *Lavine* and *Custer* (1966) using the three-point flexure test. This design was selected on the basis of the infinitely high shear stress that develops at terminating edges of porcelain. No significant difference in bond strength of Ceramco "O"-Ceramco porcelain specimens was observed between those which were not preoxidized (degassed) and those which were subjected to vacuum preoxidation (degassing) treatments of 10- or 20-minute duration. For Gemini II (a Ni–Cr–Be alloy) and Ceramco porcelain, preoxidation for 10 minutes with or without a followup Al_2O_3 sandblasting treatment produced higher bond strengths than no preoxidation, a 20-minute preoxidation treatment, a 10 minute preoxidation treatment, or a 10-minute preoxidation treatment followed by surface grinding with a Dedeco A/O Rubi stone. Based on dye penetrant examination, *Caputo* claimed that no tensile failures were observed in the porcelain structure.

The majority of three-point and four-point flexure tests produces significant

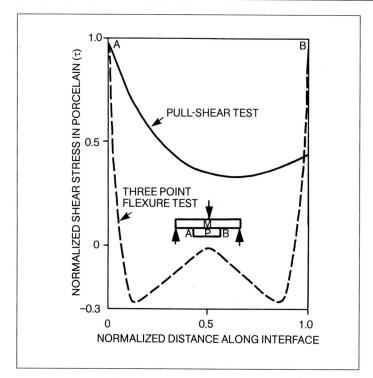

Fig. 3 Normalized shear stress in porcelain along porcelain-metal interface (A–B) in 3-point flexure bond test specimen.

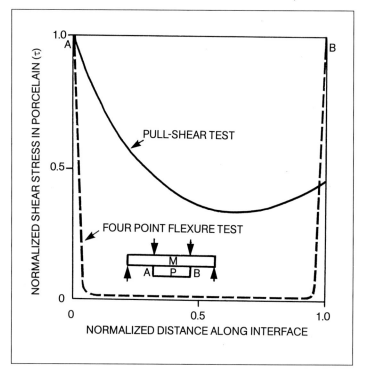

Fig. 4 Normalized shear stress in porcelain along porcelain-metal interface (A–B) in 4-point flexure bond test specimen.

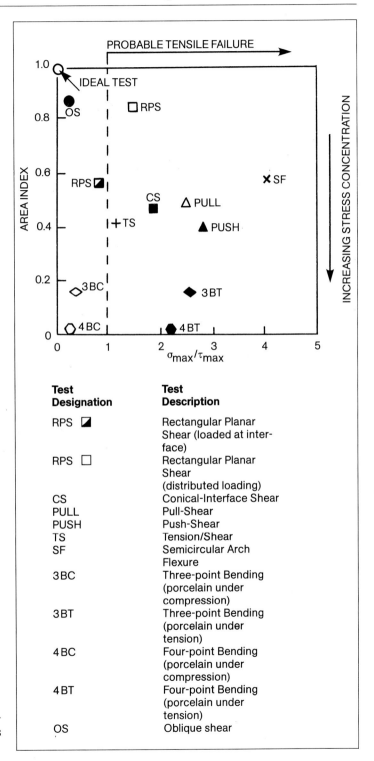

Fig. 5   Area index vs. ratio of maximum tensile stress to shear stress for 12 test configurations.

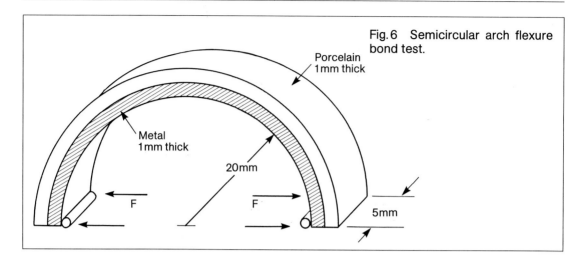

Fig. 6 Semicircular arch flexure bond test.

Porcelain
1mm thick

Metal
1mm thick

20mm

F

F

5mm

tensile stresses in the outer surface of porcelain through the application of a compressive load on the free metal surface. This loading configuration results in a high probability of porcelain tensile failure (Fig. 5). The mode of failure appears to be similar to that for the "peel test" used in other studies (*Yurenka*, 1961; *Weirauch*, 1978). In the *Weirauch* peel test study, it was concluded that adhesion between an iron-nickel alloy and a vitreous coating was primarily mechanical and that adhesion increased with increasing substrate roughness.

Finite element stress analysis (*Anusavice* et al., 1980) of three-point or four-point flexure test designs with a tensile load applied to the free metal surface (3BC and 4BC in Fig. 5) reveals a far lower probability of tensile failure than the other flexure tests. However, the stress concentration effects are just as great as in the other tests.

Stress analysis of a semicircular arch flexure test design shown in Figure 6

(*Mackert* et al., 1976) revealed a lower stress concentration effect but a very high tensile stress/shear stress ratio (Fig. 5).

In a recent study, *DeHoff* et al. (1980) reported that the failure location of four-point flexure bond tests is dependent on specimen geometry. Base metal alloy strips 10mm wide, 48mm long, and either 1mm or 2mm thick, were veneered with a layer of porcelain 25mm in length and 1mm thick. Initial failure occurred at the surface of porcelain between loading points of specimens with a porcelain-metal thickness ratio of 0.5. On the other hand, failure occurred under one of the central loading points in specimens with a porcelain-metal thickness ratio of 1.0.

Planar Shear Tests

Tests of this type are characterized by a planar metal-porcelain interface unlike the push-shear or pull-shear tests, which involve a curved interfacial area.

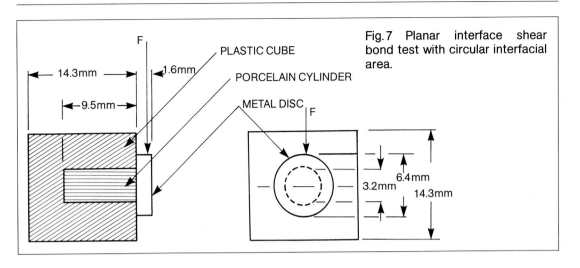

Fig. 7 Planar interface shear bond test with circular interfacial area.

Table 7 Planar Shear Test of Civjan et al. (1974)

Alloy	Alloy type	Shear Bond Strength (MPa)	
		Single Firing	Multiple Firing
Cameogold	Au–Pd–Ag	49.0 (CV = 33%)	64.9 (CV = 6%)
SMG-W	Au–Pd–Ag	56.0 (CV = 26%)	64.2 (CV = 10%)
Ceramco White	Au–Pd–Ag	48.3 (CV = 26%)	63.5 (CV = 7%)
Will-Ceram W	Au–Pd–Ag	48.3 (CV = 23%)	60.0 (CV = 18%)
Gemini	Ni–Cr–Be	40.0 (CV = 28%)	60.7 (CV = 9%)
Ticon	Ni–Cr–Be	29.6 (CV = 21%)	38.7 (CV unknown)

Civjan et al. (1974) utilized a planar shear test with a circular cross-sectional area (Fig. 7) to determine the bond strength of four Au–Pd–Ag alloys and one Ni–Cr–Be alloy with Ceramco porcelain. Another Ni–Cr–Be alloy (Ticon) was tested with Vita porcelain. However, rather than gripping an alloy cylinder and shearing off a porcelain disc, this test design involves the application of a force to metal disc approximately 6.4 mm in diameter and 1.6 mm thick bonded to a porcelain cylinder about 3.2 mm in diameter, which is embedded in an acrylic resin cube. The data are summarized in Table 7 for single-firing and multiple-firing cycles.

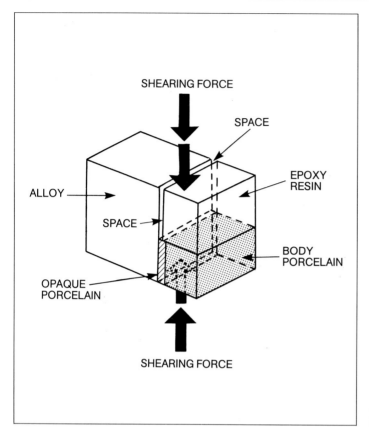

Fig. 8 Planar interface shear bond test with rectangular area.

The low values for Ticon-Vita porcelain specimens probably reflect the poor adherence of metal oxide to the metal substrate since only 6 of 30 specimens fabricated did not exhibit interfacial separation on cooling. A black scale remained attached to the porcelain cylinders after testing. Specimens that exhibited failure within porcelain were discarded from the analysis.

Susz et al. (1980) and other researchers have employed a planar shear test with a rectangular cross-sectional area to determine the effect of surface treatment of a Au–Pt–In alloy on bond strength. This test design is represented schematically in Figure 8. The block of epoxy resin adheres to the porcelain but is isolated from the alloy. Maximum bond strength was achieved by preoxidation of the alloy followed by pickling with hot diluted sulfuric acid. This improved adherence is thought to result from a reduction in indium content at the surface, thereby providing a more homogeneous indium distribution. In addition, these investigators believe that the alloy and porcelain coefficient of thermal expansion are balanced to contribute to the higher and more consistent bond strength values.

Chong and *Beech* (1980) reported that the planar shear test can discriminate poor bonding from excellent bonding systems. Also the bond strength differences for the porcelains studied are significant. Although the planar shear test design is not free of the complicating effects of residual stress, the test is easy to perform, allows for discrimination between surface roughness effects (polished versus abraded surface), and produces a relatively uniform stress distribution (Fig. 5). It is probably the most ideal test developed to date for evaluating porcelain-metal adherence. The concentrated load applied at the interface, compared to a distributed loading configuration, should reduce the probability of porcelain tension failure. The effect of the modulus of elasticity difference between alloys should also be minimal.

Tensile Tests

The typical bond strength test design consists of a layer of porcelain placed on one flat surface or between the flat surfaces of two metal rods: tensile force is applied along the long axis of the rod (or rods) until tensile failure of the adherence zone or the porcelain occurs. From a finite element stress analysis point of view, this type of test design is associated with a very high probability of porcelain tensile failure. Because of the alignment difficulties of the two-rod specimens and the presence of generalized stress raisers on the external surface of porcelain, failure within porcelain may be due to nonuniform stress distribution and one

should not summarily assume that the adherence strength is greater than the tensile strength of dental porcelain.

Conical Interface Shear Test

This test design shown schematically in Figure 9 represents the adhesion test proposed in the British Standard Institute Specification No. BS 3366 for porcelain-metal systems. Using this test, *Sced* and *McLean* (1972) determined comparable mean bond strength values for gold alloy-Vita VMK porcelain specimens, for Co–Cr alloy-Vita VMK porcelain specimens, and Ni–Cr alloy-Vita VMK porcelain specimens. The gold alloy specimen failures occurred in opaque porcelain near the conical interface, while failure in the base metal alloy specimens occurred at the interfacial region. Because of the significant decrease in the thermal expansion coefficient with increasing chromium oxide concentration, these researchers doubted that a succesful bond to porcelain could be consistently achieved with existing base metal alloys if chromium oxide is dominant.

Finite element stress analysis of the conical interface design reveals the same level of stress concentrations but slightly lower probability of porcelain tensile failure compared to the pull-shear or push-shear tests (Fig. 5). The rectangular parallel shear test with concentrated load application at the interface appears to be superior to these tests in both respects. However, a comparison of the effect of residual stress states in these test designs cannot be made at the present time.

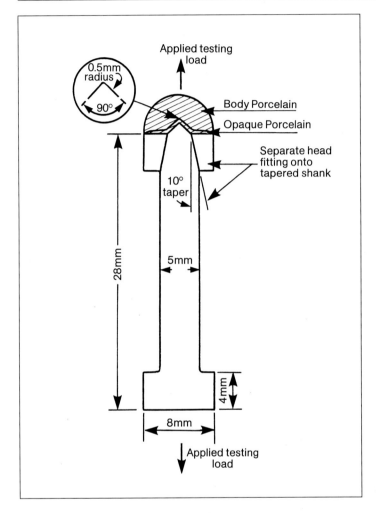

Fig. 9 Conical interface shear test.

Tension-Shear Test

In 1977, the tension-shear test was introduced by *Wight* et al. A schematic illustration of the test design is shown in Figure 10. This represents a modification of ASTM Test D 2295-72. Optimum bond strength between Ticon (Ticonium Co.), a Ni–Cr–Be alloy, and Vita porcelain resulted when the alloy was preoxidized with no hold time or when a higher firing temperature for opaque porcelain was employed.

Oblique-Shear Test

The test design shown in Figure 11 represents the most ideal test from a stress analysis point of view. A very uniform shear stress distribution develops with negligible stress concentration effects at the end points (Fig. 12). This test was

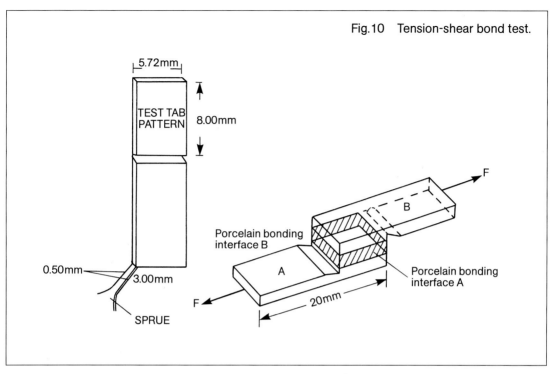

Fig.10 Tension-shear bond test.

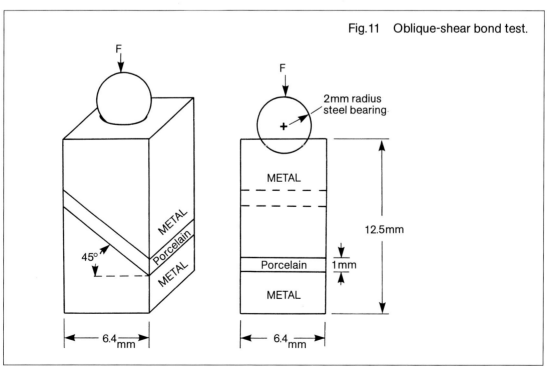

Fig.11 Oblique-shear bond test.

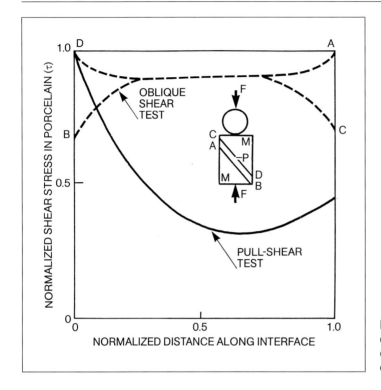

Fig. 12 Normalized shear stress distribution in porcelain along porcelain-metal interface in the oblique-shear bond test.

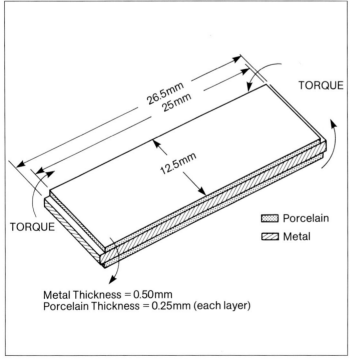

Fig. 13 Torsion bond test.

developed by *Anusavice* and *Fairhurst* in 1977. Tests with base metal alloys and Ceramco porcelain revealed consistent shear strength values in excess of 137.9 MPa (20,000 psi). However, examination of the failed interface region revealed that plastic deformation of the alloy surface frequently occurs. This results from the inability of one or both of the metal blocks to move freely in a lateral direction as fracture is initiated along the porcelain-metal interface. Unless this difficulty can be overcome, this test may lead to erroneous bond strength data.

Torsion Tests

In 1975, *Carter* (1975) proposed the torsion test represented schematically in Figure 13. A later study by *Carter* et al. (1979) using this test design revealed that, for a base metal alloy (Wiron S), sandblasting the alloy surface before porcelain application improves adherence of porcelain. Poor adherence resulted from removal of the preoxidized surface layer prior to enamelling.

Unfortunately, this test design is too complex for two-dimensional finite element stress analysis. Specimen preparation procedures and calculations of stress distributions are also fairly complex. Therefore, this test is not recommended for general bond strength evaluation.

Evaluation of Metal-Porcelain Compatibility

The term "compatibility" refers to the ability of a metal and contiguous porcelain to undergo a series of thermal expansion and contraction cycles without the generation of sufficient transient or residual stress to cause checking of the porcelain structure or deformation of the substrate metal. Some manufacturers refer to the "matched" thermal expansion coefficients of a compatible system, yet it is highly unlikely that the thermal expansion and contraction behavior of metal and porcelain will precisely coincide between the porcelain set point temperature and room temperature. Compatibility of a clinical porcelain-metal prosthesis, of course, involves not only the thermal expansion and contraction behavior of the separate components but also the restoration design, porcelain tensile strength, porcelain to metal thickness ratio, heating and cooling rates, the degree of porcelain maturation, thermal conductivity and diffusivity of the component structure, and the porcelain set point temperature or glass transition temperature.

How then can one determine with a certain degree of reliability the potential thermal compatibility of candidate porcelain-metal systems? Obviously, one cannot expect to achieve 100% compatibility, even with a nearly ideal system. Dental laboratory technicians frequently report checking of porcelain veneers in systems that have demonstrated a high degree of clinical performance over many years of service. This situation occurs because PFM restorations entail a wide range of specimen geometries and widely variable heating and cooling histories, which result in occasional catastrophic expansion and contraction differentials between the porcelain veneer and the metal substrate. Another common cause of porcelain checking in "compatible systems" is the underfiring of opaque porcelain.

An alloy should exhibit a slightly greater degree of thermal contraction than the porcelain superstructure so that upon cooling the porcelain sustains a small residual compressive stress. How can this occur if a massive pontic with full porcelain coverage is not able to cool as rapidly as the overlying porcelain structure? Can one ensure that a relatively compatible system will not experience high transient or residual tensile stresses in porcelain when non-uniform porcelain thickness is required to achieve optimum esthetics or anatomic contours? Obviously one system cannot survive the extreme range of geometry variations experienced routinely in laboratory practice. However, perhaps a 95% success rate in achieving compatibility in routine laboratory operations may be considered adequate. In any event, one should be specific with respect to transient stress compatibility, residual stress compatibility, or thermal shock compatibility. The latter refers to the relative ability of a porcelain-metal system to endure extremes in heating or cooling rates without the generation of excessively high transient stresses.

The best measure of compatibility would be to characterize the behavior of numerous crowns and bridges of representative designs subjected to extreme variations in thermal treatment. This approach would be time-consuming, inefficient, and costly. Alternative approaches are to predict the potential degree of compatibility through the development of a theory for the stress distribution that develops within a porcelain structure and to conduct laboratory evaluation of specimens designed to measure the effects of thermal contraction differentials. The theoretical analyses would then be confirmed by correlation of the predicted stress states with experimental measurements of compatibility performance. Experimental tests may entail the measurements of the degree of opening or closure of a split metal ring, determination of the resistance of systems to thermal shock conditions, evaluation of the flexure of a bimaterial strip, or the use of birefringence techniques. In this chapter, several of these experimental methods will be discussed.

One of the prerequisites for an ideal screening test is simplicity of specimen preparation and testing. Preparation of specimens and analysis of data should not require an inordinate period of time. One of the indirect methods of analysis involves the measurement of thermal expansion and contraction data for the separate components and specifying a limit to the difference that may exist between the metal and porcelain expansion or contraction curves between room temperature and some upper temperature limit such as the equivalent set point of the porcelain (*Rekhson,* 1979). Above the

Table 8   "Compatible" Metal-Porcelain Systems

ALLOY*	ALLOY TYPE	Jelenko	Ceramco	Vita-VMK	Biobond	Will-Ceram	Crystar
				PORCELAIN**			
Jelenko "O"	Au-Pt-Pd						
Artisan	Au-Pd-Ag			NR			
Olympia	Au-Pd				NR		NR
Cameogold	Au-Pd-Ag			NR			
Jelstar	Pd-Ag			NR			
Goldstar	Pd-Ag-Au			NR			
Odyssey	Ni-Cr-Be			NR	NR		NR
Genesis	Co-Cr						NR

  * All alloys are produced by J. F. Jelenko & Co.
** Jelenko porcelain is a product of J. F. Jelenko & Co.
    Ceramco porcelain is a product of Ceramco, Inc.
    Vita-VMK porcelain is a product of Vita Zahnfabrik AG.
    Biobond porcelain is a product of Dentsply International Inc.
    Will-Ceram porcelain is a product of Williams Gold Co.
    Crystar porcelain is a product of Shofu Dental Corp.

set point temperature, the stresses within the porcelain are assumed to relax instantaneously. Below this temperature, the porcelain or glass is a perfect elastic solid in which no stress relaxation can occur. Some manufacturers arbitrarily establish a limiting value that may exist between the two expansion or contraction curves at one specific temperature, for example 500° C. In the glass industry, expansion curves of the two materials are superimposed so that they coincide at the set point temperature and the $\Delta L/L_0$ differential at room temperature is evaluated.

None of the existing theories for compatibility in the dental literature have adequately explained the incompatibility of certain porcelain-metal systems. The screening tests to be described offer an alternative approach to this problem.

Dental alloy and porcelain manufacturers frequently provide information on potentially incompatible metal-porcelain systems. For example, in the January, 1982 edition of the Thermotrol Technician (J. F. Jelenko & Co.), a list of compatible metal-porcelain systems and those not recommended (NR) for use were presented (Table 8).

Bimaterial Strip Method

In 1925, *Timoshenko* presented a theory to predict the bending stress σ that results in a bimetallic thermostat strip on cooling. This resultant stress equation may be applied to a metal-ceramic system and is represented by:

$$\sigma = k\Delta\alpha\Delta T$$

where k is a constant representing the geometry and elastic characteristics of the ceramic and metal, $\Delta\alpha$ is the differential in thermal contraction coefficients, and ΔT is the temperature differential of interest. One of the inherent assumptions used is that the coefficient of contraction is not affected by the reaction of the ceramic with the metal substrate or by the formation of an intermediate metal oxide layer during preoxidation.

Tuccillo and *Nielsen* (1972) measured the deflection and radius of curvature change of Ceramco 'O'–Ceramco opaque porcelain strips of varying porcelain-metal thickness ratios. They theorized that the difference between the initial and final curvature was proportional to the interfacial shear stress. Radius of curvature measurements were used to calculate the tangential stress in porcelain as a function of porcelain-composite (P/C) thickness ratio. Compressive stress was produced in porcelain when P/C was less than 0.70. Tensile stress developed in porcelain when P/C ratios fell within the range of 0.55 to 0.70.

Bertolotti (1980) used Biobond C & B base metal alloy strips (60 x 7.8 x 0.508 mm) veneered with Ceramco opaque porcelain to determine the transient interfacial stress as a function of temperature. The experimental conditions were similar to those of *Tuccillo* and *Nielsen* except for orientation of the bimaterial strip in a horizontal position during firing. He related the curvature change during cooling to the change in shear stress between the two materials. The apparent transient bending stress during cooling at 30° C/min. increases sharply at about 600° C, passes through an inflection in the glass transition temperature range to a maximum value at about 400° C, and then decreases gradually to a negligible level at room temperature. This study shows that stress development may occur well above (600° C) the glass transition temperature calculated for a 30° C/min. cooling rate (543° C), and far above the glass transition temperature (507° C) determined at a cooling rate of 3° C/min. The maximum transient stress occurred near 400° C at a cooling rate of 30° C/min. Somewhat higher peak transient stresses may result at cooling rates higher than 30° C/min.

Tsutsumi et al. (1976) determined the residual stress state in KIK gold alloy-Ceramco porcelain plates by progressively etching away the porcelain with 50% HF and monitoring strain changes on the metal surface with strain gauges. The metal plates, 20mm long x 10mm wide x 0.55mm thick, were veneered with a porcelain thickness of 0.96mm or 1.11 mm. For a porcelain-metal thickness ratio of 1.7, a maximum tensile stress results at the porcelain surface and transforms to a compressive stress near the porcelain-metal interface. For a porcelain-metal thickness ratio of 2.0, com-

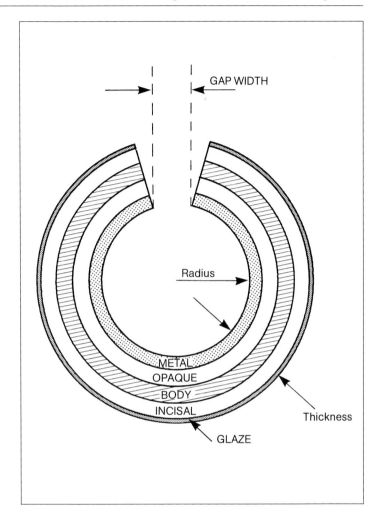

GAP WIDTH

Radius

METAL
OPAQUE
BODY
INCISAL

GLAZE

Thickness

Fig.14   Split ring test design.

pressive stress exists at the outer porcelain surface and near the interface. A tensile stress develops at a distance of 0.3 mm from the outer porcelain surface.

Split Ring Method

The use of a split metal-ceramic ring for determination of incompatibility strain has been used for many years in the porcelain enamel industry. In 1953 *Walton* and *Sweo* reported strains that developed between enamel and iron. They defined the slope of the ring movement vs. temperature curve as the coefficient of strain. This parameter and the no-strain temperature were proposed as guides to the selection of compatible materials.

Whitlock et al. (1980) introduced a porcelain-veneered split metal ring for evaluation of dental alloy-porcelain systems.

393

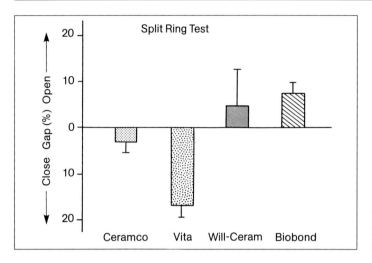

Fig. 15   Gap width change in split ring for four commercial porcelain products.

Metal (Ni–Cr–Be Alloy) rings 20 mm in diameter, 10 mm wide and 1 mm thick with a gap width of about 0.8 mm were ground to a thickness of 0.5 mm. An opaque porcelain layer, 0.67 mm thick, and a body porcelain layer, 1.52 mm thick were applied and fired through the glaze cycle. A schematic illustration of a split ring specimen is shown in Figure 14. The gap width changes for Pentillium alloy (Pentron Corp.) with each of four porcelains are shown in Figure 15. Compared to the gap width of the preoxidized state, the gap width for Pentillium alloy decreased by 2.6 ± 2.5% when veneered with Ceramco porcelain and decreased by 16 ± 2.5% when veneered with Vita porcelain.

Thermal Shock Tests

The dental industry has used thermal shock testing to a limited extent as a means of screening out grossly incompatible metal-porcelain systems. The test procedure usually involves the evaluation of fixed partial dentures with three or more units after single or multiple thermal shock cycles. The single-cycle approach consists of heat soaking the porcelain-veneered bridge at a temperature of 90° C followed by quenching in ice water. After a drying cycle at 90° C, the porcelain is examined for evidence of checking. If no failure is observed, the bridge is heat-soaked at 100° C and quenched again in ice water. This process is continued in increasing increments of 10° C until porcelain cracks are observed using fiber optic transillumination and fluorescent dye penetrant illuminated with an ultraviolet light. The temperature differential to cause failure, ΔT, is used to describe the system's thermal shock resistance.

There is some controversy regarding the usefulness of thermal shock tests. *Buessem*, in 1955, addressed the question of whether the limited usefulness of thermal shock data was of a principal nature or whether this problem was due

Table 9   Thermal Shock Resistance (ΔT) of Porcelain-Metal Systems (Anusavice, 1981)

Porcelains	ΔT (° C)										
	Alloys										
	J	S	O	CG	WC	CB	NP	JB	NM	G	CY
Biobond	130	114	97	125	129	129	129	114	110	126	110
Will-Ceram	137	143	131	140	134	142	142	136	141	148	137
Neydium	158	140	141	149	146	131	142	137	132	142	133
Ceramco	145	153	146	146	140	127	147	145	142	154	146
Vita	170	163	179	169	157	164	173	164	176	181	173

J	=	Jelenko "O" (J.F. Jelenko & Co.)
S	=	SMG–3 (J.M. Ney Co.)
O	=	Olympia (J.F. Jelenko & Co.)
CG	=	Cameogold (J.F. Jelenko & Co.)
WC	=	Will-Ceram W–1 (Williams Gold)

CB	=	Biobond C & B (Dentsply Int'l)
NP	=	Microbond N/P^2 (Howmedica, Inc.)
JB	=	Jelbon (J.F. Jelenko & Co.)
G	=	Gemini II (Kerr Mfg. Co.)
CY	=	Ceramalloy (Ceramco, Inc.)

to the use of inadequate test methods. He theorized that the prediction of performance consists of the evaluation of the performance index, P, which is defined as the ratio of the maximum stress during thermal shock to the strength of the material of interest. *Buessem* claimed that the strongest argument against the use of thermal shock tests is the fact that thermal conductivity, *Poisson's* ratio, elastic modulus, thermal conductivity, and thermal expansion coefficient are not constant but are strongly dependent on temperature. He suggested that the lack of useful thermal shock data reflects the fact that thermal shock resistance is not an intrinsic material property.

Anusavice et al. (1981) tested the thermal shock resistance of 55 porcelain-metal systems using a single crown design. All crowns were made using identical wax patterns injection molded in a split-mold assembly. The facial surface of metal, approximately 0.4 mm thick, was veneered with 0.3 mm of opaque porcelain and 1.0 mm of body porcelain. The mean ΔT values for each metal-porcelain system are given in Table 9. A Tukey HSD Multiple Range Test revealed no significant difference ($p \leq 0.05$) between the Olympia-Biobond specimens and alloys of Jelbon, Ceramalloy, Neydium, and SMG-3 with Biobond porcelain. The Olympia-Biobond thermal shock resistance was significantly lower than 50 of the systems studied.

It was found that the effect of porcelain was the most significant determinant of ΔT values although the effects of alloy and alloy-porcelain interaction were also significant. The thermal shock resistance of porcelains decreased in the order, Vita $>$ Ceramco, Neydium and Will–Ceram $>$ Biobond, where Ceramco $>$ Will–Ceram.

In another study, *Anusavice* et al. (1982) investigated possible correlations of dilatometry-derived thermal expansion data with these thermal shock ΔT values. The compatibility index (*Ringle* et al., 1978, *Fairhurst* et al., 1981), C_i, was used as a measure of metal-opaque porcelain and opaque porcelain-body porcelain compatibility. Good correlation ($r^2 = 0.900$) was found between dilatometry-derived data and thermal shock ΔT values. It should be emphasized, however, that this correlation does not establish a causal effect. The good correlation is surprising considering that an oversimplified model was used for calculation of C_i values.

One difficulty associated with thermal shock data is related to the uncertainty in determination of the origin of porcelain fracture lines. It is not an easy task to detect fracture lines in opaque porcelain. Visual, nondestructive examination for porcelain checking only reveals the crack lines present in body porcelain. Therefore, it is difficult to determine if the thermal shock-induced transient stress combined with existing residual stress is causing crack propagation primarily in body porcelain, opaque porcelain, or at the metal-opaque, or opaque-body porcelain interfacial areas.

Marginal Distortion Studies

Studies of bimaterial strip flexure and opening or closure of a split metal ring during firing have provided evidence that elastic distortion of metal copings or frameworks may result due to thermal contraction incompatibility. However, a controversy exists over the extent to which porcelain-metal incompatibility may cause localized marginal distortion or generalized distortion of PFM crowns or bridges. Complicating the analysis of incompatibility distortion of long-span bridges is the potential for alloy creep or sag during the porcelain firing cycles. This subject is discussed later in this chapter.

Ando et al., in 1972, reported that the marginal discrepancy change of open-ended castings (with and without a partial porcelain veneer) that were placed on a tapered (1:10) die was greatest after the degassing treatment. Positive shoulder gap dimensional changes of about $100\,\mu m$ and $150\,\mu m$ were observed for Ceramco No. 1 (J.F. Jelenko & Co.) and Ceramic Gold (Shofu Dental Mfg. Co., Ltd.) alloys, respectively. Negative dimensional changes of approximately $100\,\mu m$, $125\,\mu m$, and $150\,\mu m$ resulted in the KIK (Ishifuku Metal Industry Co., Ltd.), Porcelain Gold (Sankin Metal Industry Co. Ltd.), and Ceram 1 (Tokuriki Metal Co.) alloys, respectively. No significant further gap changes occurred due to porcelain firing procedures or a final hardening heat treatment at 550° C for 10 minutes.

Shillingburg et al., in 1973, published the results of facial margin opening changes of four different coping designs that re-

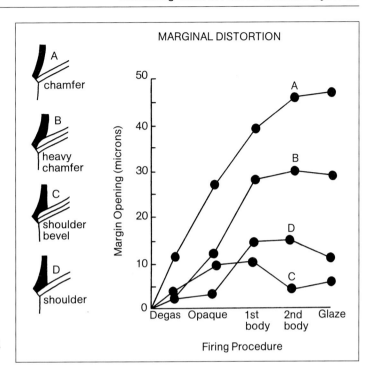

Fig.16 Marginal distortion data of *Shillingburg* et al. (1973).

sulted during each firing cycle. Specimens of Ceramco 165 metal (J. Aderer Inc.) and Ceramco porcelain were fabricated for adaptation to dies with chamfer, chamfer-bevel, shoulder and shoulder-bevel preparations. The marginal openings measured as a function of each firing procedure are shown in Figure 16. In contrast with the results of *Ando* et al. (1972), the greatest marginal opening changes occurred during those stages when porcelain was fired to the copings. All four specimen designs exhibited progressively greater marginal gap changes through the first body porcelain firing cycle. The shoulder preparations, with and without a bevel, were associated with less marginal distortion than either of the two chamfer preparations.

Iwashita et al. (1977) studied the effect of full-coverage and partial veneer designs and variable metal thickness on the marginal discrepancy. A Au–Pt–Pd alloy, Ceramic Gold-Extra Hard (Shofu Mfg. Co.), and Metal-Bond porcelain (Shofu Mfg. Co.) were used in this study. They found that the marginal discrepancy was larger and the corresponding fit was poorer for full porcelain coverage specimens. The largest gap change (187 µm) resulted from a full coverage specimen. Although the degassing procedure contributed to the marginal discrepancy, the effect of the thermal contraction differential between metal and porcelain was also found to be significant.

In a study by *Feichtinger* et al. (1973), marginal distortion changes of up to 64 µm were observed to occur during the metal oxidation treatment but not during the porcelain firing procedure.

Kulmer et al. (1978) published a paper on a technique to minimize dimensional changes that occurred routinely in gold alloy-ceramic crowns during oxidation. To minimize the oxidation cycle dimensional changes, *Kulmer* employed twenty well-fitting, gold alloy crowns reinvested and heat treated at 850° C for 30 minutes. To avoid distortion contributions due to devesting, the investment was dissolved from the crowns using hydrofluoric acid. The greatest dimensional change of any crown following the invested heat treatment procedure was 19.2 μm. No additional changes were observed after a subsequent free oxidation process.

Faucher and *Nichols* (1981) introduced a technique for monitoring marginal changes that occurred during a series of firing procedures. The external surface of the margin was traced and profiled in two dimensions. Profiles were analyzed after preoxidization, opaque, first body-incisal, second body-incisal, and glaze firing procedures. Using Jelenko "O" (J. F. Jelenko & Co., Inc.), a Au–Pt–Pd alloy, and Biobond porcelain (Dentsply International), castings were fabricated for maxillary central incisor dies with chamfer, shoulder and shoulder-bevel preparations. A full porcelain design was used in each case.

In general, there was an increase in the mesiodistal dimensions (Fig. 17) and a decrease in the faciolingual dimensions (Fig. 18). Although most of the distortion occurred during the preoxidation ("de-gassing") cycle, additional dimensional changes occurred during subsequent firing procedures. The chamfer specimens exhibited significantly greater ($p \leq 0.01$) distortion than the shoulder or shoulder-bevel designs. No significant difference was detected between shoulder and shoulder-bevel specimens.

A distortion study of fixed partial dentures was reported by *Bridger* and *Nichols* in 1981. Anterior six-unit bridges with four terminal retainers and two pontics were monitored for three-dimensional changes resulting during the firing cycle and after porcelain deveneering. The alloy and porcelain used were not specified. The largest distortions occurred during the preoxidation (degassing) stage and the glazing cycle. The anterior or pontic region moved anteriorly approximately 50 μm and the most posterior retainers moved toward each other about 27 μm. This overall distortion is expected to result in a marginal distortion of about 150 μm. Vertical distortion was relatively small. When the porcelain was chemically removed, elastic recovery of the framework to the approximate geometry resulting during the preoxidation cycle was observed.

The original oxidation cycle distortion was attributed to the relief of stresses that developed during casting solidification. The larger dimensional change during the glazing cycle compared to the body porcelain firing cycles was explained on the basis of the slower heating and cooling rate for the body porcelain firing cycle possibly contributing to some stress relief during cooling.

Strating et al. (1981) investigated possible

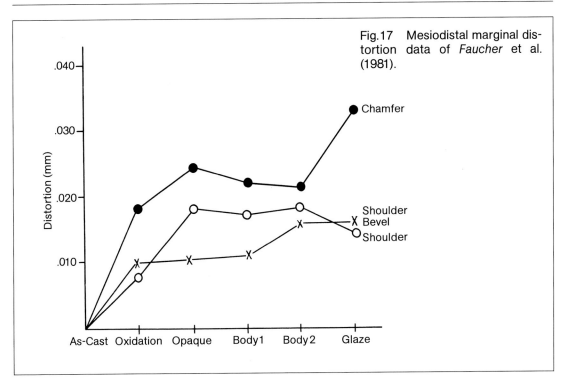

Fig.17 Mesiodistal marginal distortion data of *Faucher* et al. (1981).

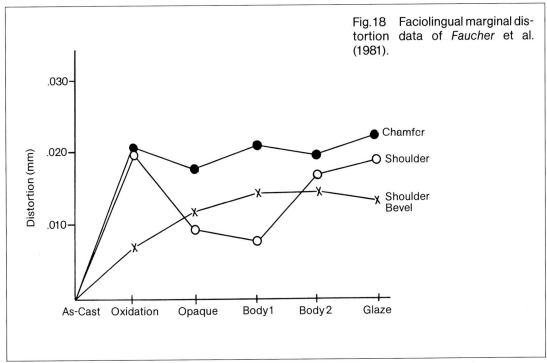

Fig.18 Faciolingual marginal distortion data of *Faucher* et al. (1981).

399

metal distortion of crowns with and without 0.5 mm cervical metal collars, and another group with facially butted porcelain margins. Castings approximately 0.4 mm thick were made using Jelenko "O" (Au–Pt–Pd), Olympia (Au–Pd), and Jelbon (Ni–Cr) alloys. Ceramco porcelain was used in each case. Each crown was cemented with zinc polycarboxylate cement onto the dies used for pattern fabrication and the cement thickness was measured along a mid-sagittal plane at several points along the interface. No significant metal distortion was observed in collarless or collar-type coping designs. No difference was detected among the three alloys with respect to casting fit and metal distortion.

In contrast to the previous study, *Buchanan* et al. (1981) reported greater marginal distortion of the base metal alloy, Jelbon, compared to the Au–Pt–Pd alloy, Jelenko "O", when fired with Dentsply Biobond VF porcelain. The metal conditioning procedure resulted in a marginal opening change of about 70 μm for Jelbon and 7 μm for Jelenko "O". Subsequent firing procedures produced little change from the conditioning cycle. The larger discrepancy for the base metal alloy was explained on the basis of the formation of a layer of oxide on the internal surface of these copings.

Castability of PFM Alloys

The marginal approximation of a cast alloy to the preparation finish line is dependent on alloy castability, mold expansion, casting force, metal-investment contact angle, solidification shrinkage, surface smoothness, and burnishability. Several studies have been made on the evaluation of castability and fit. However, there is no simple screening test for evaluating these variables simultaneously. Most studies evaluate the marginal discrepancy of full crowns or onlays with respect to split dies or one-piece dies. The one-piece dies with cervical chamfer or shoulder do not provide the capability for measurement of oversize castings. Many screening test designs have been developed to evaluate alloy castability. The remainder of this section will concentrate on these studies.

One of the most frequently used castability test specimens is a tapered blade or wedge design such as those used by *Mackert* et al. (1975), *Nielsen* et al. (1977), *Barreto* et al. (1978, 1980), and *Sutow* et al. (1981). The *Barreto* et al. study (1978) revealed that several base metal alloys cast as well as selected noble metal alloys. It was found that the castabilities of Jelenko "O" (Au–Pt–Pd) and Jelbon (Ni–Cr) were essentially equivalent and that these alloys were superior in castability to Cameogold (Au–Pd–Ag), Ceramalloy (Ni–Cr), and Microbond N/P (Ni–Cr). All of these alloys exhibited better castability performance than Microbond N/P. In 1980, *Barreto* et al. reported the order of decreasing castability as SMG–3 (Au–Pt–Pd alloy), Jelbon (Ni–Cr alloy),

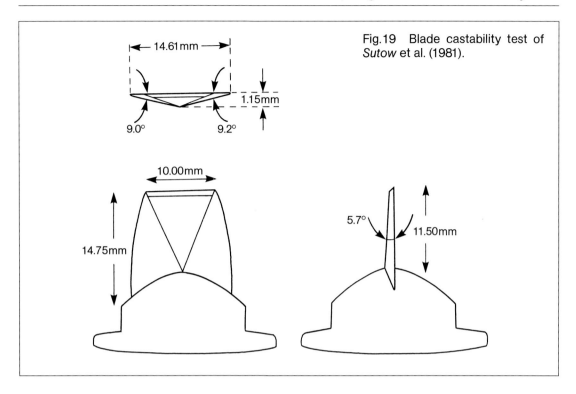

Fig.19 Blade castability test of *Sutow* et al. (1981).

Wiron S (Ni–Cr alloy) and Biobond C & B (Ni–Cr alloy). The brand of casting investment used was found to significantly affect castability values.

The blade pattern of *Sutow* et al. (1981) is shown in Fig.19. This design consists of three major bevels and one secondary bevel on one surface and a flat, non-tapered geometry on the other surface. The pattern was cast as a Co–Cr blade that was subsequently polished through 3 μm alumina abrasive. The blade was removed from the investment three minutes after the loss of gloss stage. A horizontal orientation was employed during the casting procedure. No significant difference was found between a gold alloy (Will–Ceram Y) and eleven base metal alloys.

The best method for simultaneous evaluation of castability and fit is to evaluate the marginal discrepancy of simulated clinical crowns. Duncan (1980) reported that the marginal discrepancy of four Ni–Cr alloys was generally greater than that of a Au–Pt–Pd alloy (Jelenko "O"). Omega and Microbond N/P[2] exhibited marginal discrepancies ranging from 0.25 mm to about 0.70 mm. Ultratek, a Ni–Cr–Be alloy, demonstrated discrepancies ranging from approximately 0.12 mm to 0.33 mm compared to a range of from 0.04 mm to 0.19 mm for Jelenko "O". The relatively poor performance could be due to inadequate mold expansion, poor

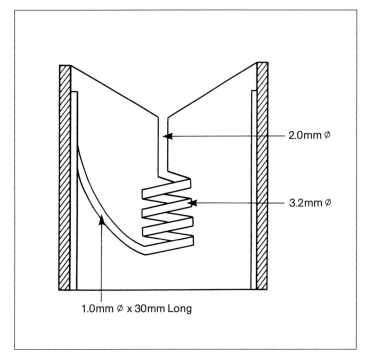

2.0mm Ø

3.2mm Ø

1.0mm Ø x 30mm Long

Fig. 20 Typical spiral castability test design.

castability or a combination of these factors.

Smith et al. (1980) attempted to differentiate between castability factor, a size factor, and the total marginal discrepancy of seven PFM alloys. It was observed that the gold-base alloys, Olympia (Au–Pd) and Will–Ceram Y (Au–Pt–Pd), were superior in castability performance to the Ni–Cr alloys, Biobond C & B, Ceramalloy II, and Microbond N/P[2]. Olympia showed a tendency to cast more complete margins than all alloys except Will–Ceram Y. The base metal alloys Jelbon and Rexillium III seemed to show better castability performance than Microbond N/P[2] but not significantly better than Biobond C & B and Ceramalloy II alloys.

The seating capability of Rexillium III appeared to be better than that of Olympia and Jelbon alloys, but there was little difference between Rexillium III and Ceramalloy II, Microbond N/P[2], Will–Ceram Y, and Biobond C & B. Obviously, these variables are sensitive to changes in investing, burnout, and casting conditions and the rank order of some alloys could change markedly if optimum conditions were selected.

Several studies have used a spiral-type design to measure castability. A typical design such as used by *Daita* (1975) is shown in Figure 20. Although this approach may provide useful information, the wax patterns are rather difficult to duplicate and the coefficient of variation associated with the castability data may be relatively high.

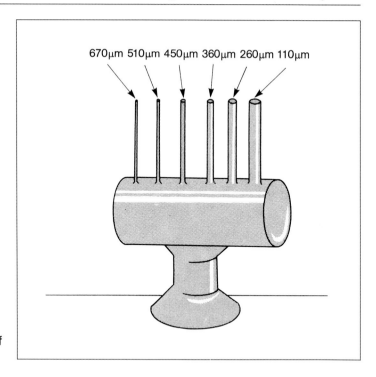

670μm 510μm 450μm 360μm 260μm 110μm

Fig. 21   Fiber castability test of *Vincent* et al. (1977).

One of the difficulties often experienced with the use of base metal alloys is the tight fit of these castings on prepared teeth. This result may be confused with the potential poor castability performance of these alloys. A study by *Eden* et al. (1979) revealed that although undersized base metal castings are routinely experienced when following manufacturers' directions, oversize castings can be produced by employing a modified investing technique and the use of more resilient and thicker ring liners.

In the *Mackert* study (1975), the thickness of the cast replica of an invested (but removed) utility knife blade was measured at the meniscus area. The mean thickness of a Ceramco "O" (Au–Pt–Pd) alloy blade was 49.1±19.1 μm. In decreasing order of castability performance, the blade thickness values were 51.0 ± 29.6 μm (Gemini II), 63.5 ± 37.8 μm (Ultratek), 82.4 ± 33.6 μm (Dentillium), 117.0 ± 54.9 μm (Permabond), and 129.6 ± 49.2 μm (Omega VK).

The simple wedge castability monitor appears to satisfy most of the criteria for an ideal test. However the measurement of blade thickness requires alignment of each blade in mounting resin, subsequent sequential polishing, microscopic measurements, and photography of the blade profiles.

In a search for a simple castability method, *Vincent* et al. (1977) introduced a specimen geometry consisting of a series of six nylon fibers with diameters ranging from 110 μm to 670 μm. A sche-

403

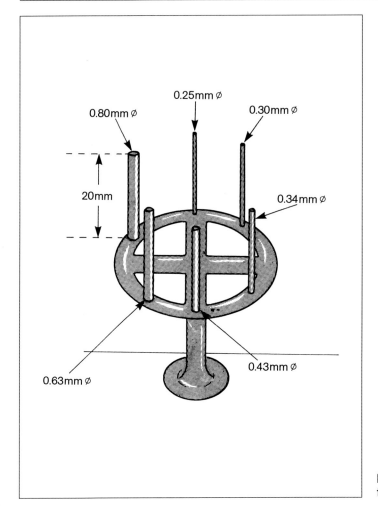

Fig. 22 Filament-ring castability test of *Howard* et al. (1980).

matic illustration of this test design is shown in Figure 21. The lengths of the projections were measured using a microscope. Thermocraft and Degudent Universal, both precious alloys, and Wiron S, a Ni–Cr alloy, exhibited superior casting performance to the base metal alloys Ultratek and Victory.

A modification of the filament design of Vincent was proposed by *Howard* et al. in 1980. Six gauges of nylon fishing line, each approximately 20 mm long, were attached to a ring with four spokes as shown in Fig. 22. A significant disparity was observed between the casting performance of the low gold crown and bridge alloys and the gold-base PFM alloys evaluated. The mean cylinder lengths for the largest diameter (0.40 mm) and the smallest diameter (0.25 mm) cast filaments are summarized in Table 10. The low gold crown and

Table 10 Castability Data of Howard et al. (1980).

Alloy	Manufacturer	Mean Cylinder Length (mm)	
		0.252 mm Dia	0.800 mm Dia
Firmilay	J. F. Jelenko & Co.	9.2± 4.8	20±0
Tiffany	Sterngold, Inc.	18.9± 1.6	20±0
Neycast III	J. M. Ney Co.	11.7± 4.0	20±0
Midas	J. F. Jelenko & Co.	6.7± 2.2	20±0
Stabilor NF	Degussa, Inc.	10.2± 4.5	20±0
Midigold 50	Williams Gold Co.	12.3±10.0	20±0
Galaxy	Sterngold, Inc.	1.5± 0.5	18.5±2.6
Vista	Sterngold, Inc.	1.7± 0.3	7.2±2.9
Eclipse	J. M. Ney Co.	2.3± 0.6	20±0
Olympia	J. F. Jelenko & Co.	1.8± 0.3	18.8±1.6
Deva	Degussa, Inc.	1.7± 0.3	20±0
Will–Ceram W–3	Williams Gold Co.	2.0± 0	16.8±3.6
Cameogold	J. F. Jelenko & Co.	1.8± 0.4	20±0

bridge alloys cast the full 20 mm length of the 0.80 mm diameter filament while only Eclipse (Au–Pd) and Cameogold (Au–Pd–Ag) cast complete filaments among the seven PFM alloys studied.

As the authors of this paper have stated, the potential clinical significance of these data cannot be determined from this study.

A recent study by *Whitlock* et al. (1980) was focused on the percent castability of a mesh screen pattern using fourteen PFM alloys. A schematic illustration of the test pattern is shown in Figure 23. The principal results of this study are summarized in Figure 24. The highest castability percentages (92.0±7.3%) were recorded for Rexillium III (or Pentillium) which are Ni–Cr–Be alloys. Jelenko "O", a Au–Pt–Pd alloy, had a castability value of 74.4 ± 10.3% followed by Ceramalloy I, a Ni–Cr alloy, with a 73.8±5.4% castability

405

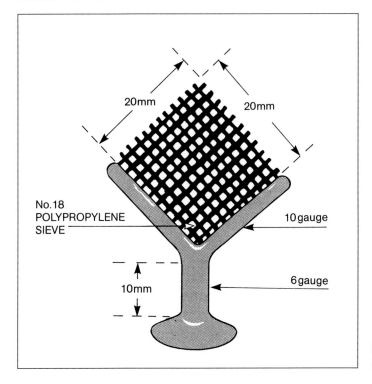

Fig. 23 Castability test of *Whitlock* et al. (1980).

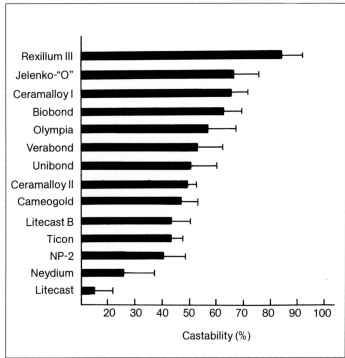

Fig. 24 Castability data of *Whitlock* et al. (1980).

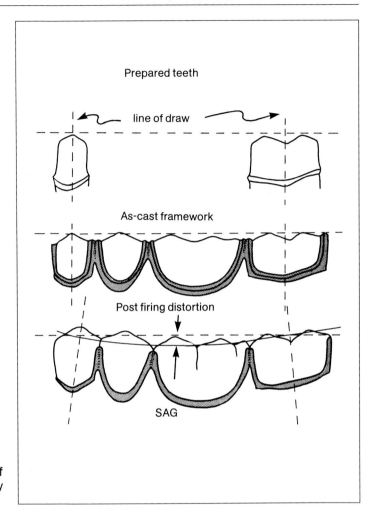

Fig. 25 Schematic illustration of framework distortion due to alloy sag.

value. The lowest castability values were associated with the base metal alloys, Litecast B, Ticon, Microbond N/P^2, Neydium, and Litecast. Additional data by these authors reveal that further improvement in castability may result from the use of the optimum burnout temperature, casting temperature, and casting investment.

Sag Resistance of PFM Alloys

Studies of fixed partial denture distortion that may result from porcelain veneering procedures are complicated by the alloy flexural creep or sag that may occur at elevated temperatures. A schematic illustration of the effect of sag on prosthesis fit is shown in Figure 25. After sag has occurred, the occluso-gingival axes of the retainers are no longer parallel and

407

the casting fit on prepared teeth may become clinically unacceptable. Although the laboratory measurement of the sag rate of PFM alloys is fairly straightforward, clinical cases may also experience significant distortion due to the relief of trapped stresses resulting from the casting process. This effect is analagous to the significant distortion that results in single unit crowns after the preoxidation process. Little data are available on this phenomenon in fixed partial dentures.

Bryant and Nicholls (1979) investigated the three-dimensional distortion changes in simulated bridges during the preoxidation cycle. Each specimen consisted of a 3.4 mm diameter rod with five 6.5 mm diameter x 6.0 mm cylinders distributed along a span of 50 mm. The total deformation of Jelenko "O" alloy specimens with and without solder joints was measured after removal from the furnace chamber. No significant difference was found between specimens with cast connectors or soldered connectors. Although custom-made sagger trays were recommended for support of long-span prostheses, these investigators actually observed a rise of the midpoint of the span when intermediate support was provided.

Bridger and Nicholls (1981) measured the distortion that occurred in six-unit bridges with four terminal retainers. During all firing procedures, the specimens were supported with custom sagger trays. The alloy used was not specified. Specimen distortion occurred primarily during the preoxidation (degassing) and glazing cycles. The net result was usually a narrowing (closure) of the bridges toward the midline and corresponding maximum anterior displacement of the pontic area of the bridges. An elastic recovery of deformation occurred following dissolution of porcelain.

From a clinical point of view, clinicians and laboratory technicians are concerned with the fit of a PFM fixed partial denture after the final glazing cycle. It is apparent that the distortion of metal frameworks may result from one or more of three effects; alloy creep (sag), release of residual as-cast stresses, and the porcelain-metal contraction differential. The combined contribution of these factors to framework distortion is of primary importance but the individual contribution should be investigated to fully characterize each porcelain-metal system. The remainder of this section will focus on investigations of alloy sag resistance.

Moffa et al. in 1973 determined the sag potential of two base metal alloys, Jel-Span and Ultratek, and Ceramco "O", a gold base alloy. After four simulated porcelain firing cycles, no detectable sag deformation was evident in the base metal specimens while the mid-span deflection of the Ceramco "O" alloy was approximately 2.28 mm.

In 1979, Anusavice et al. employed a bending beam viscometer to measure the sag properties of three gold base alloys, a Pd–Ag alloy, and nine base metal alloys. Alloy strips were subjected to midspan load of 60 g at a heating rate of 11° C/min. from room temperature to 1000° C. The initial sag temperature was found to range from 750° C to 843° C for

Table 11   Alloy Sag Data of Bertolotti and Moffa (1980).

Alloy	Alloy Type	Activation Energy (kcal/mole)	Creep Rate 600° C (μm/min.)
SMG–2 (AC)	Au–Pt–Pd	28.4	13.8
SMG–2 (HT)		31.3	6.0
SMG–3 (AC)	Au–Pt–Pd	34.5	9.0
SMG–3 (HT)		34.9	3.9
Eclipse (AC)	Au–Pd	42.0	0.840
Eclipse (HT)		44.4	0.132
Olympia (AC)	Au–Pd	52.5	0.060
Olympia (HT)		56.1	0.051
Jelstar (AC)	Pd–Ag	45.9	1.26
Jelstar (HT)		37.4	0.84

the gold alloys and from 925 to 990° C for the base metal alloys.

Bertolotti and *Moffa* (1980) measured the creep rates of 4 gold base alloys and a Pd–Ag alloy using a bending beam viscometer similar to that used in the Anusavice study. However, an extremely high load was applied to the specimens in this study. The resultant bending stress level was 17.8 times higher than the equivalent stress of the *Anusavice* study. The rationale for this high stress level was the development of residual stress levels of this magnitude during typical porcelain firing cycles. This stress level may be appropriate for sag measurements below 600° C, but would be excessive at higher temperatures because of the stress release that occurs above the porcelain set point temperature.

For sag rate measurements, *Bertolotti* used 16 gauge cylindrical specimens with a span length of 45mm. Measurements were made in the as-cast (AC) condition and a heat-treated (HT) condition. The heat-treated state represented the firing of specimens through preoxidation, opaque, body, and glaze firing cycles. The sag rate data for the five alloys studied are summarized in Table 11.

It is surprising that the sag rate for Eclipse at 600° C in the as-cast state is approximately 14 times greater than that for Olympia. The gold and palladium contents of these alloys are nearly the same. In the heat-treated state the sag rate for Eclipse is only 2.6 times greater. The sag rate ratios (as-cast to heat-treated) for Eclipse and Olympia are about 6.4 and 1.2, respectively. The authors did not provide an explanation for this difference between the two alloys.

Possible phase changes or a modification in the number or location of atomic defects were cited as possible explanations for the improvement between the as-cast versus heat-treated sag rates for each of the alloys studied.

Additional studies are needed to identify the magnitude of sag that occurs under clinically relevant conditions. The differentiation between dimensional changes due to relief of as-cast stresses, sag, and the porcelain-metal contraction differential should be identified so that optimum design and heat-treatment procedures may be recommended to minimize prosthesis distortion.

Summary

The planar shear test represents the most ideal design for measurement of porcelain-metal bond strength. For a practitioner, such a test would not be useful. Several simpler qualitative tests may be used. One of these involves compressing a pair of wire cutter blades perpendicular to a porcelain until fracture occurs. Another approach is to cut a narrow slot through the porcelain just into the metal surface. Place a screwdriver in the slot and twist until porcelain fracture occurs. The alloy fracture surface should then be examined under 10X–20X magnification in areas near the applied force. The absence of uniformly distributed fragments of porcelain or the appearance of a shiny metal surface devoid of metal oxide indicates potentially poor adherence.

A more critical test would involve the use of a highly polished flat metal plate veneered with porcelain. This specimen reduces the effect of porcelain adherence due to mechanical retention. This effect may occasionally occur with some Pd–Ag alloys and certain base metal alloys.

Porcelain-metal compatibility may best be determined by means of thermal expansion data. Although these data have not been generally reliable in predicting incompatibility, comparison of these data with technician reports of clinical case failures provide adequate evidence of the checking potential of various systems.

The thermal shock tests may allow detection of grossly incompatible systems but may not be useful for ranking all systems. Further research is needed to demonstrate the reliability of this approach.

For castability evaluation, the mesh screen test is a convenient approach for predicting optimum casting conditions and performance. Clinicians may also choose to evaluate the castability and fit of full crown patterns with knife-edge margins on silver-plated dies. However, it should be noted that the reproducibility of data is sensitive to technique variables such as burnout temperature, casting temperature, and wax pattern orientation.

In general, research data indicate that

yellow-gold crown and bridge alloys exhibit superior castability to most available types of PFM alloys. Furthermore, lower gold content PFM alloys appear to exhibit inferior casting performance compared to ADA Specification No. 5 gold alloys. These results indicate that more precise control of the variables associated with the casting and fit of PFM alloys compared to conventional non-ceramic Type III gold alloys is indicated to produce clinically acceptable prostheses.

References

Ando, N., Nakamura, K., Maniki, T., Sugata, T., Suzuki, T., and *Moriyama, K.* (1972): Deformation of porcelain bonded gold alloys. J. Japan Soc. Appar. Mat. 13:237.

Anusavice, K. J., Ringle, R. D., and *Weber, R.* (1979): Dynamic measurement of porcelain-fused-to-metal alloy sag resistance. J. Dent. Res. 58A: Abstract No. 686.

Anusavice, K. J., DeHoff, P. H. and *Fairhurst, C. W.* (1980): Comparative evaluation of ceramic-metal bond tests using finite element stress analysis. J. Dent. Res. 58:608.

Anusavice, K. J., Ringle, R. D., Morse, P. K., Fairhurst, C. W. and *King, G. E.* (1981): A thermal shock test for porcelain-metal systems. J. Dent. Res. 60:1686.

Anusavice, K. J., Twiggs, S. W., DeHoff, P. H., and *Fairhurst, C. W.* (1982): Correlation of thermal shock resistance with thermal compatibility data for porcelain-metal systems. J. Dent. Res. 61:419.

Asgar, K., and *Giday, Z.* (1978): Refinement on testing of porcelain to metal bond. J. Dent. Res. 57A: Abstract No. 870.

Barreto, M. T., Mumford, G., and *Goldberg, A. J.* (1978): Castability of high-fusing non-precious alloys for fixed restoration. J. Dent. Res. 57A: Abstract No. 500.

Barreto, M. T., Goldberg, A. J., Nitkin, D. A., and *Mumford, G.* (1980): Effect of investment on casting high-fusing alloys. J. Prosthet. Dent. 44:504.

Bertolotti, R. L., and *Moffa, J. P.* (1980): Creep rate of porcelain-bonding alloys as a function of temperature. J. Dent. Res. 59:2062.

Bertolotti, R. L. (1980): Calculation of interfacial stress in porcelain-fused-to-metal systems. J. Dent. Res. 59:1972.

Bridger, D. V., and *Nicholls, J. I.* (1981): Distortion of ceramometal fixed partial dentures during the firing cycle, J. Prosthet. Dent. 45:507.

Bryant, R. A., and *Nicholls, J. I.* (1979): Measurement of distortions in fixed partial dentures resulting from degassing. J. Prosthet. Dent. 42:515.

Buchanan, W. T., Svare, C. W., and *Turner, K. A.* (1981): The effect of repeated firings and strength on marginal distortion in two ceramometal systems. J. Prosthet. Dent. 45:502.

Buessem, W. R. (1955): Thermal shock testing. J. Am. Ceram. Soc. 38:15.

Caputo, A. A. (1977): A flexural method for evaluation of metal-ceramic bond strengths, J. Dent. Res. 56:1501.

Carpenter, M. A., and *Goodkind, M. S.* (1979): Effect of varying surface texture on bond strength of one semiprecious and nonprecious ceramo-alloy. J. Prosthet. Dent. 42:86.

Carter, J. M. (1975): An investigation into the porcelain enameling of metal surfaces, Thesis, State University of New York at Buffalo.

Carter, J. M., Al-Mudafar, J., and *Sorensen, S. E.* (1979): Adherence of a nickel-chromium alloy and porcelain. J. Prosthet. Dent. 41:167.

Chong, M. P., and *Beech, D. R.* (1980): A simple shear test to evaluate the bond strength of ceramic fused to metal, Austral. Dent. J. 25:357.

Civjan, S., Huget, E. F., De Simon, L. B., and *Reisinger, P. J.* (1974): Determination of apparent bond strength of alloy-porcelain systems. J. Dent. Res. 53 Special Issue: Abstract No. 742.

Daita, K. (1978): Castabilities with various kinds of dental alloys and investments. Dissertation, Osaka University, Osaka, Japan.

DeHoff, P. H., Anusavice, K. J., and Hathcock, P. W. (1980): Evaluation of four point flexure test as a measure of metal-ceramic bond strength, J. Dent. Res. 59 B: Abstract No. 34.

Duncan, J. D. (1980): Casting accuracy of nickel-chromium alloy: Marginal discrepancies. J. Dent. Res. 59:1164.

Eden, G. T., Franklin, O. M., Powell, J. M., Okta, Y., and Dickson, G. (1979): Fit of porcelain-fused-to-metal crown and bridge castings. J. Dent. Res. 58:2360.

Fairhurst, C. W., Anusavice, K. J., Ringle, R. D., and Twiggs, S. W. (1981): Porcelain-metal thermal compatibility. J. Dent. Res. 60:815.

Feichtinger, C., Gausch, K., and Kulmer, S. (1973): Über das Randschlußverhalten bei der Fertigung von Metallkeramikkronen. Oestr, Z. Stomat. 70:430.

Faucher, R. R., and Nicholls, J. I. (1981): Distortion related to margin design in porcelain-fused-to-metal restorations. J. Prosthet. Dent. 43:149.

Hatfield, R. S. (1977): An analysis of stresses from four point loading of metal reinforced dental porcelain. Thesis, UCLA School of Engineering, Los Angeles, CA.

Howard, W. S., Newman, S. M., and Nunez, L. J. (1980): Castability of low gold content alloys. J. Dent. Res. 59:824.

Iwashita, H., Kuriki, H., Hasuo, T., Ishikawa, K., Hashimoto, K., Harada, H., Uochi, T., and Hata, Y. (1977): Studies on dimensional accuracy of porcelain fused to precious metal crown. The influence of the porcelain to the metal coping on the porcelain fusing procedure, Shigaku, 65:110.

Johnston, W. M., and O'Brien, W. J. (1980): The shear strength of dental porcelain. J. Dent. Res. 59:1409.

Kawaski, T. (1980): Studies on bonding between Ni alloys and porcelain-Effect of addition of Cr and Co to Ni alloys. Shika Rikogasku Zasshi. 21:86.

Kingery, W. D. (1960): Introduction to Ceramics. New York: John Wiley & Sons, 1960.

Koji, K. (1977): Bond strength between nonprecious metal alloy and porcelain. Part 2. Effects of Mn, Mo, Si, Sn, Ta and Ti on bond strength of 80 Ni–20 Cr Alloy. J. Japan Soc. Dent. Appar. and Mat. 18:217.

Koji, K. (1976): Bond strength between nonprecious metal alloy and porcelain. Part 1. Bond strength with press condensing method. J. Japan Soc. Dent. Appar. and Mat. 17:112.

Kulmer, S., Feichtinger, C., Gaisch, K., and Sattler, C. O. (1978): Dimensionsänderung der Kronendurchmesser von Metallkeramikkronen waknend des oxydglukens. Oestr. Z. Stomat 75:408.

Lavine, M. H., and Custer, R. (1966): Variables affecting the strength of bond between porcelain and gold. J. Dent. Res. 45:32.

Lubovich, R. P., and Goodkind, R. J. (1977): Bond strength studies of precious, semiprecious and nonprecious ceramic-metal alloys with two porcelains. J. Prosthet. Dent. 37:288.

Mackert, J. R., Moffa, J. P., Lew, P., and Jendresen, M. D. (1975): A castability test for dental alloys. J. Dent. Res. 54 A: Abstract No. 355.

Mackert, J. R., Jr., Anusavice, K. J., Ringle, R. D., and Fairhurst, C. W. (1976): A flexure-shear test for porcelain-fused-to-metal bonding. J. Dent. Res. 55 B: Abstract No. 698.

Malhotra, M. L., and Maickel, L. G. (1980): Shear bond strength of porcelain-fused-to-alloys of varying noble metal contents. J. Prosthet. Dent. 44:405.

McLean, J. W., and Sced, I. R. (1973): Bonding of dental porcelain to metal. I. The gold/porcelain bond. Trans. Brit. Ceram. Soc. 72:229.

McLean, J. W., and Sced, I. R. (1973): Bonding of dental porcelain to metal. II. The base-metal alloy/porcelain bond. Trans. Brit. Ceram. Soc. 72:235.

Moffa, J. P., Lugassy, A. A., Guckes, A. D., and Gettleman, L. (1973): An evaluation of nonprecious alloys for use with porcelain veneers. Part 1. Physical Properties. J. Prosthet. Dent. 30:424.

Moffa, J. P. (1977): Physical and mechanical properties of gold and base metal alloys. Alternatives to Gold Alloys in Dentistry, Conference Proceedings, Bethesda, Maryland. U.S. Department of Health, Education, and Welfare, DHEW Publication No. (NIH) 77:1227.

Nally, J. N. (1968): Chemico-physical analysis and mechanical tests of the ceramo-metallic complex. Int. Dent. J. 18:309.

Nielsen, J. P., and Shalita, S. (1977): Margin casting monitor. J. Dent. Res. 56 B: Abstract No. 645.

Rekhson, S. M. (1979): Annealing of glass-to-metal and glass-to-ceramic seals. Part 1. Theory Glass Technology, 20:27.

Ringle, R. D., Weber, R. L., Anusavice, K. J., and Fairhurst, C. W. (1978): Thermal expansion/contraction behavior of dental porcelain-alloy systems. J. Dent. Res. 57 A: Abstract No. 877.

Sced, I. R., and McLean, J. W. (1972): The strength of metal/ceramic bonds with base metals containing chromium. Brit. Dent. J. 132:232.

Schwickerath, H. (1980): Fusion strength of metal ceramics. Deutsche Zahnärztliche Zeitschrift 35:910.

Shell, J. S., and Nielsen, J. P. (1962): Study of the bond between gold alloys and porcelain. J. Dent. Res. 41:1424.

Shillingburg, H. T., Hobo, S., and Fisher, D. W. (1973): Preparation design and margin distortion in porcelain-fused-to-metal restorations. J. Prosthet. Dent. 29:276.

Smith, C.D., Deckman, J., and *Fairhurst, C.W.* (1980): An alloy castability and adaptation test. J. Dent. Res. 59 A: Abstract No. 328.

Strating, H., Pameijer, C.H., and *Gildenhuys, R.R.* (1981): Evaluation of the marginal integrity of ceramo-metal restorations. Part I. J. Prosthet. Dent. 46:59.

Susz, C.P., Meyer, J.M., Stoian, M., and *Sanchez, J.* (1980): Influence des traitements precedant la cusson de la porcelaine sur la resistance de la liaison ceramo-metallique. Rev. Mens, Suisse Oconto-stomatol 90:393.

Sutow, E.J., Jones, D.W., Bannerman, R.A., LLoyd, D.I., and *Haass, D.* (1981): Corrosion resistance and castability of PFM base metal alloys. J. Dent. Res. 60 A: Abstract No. 316.

Timoshenko, D. (1925): Analysis of bimetal thermostats. J. Opt. Soc. Amer. 11:233.

Trifunovic, D.M., von Fraunhofer, J.A., and *Davies, E.H.* (1976): Transverse bond strength of base metal alloy-porcelain systems. Surface Technology 4:485.

Tsutsumi, S., Miyauchi, S., Enomoto, S., Takeuchi, M., and *Yamaga, R.* (1976): Residual stress distribution measurement of porcelain fused to metal. J. Japan Soc. Dent. Mat. and Appar. 32:214.

Tuccillo, J.J., and *Nielsen, J.P.* (1972): Shear stress measurements at a dental porcelain-gold bond interface. J. Dent. Res. 57:626.

Tuccillo, J.J., and *Nielsen, J.P.* (1967): Creep and sag properties of a porcelain-gold alloy. J. Dent. Res. 46:579.

Vincent, P.F., Stevens, L., and *Basfore, K.E.* (1977): A comparison of the casting ability of precious and nonprecious alloys for porcelain veneering. J. Prosthet. Dent. 37:527.

Walton, J.D., Jr., and *Sweo, B.J.* (1953): Determination of strains between enamel and iron by means of split rings. J. Am. Cer. Soc. 36:335.

Weirauch, D.F. (1978): Mechanical adhesion between a vitreous coating and an iron-nickel alloy. Ceramic Bulletin 57:420.

Whitlock, R.P., Tesk, J.A., Parry, E.E., and *Widera, G.E.O.* (1980): A porcelain veneered split metal ring for evaluation of compatibility of dental porcelain-alloy systems. J. Dent. Res. 59 A: Abstract No. 660.

Whitlock, R.P., Hinman, R.W., Eden, G.T., Tesk, J.A., Dickson, G., and *Parry, E.E.* (1981): A practical test to evaluate the castability of dental alloys. J. Dent. Res. 60 A: Abstract No. 374.

Wight, T.A., Baumann, J.C., and *Pelleu, G.B., Jr.* (1976): Variables affecting the strength of the porcelain/non-precious alloy bond. J. Dent. Res. 59:608.

Yurenka, S. (1961): Peel testing of adhesive bonded metal. Symposium on Adhesives for Structural Applications, pp. 15–23.

Porcelain-to-Metal Bonding and Compatibility

Raymond L. Bertolotti

Introduction

The adherence of modern dental porcelains to metal castings has been studied for over twenty-five years. Although a number of theories have been advanced and our understanding has increased, several aspects of bonding and the compatibility have not been resolved. The clinical success of ceramo-metal restorations has relied largely on empirical testing without a complete understanding of the determinants of porcelain-metal compatibility. The term "compatibility" refers to many factors, including thermal expansion and porcelain-to-metal bond strength, which determine the functional and esthetic qualities of the porcelain-bonded-to-metal restorative technique. The purpose of this paper is to review the nature of the porcelain-to-metal bond and the current state of knowledge of materials compatibility.

It is generally recognized that three modes of bonding are applicable to varying degrees in porcelain-bonded-to-metal systems: mechanical interlocking, true chemical bonding, and a variant of true chemical bonding termed *Van der Waals* bonding.

When microscopic irregularities in the metal surface are created and subsequently filled with porcelain, retention of the porcelain veneer by mechanical interlocking is achieved. The fraction of the total porcelain retention provided by this mechanical interlocking may be quite high. However, very strong porcelain-metal bonds can be obtained on highly polished metal surfaces where no mechanical interlocking occurs. In these cases, chemical bonding mechanisms are responsible for the strength of the bond.

Chemical bonding is generally not as well understood as is mechanical interlocking. True chemical bonding results from electron transfer between the oxygen of the glassy phase of porcelain and an oxidized metal surface. Porcelain applied to a nonoxidized metal surface, platinum foil for example, will not exhibit evidence of chemical attachment. The addition of oxidizable elements such as tin, indium, or iron to a noble metal casting alloy

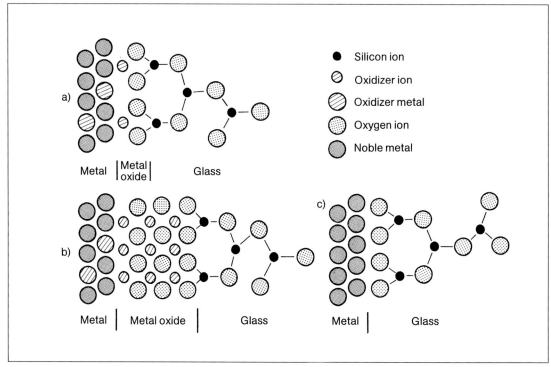

Fig. 1   Schematic illustrations of chemical bonding of glassy porcelain to metal with (a) an ideal mono-molecular oxide layer, (b) a discrete oxide layer, and (c) no oxide layer where only *Van der Waals* forces are present.

creates the potential for oxidization of the alloy and subsequent chemical bonding to the porcelain. In base metal alloys such as nickel-chromium, oxidation of the metal is easily achieved. However, excessive oxidation of these alloys can be a problem, since an excessively thick oxide layer is subject to spalling and fracture.

Van der Waals bonding results from forces of attraction between polarized atoms in close proximity to each other but without the exchange of electrons seen in true chemical bonding. Such a mechanism does not depend on an oxi-dized metal layer for adhesion; rather, the degree of adhesion observed is related to the ability of viscous porcelain to wet the metal substrate. Generally, *Van der Waals* bonding makes only a minor contribution to the overall bond strength.

Figure 1 schematically illustrates three types of chemical bonding: chemical bonding with an ideal monomolecular oxide layer; chemical bonding with a discrete oxide layer; and *Van der Waals* bonding with no oxide layer.

In reviewing the reported studies of por-celain-metal adherence in dental systems, it appears that adequate bonding of porcelain to metal is nearly always possible, although specialized and carefully controlled techniques are sometimes required. However, there is considerable disagreement as to how the bonding occurs. Much of this confusion results from the complexity of dental restorative materials. Our knowledge is not based on an understanding of simpler model systems, but rather on studies of complex systems that have been developed empirically. Future research directed at a more fundamental understanding of the basic dental materials systems would be most desirable.

This paper will discuss the chemical and physical criteria that must be met to achieve a satisfactory porcelain-to-metal bond. Variables in processing techniques can have a major effect on bonding, and these variables will also be discussed.

Chemical Factors

Chemical Bonding

Our understanding of the chemical nature of the porcelain-to-metal bond has been greatly enhanced by the investigations of *J. A. Pask* and his coworkers (1972; 1977; *Pask* and *Fulrath,* 1962). *Pask's* theory is that chemical bonding occurs when there is a balance of bond energies across the transition zone between glass and metal. The balance of bond energies is achieved by solution of the lowest valent oxide of the metal into the glass so that glass and metal at the interface are saturated with the oxide and a continuous electronic structure exists across the interface. The activity of metal oxide in both metal and glass is then equal to one. To maintain a stable chemical equilibrium, diffusion of dissolved oxide away from the interface must be slower than the rates of oxide formation and solution at the interface.

Many other researchers (*Bhat* and *Manning,* 1973; *King, Tripp,* and *Duckworth,* 1959; *Nedeljkovic,* 1975) have supported *Pask's* theory that chemical bonding occurs between glass or ceramic and metal when thermodynamically equilibrated compositions relative to the lowest valent oxide of the metal exist at the interface. Most of *Pask's* work has been on model systems, such as sodium disilicate glass on unalloyed metal substrates. With complex dental alloys and porcelains, the criteria for chemical bonding have not yet been resolved, but are likely to follow as an extension of *Pask's* theory. Work by *Borom* and *Pask* (1966) suggested that the adherence-promoting oxide in the glass should form a continuous solid solution with the metal substrate In order to maintain necessary equilibrium in the dynamic system. Other workers (*Brennan* and *Pask,* 1973; *Borom, Longwell,* and *Pask,* 1967) demonstrated that alkali oxides present in glass have an effect on metal oxide saturation at the interface. It is well known that different brands of opaque dental porcelain have markedly different effects on the oxidation and interface behavior of dental alloys systems, especially base metal alloys. This subject is presently being investigated.

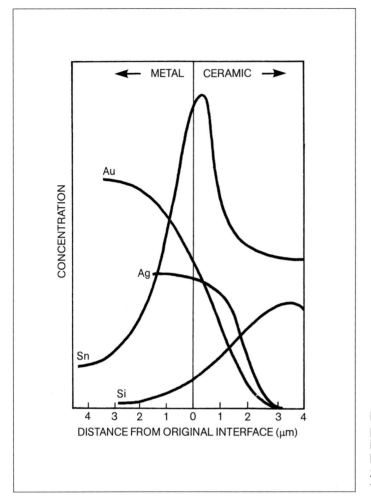

Fig. 2 Elemental concentration profiles across a porcelain-metal interface illustrating the accumulation of Sn within the interaction zone. (From *Anusavice*, et al., 1977).

One early study (*Vickery* and *Badinelli;* 1968) concluded that chemical bonding in a gold-platinum-palladium based alloy takes place by preferential formation of interstitial compounds of trace elements. This concept of localized chemical bonding is open to question because subsequent microprobe analysis (*Lautenschlager, Greener,* and *Elkington,* 1969; *Nally, Monnier,* and *Meyer,* 1968; *von Radnoth, Szantho,* and *Lautenschlager,* 1969) demonstrated a segregation of oxidizers (such as iron and tin) to within a few microns of the porcelain-metal interface. It now appears that an equilibrium of trace metal oxides across the porcelain-metal interface is responsible for chemical bonding in noble metal alloy systems.

Figure 2 shows a representative microprobe line-scan of elemental concentrations across a porcelain-metal interface after firing. Such data strongly support the theory that chemical bonding mechanisms are controlled by the oxidizing elements. Transport of the oxidizing elements to the metal surface is controlled by diffusion during the metal conditioning cycle. Grain boundaries enhance the diffusion rate, but the oxidation rate is limited by the ion diffusivities through the oxide layer. In general, the grain structure of porcelain bonding alloys is not affected by firing of the porcelain.

Anusavice, Horner, and *Fairhurst* (1977) studied the diffusion of elements in dental porcelain-metal couples subjected to a range of metal preoxidation times and porcelain firing times. An accumulation of tin atoms near the interface was noted. The source of these atoms was the opaque porcelain. Tin oxide (SnO_2) was hypothesized to provide the continuity of electronic structure necessary for chemical bonding.

Work reported by *McLean* and *Sced* (1976) revealed an optimal tin thickness for subsequent bonding of porcelain to platinum. Too thin a layer resulted in a weak porcelain bond while a thick layer resulted in fracture within the tin oxide-rich layer. Use of the tin electroplating led to development of the platinum-bonded aluminous porcelain crown.

Further support for the oxide equilibria concept is found in a series of studies of dental porcelain to metal adherence reported by *McLean* and *Sced* (1973a). Their investigations concluded that preoxidation and a rough surface, such as created by sandblasting, produced the best porcelain bond strength to a gold alloy. Pickling in hydrofluoric acid after degassing reduced bond strength. Decrease in bond strength was attributed to the removal of surface oxides, while roughness increased bond strength by increasing the surface area of the bond. The subject of surface roughness will be discussed later, but its effect on bond strength is probably not great in most dental porcelain-bonded-to-metal restorations (*Kelly, Asgar,* and *O'Brien,* 1969).

Pask's theory of bonding is further supported by observations (*Knap* and *Ryge,* 1966; *Leone* and *Fairhurst,* 1968) that oxidizing atmospheres enhance the porcelain-metal bond strengths. Under conditions promoting oxidation, even pure gold bonds to glass, although adherence is not obtained in a vacuum, in nitrogen, in water vapor, or after exposure to carbon (*Tso* and *Pask,* 1979).

The contribution of *Van der Waals* bonding in ceramo-metal systems is not well understood, and much of the reported research on this subject is not in agreement (*Ryge,* 1965; *O'Brien* and *Ryge,* 1965; *Vickery* and *Badinelli,* 1968; *McLean* and *Sced,* 1973). Bonding of the *Van der Waals* type results when wetting occurs but without an equilibrium transition zone at the interface. In general, the contribution of *Van der Waals* bonding in dental systems is thought to be relatively small. The foregoing discussion concerned noble metal alloy-porcelain bonding, but the same principles apply to non-noble or base metal alloy systems, of which nickel-chromium is the most familiar. Compared to noble metal systems research, the dental literature on base metals is relatively limited.

Because base metals are all easily oxidized, small alloying additions are made to control oxidation rather than to promote it, as in noble metal alloys. Chromium is added (usually about 20 %) to nickel-based alloys to protect against tarnish and corrosion by a phenomenon known as *passivation. Passivation* refers to the formation of a thin, tenacious, and impervious oxide that forms a barrier to further oxidation. At high temperatures, however, chromium oxide tends to form a thick, weak layer of a dark green oxide. Various alloying additions are made to control this oxidation behavior, the most common being beryllium, aluminium, niobium, and manganese. Beryllium is the most effective addition in controlling oxidation. Only about one- to two-weight percent is required to achieve a protective beryllium oxide layer, which inhibits excessive chromium oxide formation. While the remaining elements are not as toxic as beryllium, they are generally less effective in controlling oxidation. A number of other trace elements, such as silicon and zirconium, significantly improve adherence of the oxide to metal (*Lustman,* 1950) as do the rare earth metals (*Stringer, Wilcox,* and *Jaffee,* 1972).

In one study (*McLean* and *Sced,* 1973b), cobalt-chromium and nickel-chromium based alloys that had been preoxidized before porcelain application developed stronger bonds than those not preoxidized. Under conditions expected to suppress metal oxidation, extensive reaction of the alloy with the porcelain was observed. The study suggested that K_2O, Na_2O, and SnO_2 in the porcelain are reduced by chromium in the alloy, and that chromium oxide (and also nickel oxide) diffuses into the porcelain. The modified porcelain then has a reduced coefficient of thermal expansion and a state of residual stress results at the interface, which weakens adherence. *Moffa, et al.* (1973) took an opposing view, suggesting that residual stresses actually enhance bond strength.

Anusavice, Ringle, and *Fairhurst* (1977) studied interface behavior of commercial nickel-chromium alloys with porcelain and bonding agent systems. A variety of adherence zone products were found whose formation may depend on oxidation-reduction kinetics. The same investigators (*Ringle,* et al. 1979) studied the second phases present in some commercial alloys and recommended suitable techniques for assessing interface reaction zone chemistry. This study again demonstrates a complex reaction zone chemistry dependent on alloy composition.

In summarizing the studies of dental porcelain bonding to dental alloys, nearly all of the studies reviewed can be interpreted as suggesting that strong adherence develops at the porcelain-metal interface when chemical bonding occurs. Almost all of the studies of porcelain-to-metal bonding reported in the dental literature have concerned commercial porcelains and alloys. While these materials are naturally of interest to the dental profession and have immediate clinical relevance, a more basic research is needed on less complex systems. Systematic study of relatively simple systems is necessary to establish the nature of porcelain to metal bonding in order to

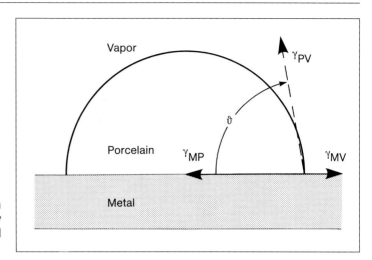

Fig. 3 Schematic diagram of an acute contact angle (ϑ) formed by porcelain drop resting on a solid alloy surface.

better understand dental ceramo-metal materials, especially the base-metal alloys.

Wetting and Spreading

Dental bake-on porcelains are composed of nearly homogeneous alkali aluminosilicate glass with relatively small additions of insoluble oxides, added principally for opaquing. At high temperatures, the glassy phase becomes a viscous liquid and takes part in the bonding process. Wetting of the metal by the viscous liquid depends on lowering the surface energy of the metal by the liquid (*Pask* and *Fulrath*, 1962). From a practical point of view, good wetting is desirable in a dental system to facilitate fabrication procedures. However, wetting alone is not sufficient to ensure a good bond, because wetting can occur with either true chemical bonding or in *Van der Waals* bonding. In the latter case, it may not

result in a good bond. When the contact angle is about 25° or less – attained when surface energy of the solid is reduced by the molten glass by an amount approaching the surface energy – a strong chemical bond usually develops (*Pask,* 1977).

In dental porcelain-metal systems, thermodynamic driving forces result in porcelain wetting an oxidized metal substrate such that an acute contact angle, ϑ, results (Fig. 3). The equilibrium contact angle is determined by horizontal components of equivalent surface tensions, γ, at the periphery of the liquid porcelain, according to *Young's* equation:

$$\gamma_{MV} - \gamma_{MP} = \gamma_{PV} \cos \vartheta$$

Here γ_{MV} is the metal-vapor, γ_{MP} is the metal-porcelain, and γ_{PV} is the porcelain-vapor equivalent surface tension. In the case of an acute contact angle, a smaller contact angle results when the metal surface has been roughened than if the metal is smooth, as described by *Wenzel* (1936). Such a phenomena may explain the increased bond strength with sand-blasted metal surfaces reported by *McLean* and *Sced* (1973a).

Little research has been conducted on wetting in dental porcelain-metal systems. The work of *O'Brian* and *Ryge* (1965) concluded that bond strengths could be explained by wetting and *Van der Waals* forces alone. That conclusion was based on comparisons of bond strength values calculated from work on adhesion and from a *Shell-Nielsen* (1962) bond strength test. Subsequent evidence for chemical bonding, as discussed above, gives reason to question *O'Brian* and *Ryge's* conclusions. The role of *Van der Waals* forces in porcelain-metal bonding remains unsolved, but its contribution is probably small.

Diffusion

Development of a chemical bond between porcelain and metal requires an equilibrium composition only at the interface. Most porcelain and metal in dental restorations are not at equilibrium and therefore diffusion will normally continue at elevated temperatures. Diffusion of metal oxides into porcelain can alter the coefficient of expansion of porcelain (*McLean* and *Sced*, 1973b), which some investigators feel will have an adverse effect on bond strength. The effects of such an altered zone remain controversial, as some investigators feel that it could enhance bond strength (*Moffa*, et al. 1973).

Diffusion of base metal oxides into porcelain can cause color changes in the porcelain. The effects of NiO and Cr_2O_3 from base metal alloys on porcelain color are well known.

With silver-containing alloys, a silver-sodium exchange mechanism is applicable whereby silver in the metal exchanges with sodium in the porcelain under suitable oxidizing conditions (*Shelby* and *Vitko*, 1982). This ion exchange does not occur under reducing conditions. However, once the silver has been transported into the porcelain, reducing conditions are required to precipitate colloidal silver, which is responsible for the yellowish to greenish-yellow color change observed with some porcelains. Different brands of porcelain show different tendencies toward the color changes (*Lacy, Lum,* and *Winters,* 1981). The reasons for the different behaviors of each brand of porcelain is unknown at present, but they are thought to be due to differing alkali and trace element concentrations in the porcelains. These questions are the subject of current research. Some porcelain and alloy manufacturers supply carbon disks that are to be fired in proximity to silver-containing alloys to prevent silver-sodium exchange. The carbon reacts to form carbon monoxide, a reducing atmosphere, in which the silver-sodium ion exchange occurs less rapidly. Reports of success with this technique are mixed.

Coupling Agents

Coupling or bonding agents for dental ceramo-metal systems have been marketed in a variety of forms. These are applied to the metal before the opaque porcelain is applied, sometimes concurrently with the metal conditioning cycle.

One of the earliest coupling agents was a colloidal gold suspension that was applied and fired to the gold point. The coating then diffused into the surface of the gold-platinum-palladium based alloy. The rationale was to "seal" the surface of the casting and provide an easier-to-mask bright gold color to the metal substrate. Resultant porcelain bond strength has been measured by several investigators using a variety of metal and porcelain systems. Results have ranged from no significant strength loss (*Leone* and *Fairhurst,* 1968) to 80% strength loss (*Anthony,* et al., 1970). Such variations are attributable to differences in materials and to the applied thickness and thermal treatment of the gold coupling agent (*Puechner,* 1971). Recently, the use of gold coupling agents has been advocated for palladium-silver alloys to reduce surface activity of the silver and the aforementioned porcelain discoloration that can result.

Another type of coupling agent is a blend of refractory spherical beads and a high-fusing solder suspension (*Kuwata,* 1980). When fired, the solder fuses the beads to the surface of the alloy, providing mechanical retention for the porcelain. While there is no doubt that mechanical retention can enhance porcelain adherence, it is believed that the beads could provide a source for stress concentrations that could lead to easier porcelain cracking.

A third type of coupling agent is a relatively high-fusing opaque porcelain, usually containing adherence-promoting oxides, specifically sold for certain alloys or for alloy/porcelain combinations. For the noble metal alloys, these coupling agents often have a pinkish color, which is purported to cancel color changes due to defects in the opaque porcelain layer. More objective research is needed in order to evaluate the effectiveness of this type of coupling agent.

A fourth group of coupling agents is used for certain base metal alloys. When alloys do not contain significant amounts of aluminum, aluminum is added in a coupling agent, usually with a glass frit, in order to control the chromium oxide color and thickness.

Physical Factors

Surface Roughness

Although it is not necessary for excellent adherence, surface roughness can improve the apparent adherence when the chemical bonding between the porcelain and the metal is relatively weak. A reduction in contact angle occurs as surface roughness increases (*Wenzel,* 1936). There is evidence that surface roughness produced by sandblasting of the metal substrate can provide mechanical interlocking and also increase the surface area for porcelain attachment (*McLean* and *Sced,* 1976; *Lugassy,* 1977).

Increasing surface roughness to an excessive degree can cause a number of problems. Stress concentrations result in decreased fracture resistance of porcelain (*Kelly,* et al., 1969). Additionally, coarse abrasive wheels can cause mechanically deformed metal tags, which act as traps for gases. In the extreme case, a "zipper" effect can result from porcelain bridging across the peaks caused by coarse abrasives.

Considerable success has been obtained with a pressure blast of aluminum oxide (approximately 25 μm) in producing a surface suitable for porcelain application. Residual aluminum oxide does not adversely affect porcelain, and pressure-blast treatment is successful in removing fins of alloy created in the grinding process (*McLean,* 1980). Experience has shown that rubber abrasive wheels also produce good surfaces for receiving porcelain.

If rubber wheels, resin bonded discs, or other sources of organic contaminants are used in the metal finishing process, it is important to thoroughly clean the metal prior to porcelain application. Organics could outgas during the porcelain firing, and they are a barrier to chemical bonding. Acid pickling solutions are generally not effective in removal of organics, but hydrofluoric acid is beneficial in removing residual investment and soldering flux. The most effective cleaning of organics is accomplished using an ammoniated low-residual detergent in an ultrasonic bath followed by ultrasonic rinse in hot distilled water.

Thermal Expansion/Contraction

Failures of porcelain-fused-to-metal res-

torations occur both during fabrication and in the mouth as a result of thermal expansion incompatibility (*Tsutsumi,* et al., 1976). Typical thermal expansion curves are shown in Fig. 4. Near room temperature, the porcelain has a thermal expansion coefficient lower than that of the alloy, as seen from comparison of the slopes of the curves.* With increasing temperatures, the expansion coefficient of the porcelain increases until it equals that of the alloy near 450° C. Near 550° C, the porcelain expansion coefficient increases rather abruptly in the so-called glass transition region. This region corresponds to the transition from glassy state to liquid state behavior. Above the transition region, a relatively high expansion coefficient continues until the apparent softening temperature is reached.

In evaluating thermal compatibility, it is perhaps more relevant to plot contraction curves than expansion curves, because the former are more directly related to the porcelain-fused-to-metal fabrication procedure. At very high temperatures, usually 100° C or more above the glass transition region, porcelain is a viscous liquid incapable of retaining stress (*Bertolotti,* 1980). As the porcelain cools, it increases in viscosity and begins to retain stress induced by thermal contraction mismatch. The temperature range in which stresses begin to be retained is dependent on the porcelain used as well as on a number of processing factors (*Tuccillo* and *Nielsen,* 1968; *Bertolotti* and

---

* The thermal expansion/contraction coefficient is the fractional change in length divided by the incremental change in temperature. Integration of the coefficient with temperature yields the fractional length change.

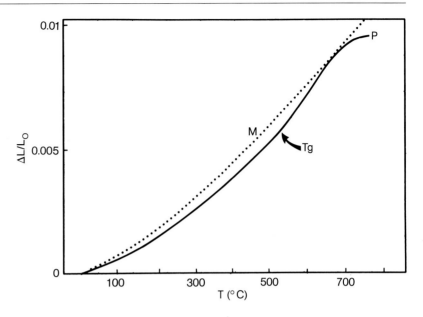

Fig. 4 Typical alloy (M) and porcelain (P) thermal expansion curves. The high temperature behavior of the porcelain is determined by its viscous flow and the plot terminates at the temperature where viscous flow rate equals thermal expansion rate under the conditions of the test. (From *Bertolotti* and *Fukui*, 1981). The approximate glass transition temperature, T_g, is indicated.

Fig. 5 Thermal contraction curves for the porcelain and metal illustrated in Fig. 4. A differential length, ΔL, results at room temperature.

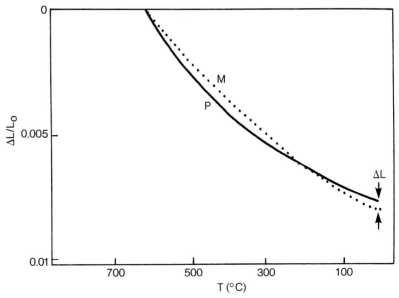

Shelby, 1979; *Bertolotti* and *Fukui,* 1981; *Fairhurst,* et al. 1981 b; *Scherer,* 1982). Figure 5 gives a plot of the thermal contraction curves for the same porcelain and metal for which the expansion data is given in Figure 4. The effective porcelain softening temperature, the temperature at which the plot was begun, was chosen by the method of *Bertolotti* and *Fukui* (1981). The reader will note that the maximum differential contraction (and consequently maximum stress) occurs at about 550° C, and with further cooling the differential is reduced. The differential length at room temperature can result in the porcelain being either in tension or compression, depending on both of the contraction coefficients and on the effective temperature for stress onset during cooling.

The appropriate temperature for beginning the contraction plots has been quite controversial and is the subject of much current research; its importance appears to have been overlooked in the past. Small changes in the upper temperature are critical, because the differential of thermal expansion coefficients are at a maximum in this region. Consequently, errors in the upper temperature limit have a maximal effect on the measured differential thermal contraction, both at room temperature and at intermediate temperatures encountered in processing.

A direct method for measurement of strain in porcelain-fused-to-metal couples has been developed by *Whitlock,* et al. (1980). The method involves observation of a split bimaterial (porcelain/metal) ring. Comparison of the split width of the ring before and after removal of the porcelain gives a direct measure of the residual strain induced by differential thermal expansion. For a single porcelain layer, residual stresses are approximately proportional to strain but an exact description of the stress state is quite complex (*Widera,* et al., 1981). The method has limitations for evaluation of complex multi-layered porcelains bonded to metal because overall strain could conceivably be zero while balancing stresses of substantial magnitude are present in the system.

Extension of *Whitlock's* split bimaterial ring specimen to measurement of strain as a function of temperature (*Bertolotti and Fukui,* 1981) provides a method for assessing stress levels encountered in processing, as well as assessment of the appropriate upper temperature limit in thermal expansion relations (*Fairhurst,* et al., 1981a, 1981b; *Bertolotti,* 1980; *Rekhson,* 1979). The method is analogous to a bimaterial thermostat where small differences in thermal expansion/contraction result in substantial changes in the specimen shape. A typical plot is given in Figure 6, showing the slit width change as a function of temperature for a porcelain/metal bimaterial ring. Above about 600° C (region c), the slit width changes are caused only by thermal contraction of the alloy, the alloy contraction being unaffected by the presence of the softened porcelain. On cooling below 600° C (region b), a rapid increase in slit width is observed to occur as the porcelain increases in viscosity and begins to retain stress. The widening of the slit with decreasing temperature is due to thermal contraction of

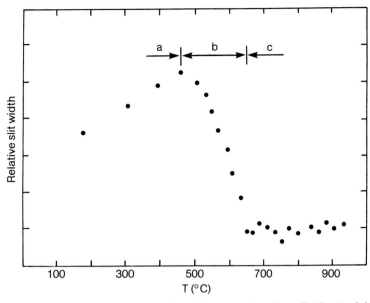

Fig. 6 Slit width as a function of temperature in a slit bimaterial ring cooled at 30° C/minute from 1000° C to room temperature. In region c, the alloy contraction is not affected by the porcelain, in region b the porcelain contraction coefficient exceeds that of the metal, and in region a the porcelain contraction coefficient is less than that of the metal.

the porcelain exceeding that of the alloy. The slit width reaches a maximum near 500° C, corresponding to the maximum differential contraction, and then decreases with further decrease in temperature (region a). The temperature at which the initial deviation of the curve from the metal-only thermal contraction curve occurs is determined by viscosity of the porcelain. As porcelain cools, its viscosity increases and the stress retention capacity increases. Eventually the porcelain becomes so viscous that it behaves like an elastic solid; bimaterial curve is determined by the differences in thermal expansion of the fused materials and is unaffected by stress relief in the porcelain. If one assumes that deviations in slit width from the metal-only behavior are proportional to differential thermal expansions or contractions of the fused materials, then a qualitative estimate of the interfacial stresses developed with temperature change can be made from the bimaterial curve. A quantitative analysis of the stress state in bimaterial rings is quite complex, and is not correctly described by a classic bimaterial thermostat equation. For a discussion of the stress state and deflection in bimaterial rings, the reader is referred to the work of *Tesk*, et al. (1981) and *Widera*, et al. (1980).

Although bimaterial rings and various

427

stress calculation methods (*Ringle,* et al. 1979; *Bertolotti,* 1980; *Whitlock,* et al., 1980) give a basis on which to evaluate thermal expansion/contraction relations in specimens of relatively simple geometry, their applicability to porcelain-fused-to-metal restorations is limited because of the complex geometries and multiple materials involved. As shown by *Rekhson* and *Mazurin* (1977) and *Scherer* (1982), a change in thickness of any one of the materials results in a change in its stiffness, and stiffness affects the rate of stress relaxation in porcelain at elevated temperatures. This explains the widely known fact that glasses of different thermal expansions are required to seal to metal parts of different sizes. Consequently, the writer rejects the widely held concept of "ideal compatibility" for porcelain-fused-to-metal materials, because the varying geometry of restorations precludes attainment of a uniform stress state. Instead, a stress state of acceptable but varying magnitude must be sought. This acceptable state will generally center around zero stress in order that neither large tensile nor compressive residual stresses will be present.

Other Stress Sources

Although considerable attention has been given to thermal expansion as a source of interface stresses, thermal gradients present an additional source of temporary stresses during the baking cycle (*Cascone,* 1979). This writer feels that these stresses, unless caused by an extreme gradient, are generally not as important as are the residual stresses due to thermal expansion/contraction mismatch, since the former occur in a dry environment. It is well documented (for example, *Wiederhorn,* 1972) that vitreous materials are much stronger in a dry condition than after exposure to 100 % humidity. Therefore stresses present during the firing cycle should generally not be as important as are residual stresses that exist under intraoral conditions. However, it should be remembered that thermal gradients can also affect the "effective" thermal expansions of the fused materials (*Cascone,* 1979) and consequently can affect the residual stress in such a manner.

Reduction of processing stresses may be achieved by the use of a coupling layer between the porcelain and metal (*Hausselt,* 1982). Plastic deformation of the bonding agent layer limits the magnitude of interfacial stresses developed at elevated temperatures encountered in processing.

Porosity in the porcelain is another source of increased stress concentration (*Jones* and *Wilson,* 1975). Porosity and its effect on strength of porcelain has been covered elsewhere in this Symposium.

Summary

The clinical success of ceramo-metal restorations depends on the compatibility of bake-on porcelains and casting alloys. However, the determinants of compatibility are largely unresolved; both esthetic and functional factors must be considered. This chapter has reviewed two of the functional factors – porcelain bonding and thermal expansion. The esthetic and additional functional factors are discussed elsewhere in this Symposium.

In reviewing the research on dental ceramo-metal materials, it is apparent that there is considerable disagreement about the nature of the porcelain-metal bond and about the bonding mechanisms applicable to particular porcelain-metal combinations. Nearly all of the reviewed studies can be interpreted to support the chemical bonding theory as the primary mechanism in successful porcelain-metal bonds. Other factors significant in determining the bond strength are surface roughness, oxidation of the metal substrate, and interface reactions.

There is also disagreement as to what constitutes thermal expansion matching of porcelain and metal. It is now clear that thermal expansion/contraction values alone are not sufficient to predict thermal expansion compatibility; equally important are thermal history, geometry, and processing variables.

In marketing of ceramo-metal materials to the dental profession, technology has preceeded science. Materials have evolved largely from empirical testing. Only relatively recently have researchers begun to critically analyze compatibility. Research has been complicated by the choice of commercial alloys and porcelains for study. While these complex materials are naturally of interest to the dental profession, research has been hampered by lack of a fundamental understanding of the principles of bonding and compatibility based on simpler model systems. Correlation of research findings is also complicated by the large number of different materials being studied and used by the dental profession. In one recent survey (CRA, 1980), for example, dentists named 233 different alloys in use for ceramo-metal restorations. Hopefully, future research will be directed toward an understanding of simpler model systems so that the principles established can be applied to the multitude of commercial products of greater complexity.

References

Anthony, D. H., Burnett, A. P., Smith, D. L., and *Brooks, M. S.* (1970): Shear test for measuring bonding in cast gold alloy-porcelain composites. J. Dent. Res. 49: 27.

Anusavice, K. J., Ringle, R. D., and *Fairhurst, C. W.* (1977): Bonding mechanism evidence in a ceramic-nonprecious alloy system. J. Biomed. Mater. Res. 11: 701.

Anusavice, K. J., Horner, J. A., and *Fairhurst, C. W.* (1977): Adherence controlling elements in ceramic-metal systems. I. Precious alloys. J. Dent. Res. 56: 1045.

Bertolotti, R. L., and *Shelby, J. E.* (1979): Viscosity of dental porcelain as a function of temperature. J. Dent. Res. 58: 2001.

Bertolotti, R. L. (1980): Calculation of interfacial stress in porcelain-fused-to-metal systems. J. Dent. Res. 59: 1972.

Bertolotti, R. L., and *Fukui, H.* (1981): Measurement of softening temperatures in dental bake-on porcelains. J. Dent. Res. 61: 480.

Bhat, V. K., and *Manning, C. R.,* Jr. (1973): Systems of Na-Fe-SiO$_2$ glasses and steel: I. Wetting and adherence. J. Am. Cer. Soc. 56: 455.

Borom, M. P., and *Pask, J. A.* (1966): Role of adherence-oxides in the development of chemical bonding at glass-metal interfaces. J. Am. Cer. Soc. 49: 1.

Borom, M. P., Longwell, M. A., and *Pask, J. A.* (1967): Reactions between metallic iron and cobalt oxide-bearing sodium disilicate glass. J. Am. Cer. Soc. 50: 61.

Brennan, J. J., and *Pask, J. A.* (1973): Effect of composition on glass-metal interface reactions and adherence. J. Am. Cer. Soc. 56: 58.

Cascone, P. J. (1979): Effect of thermal properties on porcelain to metal compatibility. IADR Progr. and Abst. 58.

CRA, (1980): Clinical Research Associates Newsletter, Provo, Utah, Vol. 4, May 1980.

Fairhurst, C. W., Hashinger, D. T., and *Twiggs, S. W.* (1981 a): Glass transition temperatures of dental porcelain. J. Dent. Res. 60: 995.

Fairhurst, C. W., Anusavice, K. J., Ringle, R. D. and *Twiggs, S. W.* (1981 b): Porcelain-metal thermal compatibility. J. Dent. Res. 60: 815.

Hausselt, J. H. (1982): Improvement of porcelain-to-metal compatibility by a new bonding agent. IADR Progr. and Abst. 1366.

Jones, D. W., and *Wilson, H. J.* (1975): Porosity in dental ceramics. Brit. Dent. J. 138: 16.

Kelly, M., Asgar, K., and *O'Brien, J. J.* (1969): Tensile strength determination of the interface between porcelain fused to gold. J. Biomed. Mat. Res. 3: 403.

King, B. W., Tripp, H. P., and *Duckworth, W. H.* (1959): Nature of adherence of porcelain enamels to metals. J. Am. Cer. Soc. 42: 504.

Knap, F. J., and *Ryge, G.* (1966): Study of bond strength of dental porcelain fused to metal. J. Dent. Res. 45: 1047.

Kuwata, M. (1980): Theory and practice of ceramo metal restorations, Chicago: Quintessence Publishing Co., Inc.

Lacy, A. M., Lum, L. B., and *Winters, S.* (1981): personal communications, to be published.

Lautenschlager, E. P., Greener, E. H., and *Elkington, W. E.* (1969): Microprobe analysis of gold porcelain bonding. J. Dent. Res. 48: 1206.

Leone, E. F., and *Fairhurst, C. W.* (1968): Bond strength and mechanical properties of dental porcelain enamels. J. Prosthet. Dent. 18: 155.

Lugassy, A. A. (1977): Characterization of surface properties of porcelain-fused-to-metal alloys. Dental Porcelain. The State of the Art. Eds. H. Yamada and P. Grenoble. University S. California. Conference proceedings.

Lustman, B. (1950): The intermittent oxidation of some nickel-chromium base alloys. Trans. AIME 188: 995.

McLean, J. W., and Sced, I. R. (1973a): Bonding of dental porcelain to metal. I. The gold alloy porcelain bond. Trans. and J. Brit. Cer. Soc. 72: 229.

McLean, J. W., and Sced, I. R. (1973b): Bonding of dental porcelain to metals. II. The base-metal alloy/porcelain bond. Trans. and J. Brit. Cer. Soc. 72: 235.

McLean, J. W., and Sced, I. R. (1976): The bonded alumina crown. I. The bonding of platinum to aluminous dental porcelain using tin oxide coatings. Austr. Dent. J. 21: 119.

McLean, J. W. (1980): The Science and Art of Dental Ceramics. Chicago: Quintessence Publishing Co., Inc.

Moffa, J. P., Lugassy, A. A., Guckes, A. D., and Gettleman, L. (1973): An evaluation of nonprecious alloys for use with porcelain veneers. Part I. Physical properties. J. Prosthet. Dent. 30: 424.

Nally, J. N., Monnier, D., and Meyer, J. M. (1968): Distribution topographique de certains éléments de l'aliage et de la porcelaine au riveau de la liaison céramo-métallique. Schweizerische Monatsschrift für Zahnheilkunde. 78: 868.

Nedeljkovic, A. I. (1975): Role of nickel in the adherence of direct-on cover coats. Proc. Porc. Enam. Inst. 36: 15.

O'Brian, W. J., and Ryge, G. (1965): Contact angles of drops of enamels on metals. J. Prosthet. Dent. 15: 1094.

Pask, J. A., and Fulrath, R. M. (1962): Fundamentals of glass to metal bonding: VIII, Nature of wetting and adherence. J. Am. Cer. Soc. 45: 592.

Pask, J. A. (1972): Chemical reactions and adherence at glass-metal interfaces. Proc. Porc. Enam. Inst. 33: 1.

Pask, J. A. (1977): Fundamentals of wetting and bonding between ceramics and metals. Alternatives to gold alloys in dentistry. NIH. Conference Proceedings. Valega, T M. cd.

Puechner, J. (1971): Der Einfluß der Brennertemperatur auf die Haftfestigkeit von zahnärztlichen metallkeramischen Verbindungen, Med. Diss. F.U., Berlin.

Rekhson, S. M. (1979): Annealing of glass-to-metal and glass-to-ceramic seals. Part. I. Theory. Glass Technology 20: 27.

Rekhson, S. M., and Mazurin, O. S. (1977): Stress relaxation in glass and glass to metal seals. Glass Technology 18: 7.

Ringle, R. D., Fairhurst, C. W., and Anusavice, K. J. (1979): Microstructures on non-precious alloys near the porcelain-metal interaction zone. J. Dent. Res. 58: 1987.

Ringle, R. D., Hashinger, D. T., Anusavice, K. J., and Fairhurst, C. W. (1979): Thermal contraction behavior of alloy-opaque porcelain-body porcelain systems. IADR Progr. and Abst. 58.

Ryge, G. (1965): Current American research on porcelain-fused-to-metal restorations. Int. Dent. J. 15: 385.

Scherer, G. W. (1983): Viscoelastic Analysis of the Split Ring Seal. J. Am. Ceram. Soc. 66: 135.

Shelby, J. E. and Vitko, J. (1982): Colloidal Silver Formation at the Surface of Float Glass. J. of Noncrystalline Solids 50: 107.

Shell, J. S. and Nielsen, J. P. (1962): Study of the bond between gold alloys and porcelain. J. Dent. Res. 41: 1424.

Stringer, J., Wilcox, B. A., and Jaffe, R. I. (1972): The high temperature oxidation of nickel–20 wt. % chromium alloys containing dispersed oxide phases. Oxidation of Metals 5: 11.

Tesk, J. A., Hinman, R. W., Whitlock, R. P., Holmes, A., and Parry, E. E. (1981): Temperature dependence of shear viscosity for several dental porcelains. IADR Progr. and Abst. 60.

Tso, S. T., and Pask, J. A. (1979): Wetting and adherence of Naborate glass on gold. J. Am. Cer. Soc. 62: 543.

Tsutsumi, S., Miyauchi, S., Enomoto, S., Takeuchi, M., Yamaga, R. (1976): 日本歯科材料器械学会雑誌 32 巻 4 号 (1976). Residual stress distribution measurement of porcelain fused to metal.

Tuccillo, J. J., and Nielsen, J. P. (1968): Thermal and firing effects in porcelain-metal restorations. IADR Progr. and Abst. 47.

Vickery, R. C., and Badinelli, L. A. (1968): Nature of attachment forces in porcelain-gold systems. J. Dent. Res. 47: 683.

von Radnoth, M. S., Szantho, M., and Lautenschlager, E. P. (1969): Metal surface changes during porcelain firing. J. Dent. Res. 48: 321.

Weiderhorn, S. M. (1972): A chemical interpretation of static fatigue. J. Am. Cer. Soc. 55: 81.

Wenzel, R. N. (1936): Resistance of solid surfaces to wetting by water. Ind. Eng. Chem. 28: 988.

Whitlock, R. P., Tesk, J. A., Parry, E. E., and Widera, G. E. O. (1980): A porcelain veneered split metal ring for evaluation of compatibility of dental porcelain-alloy systems. AADR Progr. and Abst. 59.

Widera, G. E. O., Test, J. A., Whitlock, R. D., Hinman, R. W. and Parry, E. E. (1981): Theoretical/Experimental studies of stress compatibility in porcelain-veneered split metal rings. IADR Progr. and Abst. 60.

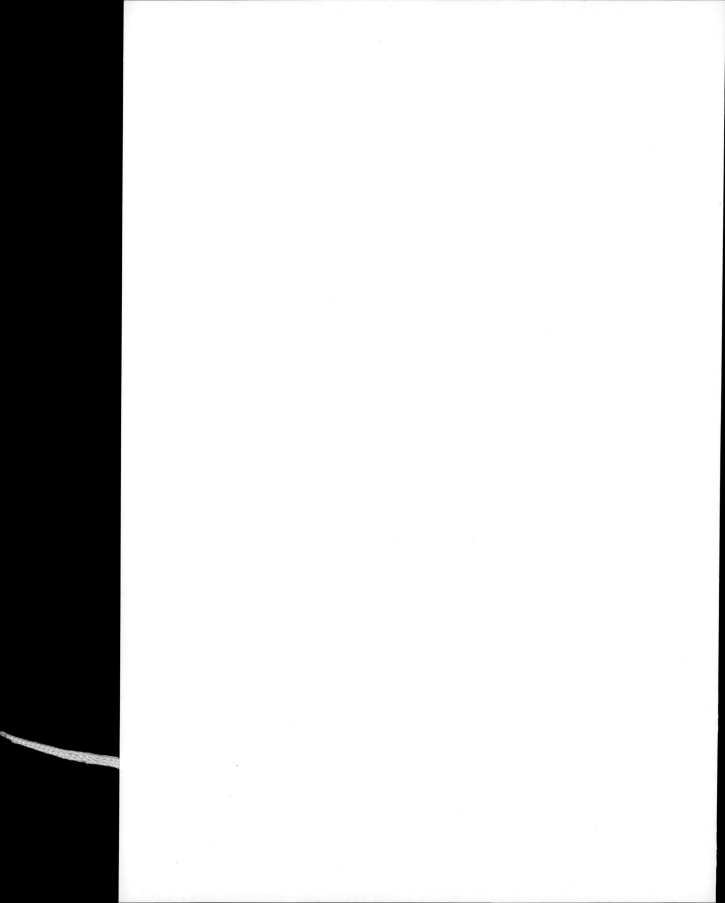

Panel of Experts: Dr. *Kenneth J. Anusavice,* Dr. *Raymond L. Bertolotti,* Dr. *Nikhil Sarkar,* Dr. *Alton M. Lacy,* Mr. *Joseph Tuccillo*

Chairman: Dr. *J. W. McLean*

Participant

Mr. *Tuccillo* mentioned that certain porcelain-metal pairs cannot tolerate slow cooling rates. You mentioned 300 degrees per minute, but yet they can presumably tolerate slow heating rates. Can you elaborate on this?

Mr. Tuccillo

Any stresses that are going to be built up in a porcelain-metal pair will occur on cooling, because porcelain softens when heated. It cannot sustain a stress until it sets as a result of cooling.

Dr. Preston

Is it not true that the addition of zinc to either the metal or the porcelain will eliminate the greening of alloys containing silver?

Dr. Bertolotti

I believe not. One of the currently marketed alloys, a palladium-silver alloy that contains about 4 % zinc, greens porcelain quite nicely. At least in limited concentrations, zinc does not seem to help. Zinc is put in these alloys to increase the thermal expansion coefficient and the casting fluidity. I think some patents limit other metal additions, so that at least some manufacturers put in zinc to achieve a balanced alloy.

Dr. Sarkar

I don't know why anybody would want to put zinc into the metal. I think palladium-silver is the optimum system in this case, and if zinc is added, palladium is replaced. I don't see any justification in using zinc for silver, except to lower the

433

melting point. Silver would also lower the melting point, and this is also undesirable.

Dr. Simmons

With so many alloy systems available, why spend so much time and research to get silver in an alloy? Is it important to have silver in a PFM system?

Mr. Tuccillo

A periodic table shows that there are very few precious metals with which to work. The elements are very limited because certain characteristics are required. The coefficient of expansion, melting point, and many other factors set limits. If you use palladium, its coefficient of expansion is too low to work with the porcelain, so you must raise the coefficient of expansion and lower the melting point. There are very few elements with which you can do this. Silver happens to be a very effective element for the purpose. If palladium is added to an alloy, the more palladium, the higher the melting point. Adding silver lowers the melting point so that the alloy can be manipulated with a gas-oxygen torch. The higher the palladium, the lower the coefficient of expansion. To raise it to match the porcelain, add silver – and you will achieve a very nice metallurgical balance. Very few other elements are suitable. There simply is no choice.

Dr. Bertolotti

In large concentrations, silver causes greening, but a small quantity of silver is present even in the well known gold alloy Jelenko 0, and it is there for very good reason. It balances the melting temperature, the castability, and the thermal-expansion. As a matter of fact, most of the "silver-free" palladium alloys would be improved by 2–5% silver, but then obviously they could not be marketed as "silver-free" alloys. However, if you want to cut costs, silver is a good solution because it's cheap, and it will do everything you need. The only problem with it is that it greens most brands of porcelain.

Participant

The point must be made that well over 400 alloys for porcelain bonding are presently available. Class characterization should not and cannot be made. The alloys within the various artificial groupings are very heterogeneous. Each alloy must be evaluated on its own merits, not as a member of a class. I am disappointed that specific parameters for alloy evaluation have not been addressed.

Dr. Anusavice

I think that the problem with classification of alloys sometimes is that they are included in presentations to simplify the selection process for dentists and technicians. We are oversimplifying the wide range of alloys available commercially by going to a simple classification system, for example, five types of alloys. It presents a convenient means of communication between dentists and dental technicians. If we talk about a gold-palladium, no-silver alloy, most of us generally understand. If we talk about a palladium-silver, no-gold type of alloy, we know the range of alloys meant. Others may fall outside of those five classifications, and eventually somebody will have to come up with a more sophisticated classification. No one yet has come up with a universally-acceptable classification system for PFM alloys.

Participant

What solutions would you consider for the problem of pontic checking on long-span bridges? Does the Ceramosonic condenser magnify the problem?

Mr. Tuccillo

I suppose that I would advise you to use metal/porcelain combinations that are recommended. I would not recommend slow cooling. When the porcelain firing temperature is reached with two materials that are recommended for use together, take the material out and let it cool on a bench naturally. As to your second question, I cannot answer that. I just don't know whether the Ceramosonic condenser helps.

Dr. Anusavice

Obviously, if we had complete porcelain coverage, most alloys would not be able to cool rapidly enough to avoid the build up of high tensile stress in porcelain. The best approach, at least superficially, would be to use as much metal cooling area on a pontic as you possibly could without sacrificing anything else. Some technicians empirically use cooling fins on pontics. They cast with fins, and during the porcelain firing procedure they remain on the pontic until after the final glaze operation, when they are cut off. This seems to work in some hands. It minimizes checking in pontics.

Dr. Bertolotti

Dr. *Anusavice's* work has shown conclusively that the little bit of metal showing in metal copings, for example in pontics, will increase the cooling rate of the metal sufficiently to avoid high internal stress. Cascone's work has shown the same thing.

The Ceramosonic condenser probably does not have anything at all to do with thermal cracks or checking. However, when a Ceramosonic condenser is used with certain porcelains, overcondensation of the porcelain may occur, which does not allow the steam and gases to escape, so a crack can arise from this totally different source. It depends on the porcelain being used and the ultrasonic amplitude as well.

Participant

Did you control ring position (leading/trailing edge) in your castability test? Did you vary other factors (burn-out time, temperature, casting temperature, investment, etc.)? Have you pursued the effect of argon atmosphere on physical properties? The advent of vacuum casting, argon atmosphere, argon pressure-assisted gravity feed casting using an induction heating (Shofu) system seems to be a great improvement over traditional casting methods.

Dr. Anusavice

In our studies with the polystyrene sieve screen, we controlled the location of the pattern from the end of the casting ring. Our pattern was a little asymmetrical compared to that proposed by the National Bureau of Standards group. We therefore oriented those in the same position and the patterns were placed in the vertical plane in the casting arm before casting. We have looked very briefly at the effect of argon gas on castability success with some base metal alloys about four or five years ago, and under those conditions we did not find a great benefit. However, with some of the pressure-assisted casting techniques that are now available, we think that there is a great benefit in using pressure-assisted casting to increase the castability performance of alloys. I have seen specimens of mesh screen that were cast with alloys such as Rexillium III using air-assisted casting that never could be completed to the same extent with conventional casting, procedures with or without an argon atmosphere. Thus, there are some definite improvements in new casting machines. We just don't have enough information presently to make any direct recommendations.

Probably the most inaccurate part of this whole castability process is the use of the induction casting machine. The precise casting temperature is not easy to determine. We have an optical pyrometer that determines the so-called casting temperature by emission of light from the heated ingots. Depending upon the size of the mass that the pyrometer is viewing, for example, either one ingot or a large area of metal, the indicated casting temperature will vary. The pyrometer may be calibrated to a known casting temperature and a known emissivity value for a given alloy. If you are using a nickel-chromium alloy with 75% nickel or one with 70%, there may be a difference. There is also a difference in emissivity values between oxidized and nonoxidized alloy ingots that will also affect the casting temperature.

Participant

Which automatic porcelain ovens cool too slowly?

Mr. Tuccillo

Any furnace that has a controlled cooling cycle does not permit removal of the restoration. The critical cooling occurs in the first 10–15 seconds, and if the restoration is not removed so that its cooling rate is down to about 500° F/min, problems may arise.

Prof. McLean—written question

Is bubbling of porcelain caused by thermal incompatibility or surface contaminants?

Participant

It results from surface contamination, usually the volatilization of organics.

Mr. Tuccillo

It also could be caused by surface porosity. Surface porosity generally is a round bubble with a very small opening. When porcelain Is fired on top of that, it bridges over, and inside that hole is air. As you heat it, the air expands and it rises into the porcelain, so you can get bubbling that way as well. This is one of the reasons that Britecoat was originally introduced: to seal off porosity.

Prof. McLean

If you are glazing at a high temperature under vacuum, you can actually cause bloating of the material.

Dr. Bertolotti

Many technicians want to use some kind of acid to clean the surface of supposedly contaminated metal. Acid does not remove organic matter, and this organic matter is often the source of contamination. This must be burned off, or washed with a surgical detergent, but acid will not eliminate the problem.

Participant

When using a metal conditioner on silver-palladium alloys, how do you prevent silver vapor escaping from the inside of the coping and attacking the porcelain during the firing cycle? Does carbon attack porcelain during firing when used in conjunction with silver-palladium alloys?

Dr. Bertolotti

Unless the carbon is in contact with the porcelain, there is no problem, because the carbon just forms carbon monoxide, which is harmless to the porcelain, and helps to inhibit the silver-sodium exchange process. Vapor transport is not the only problem. Silver is also transported through the opaque, but I don't know the transport mechanism. When porcelain is baked on a silver-free alloy and placed in the same furnace as a porcelain baked on an alloy containing silver, the silver will be transported to contaminate the porcelain on the silver-free alloy, obviously by vapor transport.

Prof. McLean

It interests me that we go through all of these procedures to use high silver content alloys. Ethically I think you should offer the patient the alternative of paying for the actual cost of the metal. My system is that I charge for the crown or bridge plus the metal at cost, thus I avoid the problem of using alloys which are not ideal in relation to discolouration of porcelain.

Dr. Lacy

The problem with that is the patient might opt for nickel-chrome alloys, which are particularly hard. A patient might opt for an occlusally incompatible alloy from economic and not biologic considerations.

Prof. McLean

The alternative I give them is of the optimum alloy that I prefer to use or something cheaper, but specifically correct in that clinical situation. I would never use a nickel-chromium on an occlusal, so they have no opportunity of actually deciding the type of treatment. At the moment, the patient is neither given the choice of metal nor, in fact, charged the proper price for it.

Participant

Please comment on the value, if any, of a heat treatment cycle before the application of opaque on base metals.

Mr. Tuccillo

Follow the manufacturer's recommendation. Some metals, base metals especially, produce a better bond if you oxidize them first and then remove that oxidized surface, because the first time you heat up the metal, one type of oxide forms and the next time, another type forms. The manufacturer's instructions lead to development of the type, amount, or quality of the oxide found to be best in bonding with porcelain.

Dr. Sarkar

Heat treatment might adversely affect the mechanical properties of the material. It might soften some of the base metal alloys and care must be taken.

Dr. Bertolotti

If copings are tried in before the porcelain application, they certainly should be degassed, (degassed is a bad word; heat treated is better) because the base metal alloys do stress relieve at around 1400° F. If you are trying them to assess the fit, they should be stress relieved first, and once you have contaminated them, it is better to heat treat them again before applying the porcelain. Dimensional changes in the second heat treatment are then negligible.

Participant

Based on your current knowledge, is there an optimum pressure and grit size that should be used to abrade the surface of base metal alloys prior to the application of the opaque?

Dr. Anusavice

The manufacturer usually specifies abrasive particles in the range of 50–500 µm and there has been no specific evidence that indicates that 500 µm is better than 50 µm. It has been reported that 500 µm particles did improve adherence of porcelain to base metal alloys, but so did sandblasting with 50 µm abrasive particles. The effect of air pressure has not been evaluated. Creating surface irregularities seems to be the main benefit and bond strength has not been shown to be highly affected by abrasive particle size as long as the porcelain wets the additional surface area.

Dr. Miller

I would like to raise an intense objection to the patient selecting modes of treatment or selecting the materials. I don't want it put on the record that we are going to recommend that the patient select the porcelain, the laboratory, or the metal. I want to provide a professional service, and I want to be completely responsible for it.

Measurement of Colour of Human Teeth

Frank J. J. Clarke

Introduction: Light and Colour

Light is electromagnetic radiation in the optical region that is capable of stimulating the eye; the term covers one octave of the spectrum, the range of wavelengths being 380 nm to 760 nm. When light stimulates the eye, a pattern of physiological activity is aroused, resulting in a perception, which is a pattern of sensations together with any immediately evoked interpretations. The perception is related to the distribution of light in the retinal image in terms of space, time, and spectral power distribution. The corresponding perceptual attributes are, respectively, space sense–such as form, texture and depth, time sense–including flicker and movement, and colour. These attributes are not simply functions of the corresponding physical properties of the stimulus (the field of view). However, it is true that the spatial distributions in the retinal image largely determine the spatial attributes, the time distributions determine the temporal attributes, and the spectral power distributions determine the sensations of colour.

In considering colour only, it will be clear that in order to disregard the other attributes of perception we must refer to some particular region of space and time in the field of view of the observer. The light coming from the region must therefore be treated as coming from a uniform element of area and as constant in respect to time. This is why it is legitimate for the viewing fields of colorimeters, photometers, and spectrophotometers, as well as the samples in colour atlases to be made uniform. They can also be measured or viewed for a significant length of time, in spite of the restriction implied in comparison with everyday viewing conditions. However, when an object, such as a tooth, has an awkward three-dimensional shape, with texture or markings and differences in gloss or size from a comparison standard, then it is not only human observers who have difficulty in colour matching: even photoelectric instruments may not be capable of giving a valid colour specification.

Colour has quantity and quality. The quantity of the causal stimulus is the psychophysical property dealt with in photometry, and is the amount of light involved, for some relative spectral power distribution. The common units used in photometry are the *lumen* for luminous flux, the *candela* for luminous intensity of a small or distant source, the *lux* (lumen per sq m) for illuminance on a surface, and the *candela per sq m* for the luminance or objective brightness of a surface. The perceptual attribute corresponding to luminance is *luminosity* or subjective brightness if the object is a source of light, or *lightness* if the object is not a source of light but a surface colour judged in relationship to its surroundings. In this latter case, the luminance arises from the product of the illuminance and the reflectance, and the lightness is the sensory correlate of the diffuse reflectance of the surface colour for visible radiation.

The quality of colour needs a pair of concepts or variables to describe it. This arises because of the trivariance of normal human colour vision (to be discussed later), but in respect to colour sensation we need only note here that any large collection of variously coloured samples of all possible colours cannot be arranged in a systematically graded manner in a two-dimensional array: three dimensions are needed. One method of dealing with this is to sort out all samples of a given lightness (eliminating luminance as a variable), when it is found that they can always be arranged systematically in a two-dimensional array. Such a two-dimensional arrangement of samples of a given lightness varying only in colour quality will have a neutral grey or white sample somewhere in the middle, and samples of increasing *saturation* (strength of coloration) going radially outwards. The most strongly coloured or least grey samples at the periphery of the array will be found to vary with *hue* as one passes tangentially from sample to sample, going round continuously through the hues of the spectrum: red, orange, yellow, green, cyan, blue and violet; and then, with a gradation of purples not found in the spectrum, going round to the red hue again. The sensory concepts of saturation and hue have psychophysical correlates in *purity* and *dominant wavelength*.

The arrays of samples considered above, one array for each distinct level of lightness, could be placed on stiff cards and assembled with spacers one above another with progressive increase in lightness. The complete set of samples would now exist, set out in three dimensions, to delineate what is called a colour solid or colour space. Such a colour solid could be formed from the same large collection of samples in a different fashion by selecting all nongrey samples of a given hue and arranging these systematically on a vertical card with variations of lightness increasing upwards and variations of saturation increasing outwards. If the grey scale samples are assembled vertically to form a central vertical axis varying from black at the bottom to white at the top, then the cards of samples for each distinct hue can be attached to the gray scale like the leaves of a book to the spine. This second method of arranging all possible colours of samples to make a systematic colour solid has been much more popular than the one described first, and forms the basis of most types of colour atlas.

Colour Atlases

A colour atlas is a systematic arrangement of a large range of coloured samples, usually surface colours, as described above, but with an important additional feature: the colours will have been spaced out regularly according to some stated criterion or requirement. Its basic purposes are to allow a colour to be given a systematic designation in place of a vague and often ambiguous name, and to allow relationships between colours to be assessed. Because of the three-dimensional nature of colour space, all colour atlases consist of a collection of charts that each represent a two-dimensional section through the colour space. The particular colour solid represented by the samples in a colour atlas is a *colour order system*. It is important to realize that the colour gamut that can be covered depends on the glossiness of the samples: the higher the gloss the more saturated or dark a sample can be. Further, the value of an atlas depends on the permanence of its specimens. The number of discriminable surface colours is very high, of the order of ten million. This is due to the fine discrimination possible with colours of the same lightness where the chromatic difference visible to the eye can only just be measured reliably with a modern photoelectric colorimeter.

Practical colour atlases, for reasons of cost, can only contain some hundreds or thousands of samples. It is also desirable that samples of given colour designations in all the copies of a particular atlas should match, even if purchased many years apart. Therefore, the samples in a colour atlas can only provide a skeleton coverage of all possible discriminable colours. The criterion of colour spacing between samples and the uniformity with which the sampling actually follows the required criterion of spacing is important: irregular sampling would make any interpolation between samples quite meaningless. There are three basic ways of spacing the samples in terms of colour difference in a colour atlas: by colorant mixture variations, by additive mixture variations, and by sampling to obtain perceptual uniformity of colour spacing.

Atlases based on Subtractive or Additive Colour Mixture

Colorant mixture spaced atlases have been made to demonstrate the coloration produced by systematic admixture of certain base colorants, for example, using subtractive colour mixture (Plate 1). These are of value to dyers and users of pigments in paint, plastics, printing etc. The Nu-Hue Custom Color System (1946) has 1,000 matte painted cards developed from a white, a black, and six chromatic single-pigment paints. The Colorizer (1947) has 1,322 matte painted chips developed from a white, a grey, a black, and twelve chromatic base paints, as well as 648 "deep tone" chips to

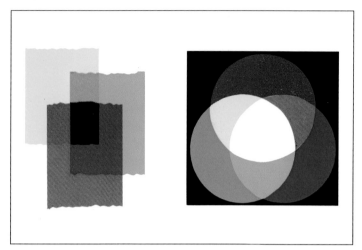

Plate 1   The left hand illustration shows the effects of subtractive colour mixture, with partially overlapping patches printed in the subtractive primary colours: magenta, yellow and cyan. The right hand illustration depicts the additive colour mixture obtained with partially overlapping light patches of some additive primary colours: red, green and blue. Results of subtractive mixture are always darker, whereas results of additive mixture are always lighter.

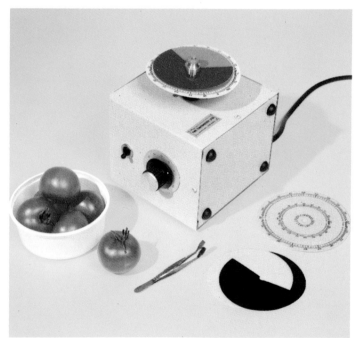

Plate 2   A Maxwell disc, for producing an additive mixture of light from surface colour samples in known proportions. In this case red and orange sectors have been adjusted to match the colour of a tomato.

(From Chamberlin & Chamberlin, 1980).

extend the colour gamut. The Plochere Color System (1948) is another example, with 1,248 matte painted cards.

The Pantone Matching System (1963, revised 1974) uses a white, a black, and eight chromatic base pigments to give 587 samples printed in both a glossy and a matte series. The colour range is extended by 56 additional saturated colours formed by making use of an extra seven saturated base pigments. The system is widely used as an aid to specifying and formulating printed colours. The ICI Colour Atlas (1969) has 1,379 opaque samples made without using black; by means of transparent neutral grey filters used as overlays, various "shades" of each opaque colour can be made, extending the total range to 27,580 surface colours. The ICI Colour Atlas thus gives the closest gradations between neighbouring colours of any atlas, and they are close enough for all commercial dyeing purposes.

Additive colour mixture spaced atlases show the sequences of colours that can be produced by additive colour mixture (Plate 1). This can be achieved by superposition of light or by rapid substitution, as with a Maxwell Disc (a rapidly spinning disc covered with different coloured sectors of varied angle, Plate 2). These are of significance to photographers and artists because they show gradations produced in surface colours by light and shade and other gradations produced by interreflection. The original conception in 1917 was that of *Ostwald* (1931), who devised a colour system with a central grey scale and radial sections containing colours of nearly the same hue. These were produced by additive light mixture, of a given full-colour (from a chromatic base pigment) with the common white and black, Figure 1. Each radial section contains sets of colours of the same white content (isotints), colours of the same black content (isotones) and colours of the same full-colour chromatic content (isochromes).

The original atlases of Ostwald had some defects and are not available for practical use, but in modern times a much better version called the Color Harmony Manual was produced. The first and second additions had 680 chips, but the third edition of the Color Harmony Manual (1948) had additional sections to improve the sampling of colour space, giving a total of 943 chips. Each chip has a matte and a glossy face and can be removed from its pocket in the section-page, and, most importantly, the CIE* colorimetric specifications are available for each face of the chips. Another additive system colour atlas is the Ridgway (1912), which is still in use, though out of print. It has about 1,000 matte painted samples, for which the Munsell renotations (see below) have been published and for which the CIE specifications can therefore be calculated.

There are two notable colour atlases that are partly based on subtractive colour mixture of colorants and partly on additive colour mixture. These are based on screen plate printing colour mixture, and are of particular value to the printing industry. The type of colour mixture is of juxtaposed small dots, normally un-

* Commission Internationale de l'Eclairage.

445

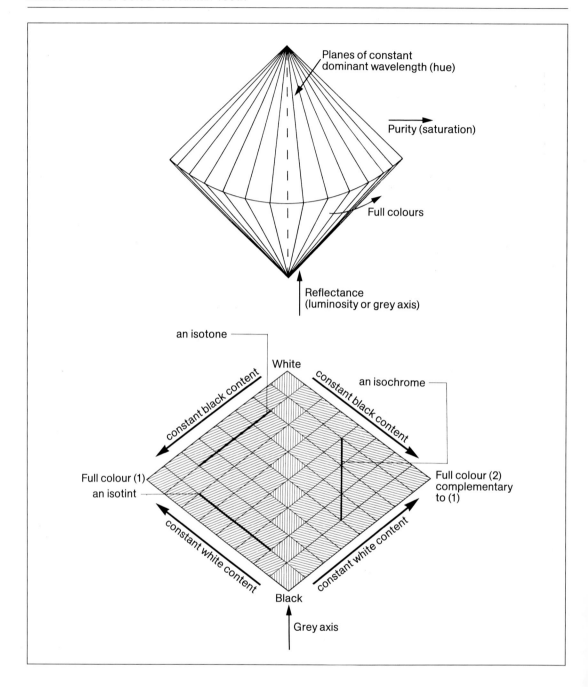

Fig. 1   Construction of the colour solid formed by the Ostwald Colour System. A central grey scale has triangular radial sections surrounding it, each with colours of a given dominant wavelength (and almost the same hue). In each radial section, the upward sloping lines give *isotints* while the downward sloping lines give *isotones*. Vertical lines give *isochromes*.

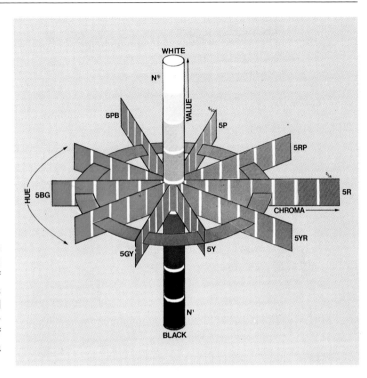

Plate 3 Arrangement of colours in the Munsell System. The central grey scale shows variations of Munsell Value. The radial arms show colours of a given hue and lightness with variations of Munsell Chroma. The ring of colours of a given lightness and chroma shows variations of hue.

resolved by the eye, the gradations of colour being produced by systematic variations in the size of dot in the screening for each of the 4 printing ink colours (3 subtractive primaries, plus black). When the dots are relatively small, they do not overlap and the overall colour effect is predicted by additive colour mixture, but for the deep and dark shades, the dots are large enough to overlap and a certain amount of subtractive colour mixture occurs as well. The Maerz and Paul Dictionary of Color (*Maerz and Paul*, 1948) has 7,056 samples printed on semi-glossy paper, and the Villalobos Colour Atlas (1947) has even more, 7,279 samples with a glossy finish.

Perceptually Uniformly spaced Colour Atlases

The final class of colour atlas is based on grading the colour spacing of the samples to produce subjectively uniform spacing with perceptually equal differences between successive samples in a sequence. Such systems are important in psychological, aesthetic, and design applications. The most famous colour atlas and system of this type is the Munsell. This was originally produced as the Munsell Book of Colour (1929, 1943), using a central vertical grey scale and 40 radial sections, each with colours of a given hue (Plate 3). The three perceptual attributes of lightness, hue, and saturation are represented by scales of value,

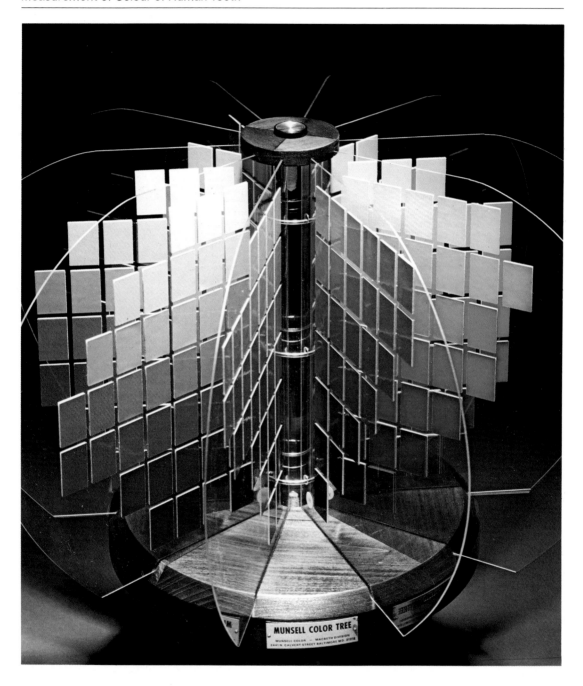

Plate 4   View of colour samples arranged in the Munsell color solid. Colours of a given hue are on separate radial sheets, each with a rectangular array of colours with columns of a given chroma and rows of a given value.

(Courtesy of Munsell Color, Macbeth Division, Kollmorgan Corp.)

hue, and chroma, respectively. Taking any radial vertical section of the Munsell colour solid (Plate 4), we see that the samples are arranged in a rectangular grid with vertical columns of colours of a given hue and chroma (saturation) but varying value (lightness), and horizontal rows of colours of a given hue and value but varying chroma. The Munsell notation of a particular bright yellow sample in the book is 5Y 8/12, that is, hue 5Y, value 8, chroma 12. The original Munsell Book of Colour had 960 matte printed samples, and it was later found that the original work on perceptually uniform colour spacing was not quite as accurate as it could be. Extensive investigations under the aegis of a subcommittee of the Optical Society of America in the 1940s allowed more accurate *Munsell renotations* to be applied to the original samples. Also, these could be converted to CIE colorimetric specifications, and vice versa. Later still, a new Munsell atlas was produced with the colours of the samples slightly adjusted to fit the regular unit intervals of the Munsell renotation system as described by *Davidson, Godlove*, and *Hemmendinger* (1957). The original 960 samples were not only replaced by better-spaced matte and also glossy samples, but the range has been extended in colour gamut and certain regions have included interpolated samples, so that about 1,500 colours are now available.

There is another perceptually uniformly spaced colour atlas and system, the DIN 6164 Colour System (1962), which was produced originally as tinted transparent gelatine filters in arrays, with surface colour versions becoming available later. In the DIN 6164 System there are three variables: farbton (hue) T, sättigung (saturation) S and dunkelstufe (darkness) D. As with the Munsell system, the hues of the DIN system are perceptually uniformly spaced round the complete gamut of hues. The scales of sättigung S and dunkelstufe D are defined by colorimetric rules, which are supposed to lead to a perceptually uniform spacing of these quantities. The line of samples of constant saturation S and hue T, but with varying darkness D, radiates from a blackpoint at the bottom of the DIN colour solid, but on the rectangular grid sectional charts of the DIN colour atlas, these samples lie in vertical columns. The DIN 6164 colours have been specified in terms of the Munsell and CIE colorimetric systems.

A very recent colour atlas, the Natural Colour System, described by *Hård* (1970), uses perceptual judgment to subdivide colour space in terms of hue, saturation, and blackness, with samples of a given hue being arranged in a triangular array with lines of equal saturation and equal blackness samples. A major defect is that the number of hue steps between the perceptually "pure" red, yellow, green, and blue hues was forced to be equal (implying that these particular hues must be arranged at 90° to each other in the space), with the result that sizes of unit steps are not equal in the four quadrants of the circle of hues.

Apart from the specific areas of interest and applications mentioned with each of the three classes of colour atlas and colour order system described above, there is a further use for a good colour atlas: it can be used for colour measurement and specification by visual comparison with the object in question. For this to be reliable and reasonably accurate, the samples of the colour atlas must be uniformly graded according to some relevant criterion, to allow interpolation. They must be spaced closely enough for only a very few just-noticeable steps to separate neighbouring samples, the samples should have known CIE colorimetric specifications in order to relate to physical colorimetry (discussed later), and they should be durable and permanent in colour.

In dentistry, the principle of colour matching and measurement by reference to a suitable colour atlas has much to commend it. The reasons for this will become clear later. However, the general-purpose colour atlases described above are not able to meet the needs of dentists for colour matching and measurement, though they could be applied to the aesthetic field such as matching gum colours in polymer. Their inherent defect is that they attempt to cover nearly all of surface colour space, and with only some hundreds (or at best a few thousand) samples practicable, the colour difference between neighbouring samples will usually be too large for reliable interpolation by visual judgment. The colours of teeth cover a very restricted region of colour space, and a special-purpose colour atlas containing perhaps 200 or 300 samples would enable neighbouring samples to be never more than three just-noticeable differences apart and usually about two. This idea is developed in the final section of this chapter.

The Coloration of Objects

The colour of opaque objects arises from the degree to which light from different parts of the visible spectrum is reflected diffusely, and the diffuse spectral reflectance distribution $\rho(\lambda)$ can be identified as the physical property that determines the colour specification with any given white illuminant. Except in the case of objects made of translucent material, like opal glass or teeth, the light diffusely reflected from opaque objects appears to come from the surface. This is, in fact, an illusion (Plate 5), for the light actually penetrates some small distance into the material of the object, where it is scattered and refracted by the microscopic structure of the substance before it emerges as the diffuse component of the reflected light. As the wavelength of light is roughly 0.5 μm (= 0.0005 mm), many tens of successive scattering events can take place within 0.1 mm, the typical thickness of a paint film or ceramic glaze.

Plate 5 Illustrations showing on the microscopic scale how light is reflected and scattered externally and internally at an opaque pigmented film. Above: a glossy orange coloured surface. Below: a matte orange coloured surface. In both cases white light is incident at 45°.

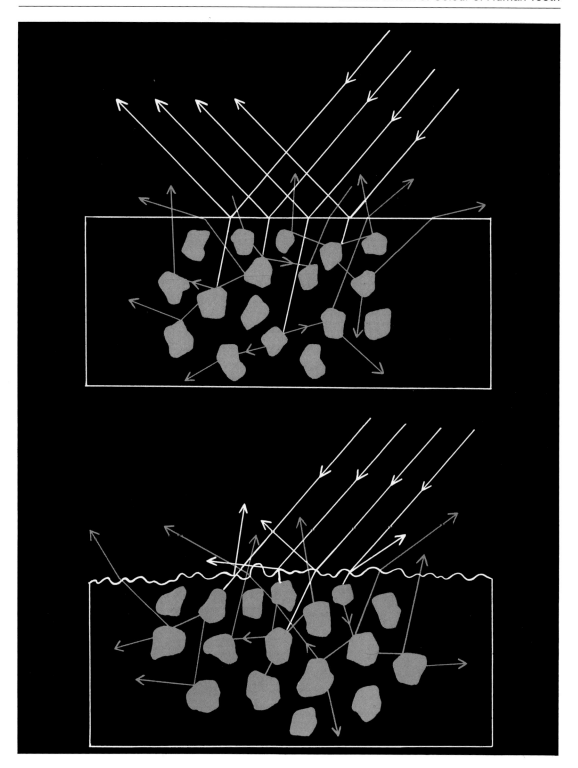

Plate 5

Objects with a microscopically smooth outer surface reflect some of the incident light specularly (Plate 5), producing an effect called *gloss*. Some objects have a less microscopically smooth outer surface and are described as semi-glossy or semi-matte, while others have a microscopically rough surface and are described as matte, with no vestige of a specular component. The spectral compositions of the light specularly reflected or scattered at the outer surface and of the light diffusely reflected from within the scattering superficial layer will generally differ markedly (discussed below), hence the colour generally varies with the angular distribution of illumination and the angle of view. This is why the CIE introduced a restricted number of recommended geometries of illumination and view for colorimetry. In everyday life, glossy samples are normally tilted to avoid the problem of specular highlights masking the diffuse component when assessing colour. It is the diffuse component of reflection that is judged, to give the "real" colour of a glossy object. This is why it would be bad practice to view teeth with directional over-the-shoulder illumination, for under this circumstance there would be numerous highlights to distract the judgment.

The diffuse spectral reflectance profile is in general determined by selective absorption and scattering processes occurring within the material. For an opaque object or layer made of uniform material with no innate directionality of its absorption or scattering characteristics, the diffuse spectral reflectance $\rho\ (\lambda)$ is given by solving the equation:

$$\frac{[1 - \rho(\lambda)]^2}{2\rho(\lambda)} = \frac{K}{S} = \frac{C_1K_1 + C_2K_2 + C_3K_3 + \ldots}{C_1S_1 + C_2S_2 + C_3S_3 + \ldots}$$

according to the simplest theory of coloration, that of *Kubelka* and *Munk*. In this equation, K is the overall absorption coefficient of the material or mixture of materials present and K_1, K_2, K_3, etc. are absorption coefficients of individual constituents. S is the overall scattering coefficient of the material or mixture of materials present and S_1, S_2, S_3, etc. are scattering coefficients of individual constituents, while C_1, C_2, C_3, etc. are the concentrations of individual constituents. The higher the value of S and the lower the value of K, the higher is the object's reflectance and hence the lighter it looks. Densely white objects therefore owe their high reflectance and opacity to having high scattering coefficients and low absorption coefficients. Materials may have innate colour or have had their colour deliberately modified by the addition of colorants, that is, colouring media. For brevity, we will assume that the colouring media are colorants rather than intrinsic to the material, but the processes are the same.

Properties of Colorants and Opaque Matrix Materials

Colorants are defined as *dyestuffs*, if present in solution, or as *pigments*, if insoluble. An ideal dyestuff works by selective absorption only, and should have no scattering. Transparent coloured media like gelatine filters or acrylic rear lamp lenses are typical applications. In textiles the scattering comes from the fibres and yarns in the cloth substrate, not the dyestuff.

In coloured glasses and a small proportion of ceramics, inorganic colorants act like the more familiar organic dyes. In many cases, the dye or dye-like colorant forms a complex and is chemically bonded to the matrix or substrate.

A pigment, however, is present in the form of numerous particles, randomly orientated and often amorphous, and the individual particles often absorb very little of the light at a single passage because of the small particle size. If the particles are large compared with the wavelength of light, perhaps of the order of 10 μm diameter, and are of different refractive index to the matrix material, then significant reflection of light takes place at the surface of the particle, either diffuse scatter from amorphous particles or specular reflection from particles with microscopically smooth surfaces such as crystallites. A proportion of the light reflected from the individual surface element of a particle eventually reaches the outer surfaces of the object after suffering multiple scattering as a result of interacting with numerous other particles. In this case, the chemical nature of the particles (giving it its characteristic absorption) and its difference of refractive index from the matrix material both play a significant role in its contribution to the diffusely reflected light. Whereas the absorption coefficient can vary markedly with wavelength, the refractive index only varies slowly with wavelength and hence the scattering coefficient only varies slowly with wavelength.

If the particle size is small compared with the wavelength of light, perhaps 0.1 μm diameter, then the light is scattered and diffracted rather than actually reflected at the particle surface, but again a proportion of the scattered light reaches the surface of the object after multiple scattering. In this case, the chemical nature plays only a small role, as the absorption coefficient will be reduced due to the short path through the particle and the low proportion of incident light that can enter the particle. However, the scattering coefficient will be significant and wavelength dependent, increasing progressively as one considers shorter wavelengths in the spectrum. This is due to the Rayleigh scattering, which occurs when particle size is rather smaller than the wavelength and the packing density is not too great. In this case, and in the absence of markedly selective absorption, the colour will be a thin bluish white and the appearance will tend to be that of a translucent material because the light penetrates further into the material since the scattering coefficient is lower than with the larger particle sizes. An example may be composite fillings containing 0.04 μm silica particles. When the particle size is comparable with the wavelength of light, an intermediate case occurs, and both the chemical nature of the colorant and the refractive index difference play significant roles: the type of scattering in this case is called Tyndall scattering.

Pigments are used widely in paints, opaque plastics, ceramic glazes, paper, and printing ink. However, some matrix materials, including opal glass, structural glasses, and solid white ceramics such as the pyroceramics are intrinsically opaque and densely scattering without any colorant being added. In these cases, the effective pigment is usually a dense dispersion of minute elements of a different phase or physical form, such as crystallites within a matrix of vitreous material, an example of phase separation. In these cases, the multiple scattering of light arises because of the difference of refractive index. If the particle size of added pigment or an intrinsic scattering element is varied, keeping the amount of such material constant, it is found that the greatest scattering coefficient, and hence the best opacity (or hiding power for a paint) is obtained when the average particle size is slightly greater than the wavelength of light. For example high covering power in porcelains can be obtained by using zirconium oxide pigment of a size range slightly greater than the wavelength of light. At larger particle sizes, the modest increase in scattering per particle is more than negated by the marked loss in multiple scattering caused by the reduction in the number of particles. At smaller sizes, the increase in the number of particles and the possible multiple scattering events is more than negated by the loss of scattering per particle. Indeed, if the particles are less than a twentieth of a wavelength in size, they cause no significant scattering at all, and a layer of the material will be described as transparent. Apart from particle size, the other physical property to optimize is the refractive index: this should be as different as possible from that of the matrix material to achieve the greatest scattering coefficient. It is worth noting that in the majority of applications, even including textiles, the scattering coefficient varies slowly with wavelength, whereas the absorption coefficient often varies rapidly with wavelength.

Specular Reflection and Thin-layer Effects

Specular reflection only occurs at surfaces that are microscopically smooth and where a discontinuous change of refractive index occurs. For any element of surface larger than several wavelengths, the specular reflection can be completely calculated by the complicated *Fresnel's* equations. For the special case of normal incidence, *Fresnel's* equations simplify to

$$\rho = (n-1)^2 / (n+1)^2$$

where n is the refractive index and for any state of polarization of the light. At oblique angles of incidence, the expressions are not only more complicated, but they depend on the state of polarization. Taking the unpolarized light that will usually be incident on teeth, the specular reflectance only increases very slowly with angle of incidence up to about 40°. The refractive index is not independent of wavelength, but it only increases very slowly as wavelength is decreased. Therefore, the specular reflectance of nearly all objects (other than those with optical thin-film coatings) is nearly independent of wavelength, so that the specularly reflected light is, for practical purposes, the same colour and spectral distribution as the light falling on the object. By contrast, the diffusely reflected light is nearly always of a different colour, because of the selectivity of the absorption and scattering processes within the material.

When a number of layers of alternating high and low refractive index are found on the surface of an object, then multiple reflection takes place. If the layers are several wavelengths thick, then very little selective interference of light occurs, and the result is a light grey pearl-like finish. If the layers are thinner, but still thicker than a wavelength of light, then weak selective interference effects are seen, and the result is a pale multi-hued mother-of-pearl finish. If, however, the layers are less than a wavelength thick, then strongly selective interference colours are seen, as on the neck feathers of pigeons or peacocks. Diffraction from periodic structures up to 4 wavelengths of light apart can cause bright colours, as seen on the wings of *morpho* butterflies. In fact, all the natural objects mentioned have just such surface structures as described above.

Colour Matching and Colorimetry

Colour Matching Properties of real Observers

The eye is rotated, almost subconsciously, by the six extrinsic muscles so as to use a highly developed area of the retina, known as the fovea, to examine the detail and colour of any object of interest in the field of view. The fovea contains cone receptors that have three photopigments responsible for colour vision. The following summary of the relevant facts of colour mixture and matching refers to foveal vision, with stimuli subtending anything between $0.3°$ and $4°$ at the eye.

Observers with normal colour vision are classed as *normal trichromats* and make up 92% of the male population and 99.5% of the female population. Colour vision deficiencies are not described here: the majority of them are congenital and involve at least one sex-linked gene. A trichromat is an observer who needs three degrees of freedom in establishing a colour match; he can, for example, match any light stimulus by an additive colour mixture of suitable proportions of any three matching stimuli, provided that these latter are chosen so that none can be matched by a mixture of the other two. Closely related to this is the trivariance of subjective colour space described earlier.

The three laws of *Grassmann* and that of *Abney* form the basis of colorimetry. *Grassmann*'s Laws state that:

1. The eye can distinguish only three kinds of difference or variation of colour (expressible as variations of brightness, hue and saturation for the sensation or as luminance, dominant wavelength and purity for the stimulus).

2. If, in a mixture, one significant component is steadily changed while the others remain constant, the colour of the mixture also steadily changes.

3. Lights of the same colour produce identical effects in mixtures, regardless of their spectral composition.

The most important corollary of these laws is: increasing or decreasing the amounts of two lights of the same colour by the same factor, keeping the relative spectral compositions of each unchanged, will not destroy the colour match. The above statements provide the basis of the additivity concept in colorimetry, which is of fundamental importance in allowing prediction of colour matches and colour specifications, as well as permitting data in terms of any triad of matching stimuli to be transformed to values in terms of any other triad of matching or reference stimuli.

Other important corollaries also follow. Lights of the same colour produce the same adapting effects. A colour match is not altered by pre-adapting the eye or by varying the colour of the surround (provided these effects are applied uniformly), in spite of the fact that the colour appearance of the matching pair can be altered considerably. Thus a red pre-adaptation or surround field will make a matching pair of yellow lights (of different spectral composition to each other) look greenish, but each looks equally greenish. This stability of colour matches is of great importance in making colorimetry useful and generally valid under diverse conditions. The last law needed is that of *Abney:* the luminance (photometric value) of a light made up of several spectral components, such as any common white illuminant, is equal to the sum of the luminances of its spectral components.

This defines photometric additivity, a complementary property to colorimetric additivity; it is a useful property of vision, not a property of visible radiation.

The laws of colorimetry and photometry stated above are valid over most of the operating range of the eye, and under all common conditions. However, at very high levels of luminance of the matching stimuli or with very bright pre-adapting lights at such levels that the eye is uncomfortable, then the laws and their corollaries start to break down. The laws apply to light entering the eye, whether it be directly from a primary source (an illuminant) or whether it comes indirectly from such a source via a secondary source (a surface colour). If the illuminant is specified and held constant, then colorimetry can be applied just as validly to surface colours as to primary sources of light.

Trichromatic Matches: The Possibility and Reality of a System of Colorimetry

If some chosen triad of matching stimuli (say a red, a green, and a blue of known composition) were used to make a trichromatic match on some sample colour, then that colour could be said to be specified in terms of the amounts of the three matching stimuli required. These three amounts (*tristimulus values*) would give a three-dimensional location of the colour in a colour space formed by axes representing the three matching stimuli. A reddish sample would give a match with a high proportion of red matching stimulus needed, and the representation of this colour would quite logically be located in this colour space towards the position of the red matching stimulus. Thus, a trichromatic system of colour measurement and specification could be created. *Newton* pointed out that colour mixtures could be predicted in such a space by the centre-of-gravity principle, which anticipated *Grassmann*'s laws.

Maxwell was the first to realise that since all white illuminants and surface colours are made up of many spectral components, as shown originally by *Newton,* then if colour matches in terms of three suitable matching stimuli could be made on all the spectral colours, it would be possible to predict the colour matches made in terms of those same three matching stimuli on any colour sample, provided its spectral composition was known. *Maxwell,* in fact, implemented the idea before 1860 and was the first to make quantitative and properly normalised trichromatic matches on a set of spectral lights covering the whole visible region.

However it was not until the late 1920s that *Guild* of the National Physical Laboratory, Teddington, United Kingdom, and *Wright* of Imperial College, London, made sufficiently rigorous independent investigations on groups of normal observers, so that an internationally accepted system of colorimetry could be formulated. For each group of observers, significant variation of colour matching was seen. Nevertheless, although carried out in terms of different triads of matching stimuli, with the data normalized quite differently and using visual colorimeters working on different principles, the mean observer data and the spread in individual observations from the two investigations agreed remarkably well when transformed mathematically to a common system of reference stimuli (*Wright* 1969).

The CIE* Colorimetric Systems

The mean data of *Guild* and of *Wright,* are shown in Figure 2 expressed in terms of the amount of each matching stimulus R, G, B needed to match each successive spectral stimulus; these *spectral tristimulus value* data were published in tabular form by the CIE (1931) as the CIE Colorimetric Standard Observer expressed in terms of real spectral stimuli R, G, B.

The data represented by Figure 2 could be used for practical colorimetry, but the system in terms of real reference stimuli has disadvantages. Suppose that the spectral power distribution of some light source is $P(\lambda)$, then the tristimulus value R, can be calculated using the additivity principle as the sum over the visible region of the spectral distribution values $P(\lambda)$ when weighted by the corresponding tristimulus values $\bar{r}(\lambda)$

$$R = \sum_{380\,nm}^{760\,nm} P(\lambda) . \bar{r}(\lambda).$$

with similar expressions for G and B in terms of $\bar{g}(\lambda)$ and $\bar{b}(\lambda)$, respectively. Now $\bar{r}(\lambda)$, $\bar{g}(\lambda)$ and $\bar{b}(\lambda)$ each have regions in the spectrum where they are negative, Figure 2, and this was considered awkward in 1931 because it would increase

* Commission Internationale de l'Eclairage.

457

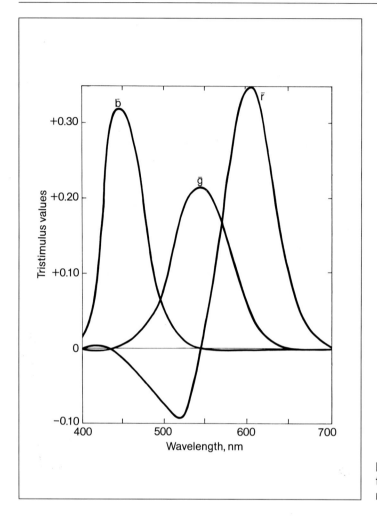

Fig. 2   CIE (R, G, B) System: spectral tristimulus values in terms of real spectral matching stimuli.

the likelihood of errors in calculations (done by hand at that time) and make it difficult to design integrator devices to automatically sum the products r̄(λ).P(λ). An all-positive system of colorimetry (X, Y, Z) was needed to aid industrial application of the new CIE system. It was also decided to exploit the fact that fully half of the spectral colours (the red-orange-yellow-green sequence) only differ from each other in respect to variations in two degrees of freedom. This meant that it was possible to transform the R G B system so as to have one of the reference stimuli, Z, represented by nonzero values in only the shortwave half of the spectrum. This has the benefit of reducing the work of calculating the summations needed to give the tristimulus values to 5/6 of what it otherwise would be. A third feature introduced into the practical (X, Y, Z) system was to have the

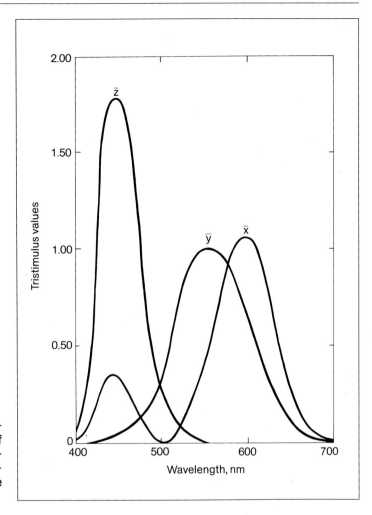

Fig. 3   CIE (X, Y, Z) System: spectral tristimulus values in terms of imaginary reference stimuli chosen to give advantageous properties for practical colorimetry (see text).

photometric value (luminance) embodied in one tristimulus value Y, with no luminance at all in the other quantities X and Z. This means that the spectral tristimulus values $\bar{y}(\lambda)$ of the (X, Y, Z) system are identical to the spectral luminosity values $V(\lambda)$ used in photometry. It has the benefit of harmonising photometry and colorimetry as well as saving computational work, since the photometric value is often needed in its own right.

The spectral tristimulus values $\bar{x}(\lambda)$, $\bar{y}(\lambda)$, $\bar{z}(\lambda)$ of the 1931 CIE (X, Y, Z) system are shown in Figure 3, and they can be regarded as the spectral responsivity curves of the CIE Standard Observer. In fact $\bar{x}(\lambda)$, $\bar{y}(\lambda)$, $\bar{z}(\lambda)$ are linear transformations of $\bar{r}(\lambda)$, $\bar{g}(\lambda)$, $\bar{b}(\lambda)$, and both these sets are linear transformations of the spectral absorption curves of the three cone pigments found in the central retina. The tristimulus value, X, for a light of spectral

459

distribution $P(\lambda)$ is calculated in the same manner as above for R:

$$X = \sum_{380\,nm}^{760\,nm} P(\lambda).\bar{x}(\lambda)$$

with similar expressions for Y and Z in terms of $\bar{y}(\lambda)$ and $\bar{z}(\lambda)$, respectively.

So far we have only considered the colorimetry of sources. In order to measure a coloured object other than a source, we need to recognise it as a secondary source with the property of modifying the spectral power distribution of the incident light $P(\lambda)$. If it is a transparent or translucent object and we are interested in the colour as seen on the opposite side to that illuminated, then its regular or diffuse transmittance $\tau(\lambda)$ will represent the modification of the incident light, and the resulting spectral power distribution becomes $P(\lambda).\tau(\lambda)$. If the object is opaque or translucent and it is to be viewed from the same side as the incident light, then the resulting spectral power distribution becomes $P(\lambda).\rho(\lambda)$ where $\rho(\lambda)$ is the diffuse spectral reflectance factor, that is, the fraction of the light incident over a stated range of angles, which is reflected within another stated range of angles. Considering this latter case of a reflecting object, the expression

$$X = \sum_{380}^{760} P(\lambda).\rho(\lambda).\bar{x}(\lambda)$$

gives the tristimulus value, X, of the reflected light, but it does not give the colour property of the surface itself, as it is essentially a product of the reflective nature of the surface taken with the inci-

dent illumination: the units and magnitude of the illumination need to be normalised out of the expression. This is done by dividing all the expressions for X,Y,Z by the luminous effect of the illuminant, so that for surface colours we have:

$$X = \frac{\sum P(\lambda).\rho(\lambda).\bar{x}(\lambda)}{\sum P(\lambda).\bar{y}(\lambda)}; \quad Y = \frac{\sum P(\lambda).\rho(\lambda).\bar{y}(\lambda)}{\sum P(\lambda).\bar{y}(\lambda)};$$

$$Z = \frac{\sum P(\lambda).\rho(\lambda).\bar{z}(\lambda)}{\sum P(\lambda).\bar{y}(\lambda)}$$

and for transparent or translucent objects viewed against the light there are similar expressions with spectral transmittance $\tau(\lambda)$ replacing $\rho(\lambda)$.

The equations given in this subsection permit the calculation of CIE colour specifications (X,Y,Z) from spectral data such as can be measured for sources with a spectroradiometer or for objects with a spectrophotometer. The conditions under which such measurements can validly be made are discussed below. However, there are other methods that can be used in colour measurement: visual colorimetry and physical tristimulus colorimetry, and these are also discussed later on page 465. The CIE Systems of colorimetry (R,G,B) and (X,Y,Z) are intended to cover a range of angles subtended at the eye of 0.3° to 4°, which covers all small and medium subtense objects. There are Supplementary 10° Standard Observer Data, which are intended to cover all objects subtending greater than 4°. These give the CIE (1964) Supplementary Colorimetric Systems (R_{10}, G_{10}, B_{10}) and (X_{10}, Y_{10}, Z_{10}), which are slightly different from the normal CIE systems in numerical values, but similar in

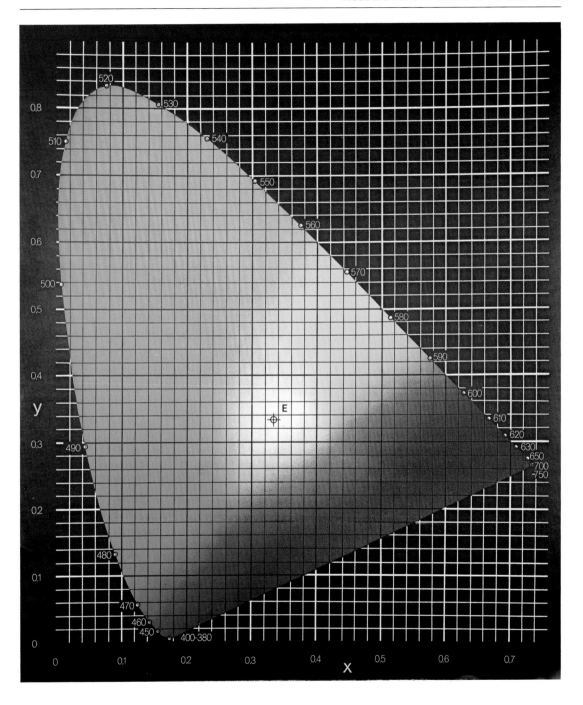

Plate 6   The CIE (x, y) chromaticity chart, showing how the colours are distributed. Colour reproduction in such a printed diagram is not accurate, due to the limitations of colour photography and printing.

construction and indeed the shape of the functions. The (X_{10}, Y_{10}, Z_{10}) System is only used for certain industrial applications such as textiles, where the samples of cloth may subtend large angles at the eye. For dentistry, the (X_{10}, Y_{10}, Z_{10}) System is irrelevant because teeth can never subtend large angles at the eye of an observer.

In the four CIE systems of colorimetry, it is advantageous for many applications to separate the photometric aspect of quantity from the chromatic aspect of colour, and in order to assess the chromatic aspect to have a chart showing relative proportions of the tristimulus values. The chromatic aspect is represented by the *chromaticity* (x,y), where the coordinates x and y are defined as

$$x = X/(X+Y+Z); \quad y = Y/(X+Y+Z)$$

with similar definitions for (r,g), (r_{10}, g_{10}) and (x_{10}, y_{10}). It should be appreciated that for a source the chromaticity (x,y) is the aspect of the colour specification that is invariant, for the amount of illumination at the measuring point (and hence the absolute magnitude of X,Y,Z) depends on the wattage of lamp or lamps and the distances and angles involved. The distribution of colours in the CIE (x,y) chromaticity diagram is indicated in Plate 6.

Standards Needed for Practical Colorimetry

The CIE Standard Observer data represent the most fundamental standards in colorimetry, and they are sufficient in principle to cover the colorimetry of light sources. Measurements on secondary sources such as surface colours require other standards to be specified: standard illuminants, standards of reflection, and recommended geometries of illumination and view. These are described in the following subsections.

However, modifications are needed to the Standard Observer data to make them more useful; namely a transformation of the (X,Y,Z) System to a more nearly perceptually uniform system with the property that equal increments of distance in any direction or for any colour will represent equally perceptible differences of colour. The need for this arises from the subjective nonuniformity of the (R,G,B) and (X,Y,Z) Systems. For industrial use a system is needed to enable measured colour differences to be expressed in terms of perceived differences. There are two CIE recommended systems in use: (L*, u*, v*) and (L*, a*, b*). These are nonlinear transformations of (X,Y,Z), and the reader is referred to recent textbooks such as those by *Grum* and *Bartleson* (1980) and by *Billmeyer* and *Salzman* (1981) for details. Of the two systems, (L*, u*, v*) is only used in television and photographic science, whereas (L*, a*, b*) is widely used in all the colour industries concerned with producing surface colours.

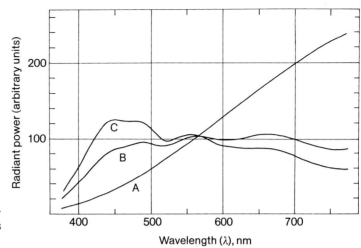

Fig. 4 Spectral power distributions of CIE Standard Illuminants A, B and C.

Standard Illuminants

Because a secondary source object has the property of modifying the light incident on it, it is obvious that its colour specification will be influenced by the choice of illuminant. As there are many types of illuminant, natural and artificial, the CIE (1931) restricted the choice of reference illuminant to three: Illuminant A, representative of incandescent electric lamps; Illuminant B, representative of direct noon sunlight; and Illuminant C, representative of overcast whole sky Illumination (Fig. 4). Reliable data on the spectral power distribution of natural daylight were not available in 1931 and Illuminants B and C were each intended to be of the correct chromaticity and only roughly of the right spectral composition.

Only recently has an adequate range of measurements been made in a number of countries, *Henderson* (1977), and CIE (1964) has recommended three more illuminants, namely D_{55}, D_{65} and D_{75}

(Fig. 5). Of these, D_{65} is intended to represent the most average daylight conditions and is coming into widespread use. D_{65} is a good representation of the average spectral composition found with both fully overcast daylight conditions and a mixture of direct sunlight with the light from a large area of blue sky. Whereas Illuminants A, B, and C have associated standard sources (specifications of practical realisations of them, using an incandescent lamp and certain optical filters), the new Illuminants D_{55}, D_{65} and D_{75} do not. In fact, these new daylight illuminants are impossible to simulate accurately with any known light sources and filters, due to their unsmooth spectral distributions (Fig. 5). At the present time, Illuminants A, C and D_{65} are the only ones in widespread use; of these D_{65} cannot be physically realised accurately, though it can be validly employed for colorimetric computation from spectrophotometric data if the sample is not fluorescent.

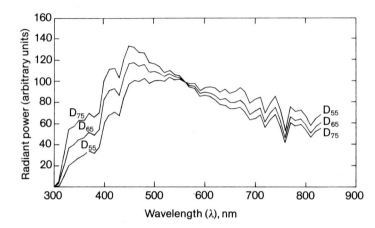

Fig. 5 Spectral power distributions of CIE Standard Illuminants D_{55}, D_{65} and D_{75}, which represent the spectral compositions of daylight of moderately low, average, and moderately high colour temperature, respectively. Colour temperature is a measure of the degree of blueness of white illuminants.

Recommended Geometries for Illumination and View

In normal use, objects seen by reflected light may be illuminated predominantly directionally from a variety of directions, varying from 0° (normal incidence) to almost 90° (grazing incidence) or in a diffuse manner over a large solid angle of approaching 2π steradians (a complete hemisphere). Furthermore, they may be viewed from a variety of angles: considering one plane element of surface, viewing angles may range from 0° (normal viewing) to 90° (grazing oblique viewing). If the colorimetry of surface colours took place variously under all these possible conditions, then there would be diverse colour specifications for a given sample, and no agreement between laboratories or companies could be established. This is because no real sample behaves like the *perfect reflecting diffuser,* which is the only object for which all reflectance factors are equal, regardless of geometry.

Reflectance factor is a generic term for all the quantities that indicate the fraction of light reflected for any geometry. To meet this problem, the CIE has recommended basic geometries of illumination and view: normal or near-normal incidence with hemispherical collection of the reflected light (commonly called 0°/ diffuse reflectance) and 45° incidence with normal viewing (commonly called 45°/0° radiance factor). These are selected to represent the commonest modes of illumination and view, bearing in mind that by the Helmholtz Reciprocity Principle the reciprocal geometries of hemispherical illumination with near-normal viewing (diffuse/0°) and near-normal illumination with hemispherical collection of light (0°/diffuse) have the same value of reflectance factor. Equally, the reciprocal geometries of 45° incidence with normal viewing (45°/0°) and normal incidence with 45° viewing (0°/45°) have the same value of reflectance factor. The four resulting recommended geometries are

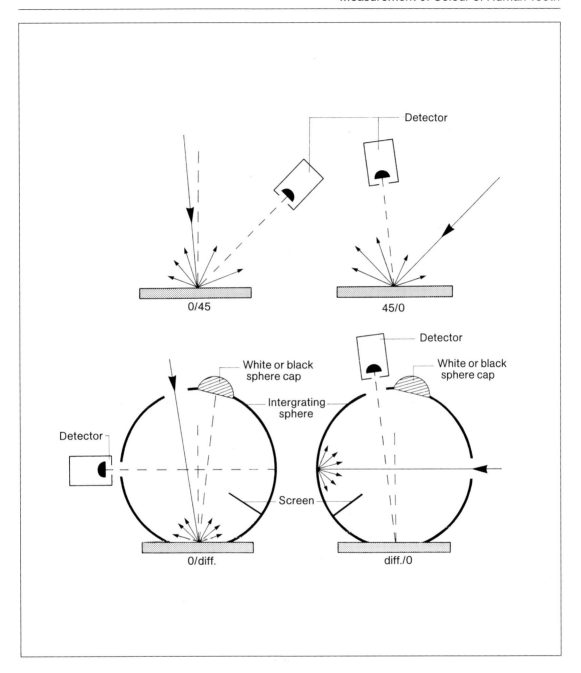

Fig. 6   Geometries of illumination and view recommended by CIE in CIE Publication No. 15 (1971). In the cases of diffuse illumination or diffuse collection of reflected light, the specular component will be either included or excluded according to whether the sphere cap shown is white like the sphere wall or black. These diagrams are only illustrative; many variations of design are possible, and in particular the 45° beam may be in the form of an annular cone.

465

shown in Figure 6. The 0°/diffuse and diffuse/0° geometries each have two cases, namely, whether the specular component of reflection is included or not. When measuring rigid glossy samples, the specular component needs to be excluded if measurement is to correlate well with how one judges the colour, for in normal life one tilts a glossy sample to avoid the specular highlight when appraising colour. With textiles, the specular component is often included, to correlate with an "average" impression of colour with draped or pleated material presented at various angles.

It remains to indicate the special names for the various reflectance factors under different geometries. Whenever a sample has light collected at one angle of reflection (and a narrow range of angles about this angle), the quantity is a *radiance factor or luminance factor.* Whenever the light is collected over the whole hemisphere of possible solid angle, the quantity is called *reflectance.* In all other cases, the only correct term is the generic *reflectance factor.* Real colour measuring equipment cannot strictly achieve the ideal geometries needed for radiance factor or reflectance, but the quantity measured is usually referred to as the quantity to which it approximates.

Standards of Reflectance and Radiance Factor

In 1931, CIE recommended that a thick layer of freshly smoked magnesium oxide should be the reference standard against which all surface colours should be measured. At the time this was the nearest practicable surface that could be produced to represent the *perfect reflecting diffuser.* This last is an idealised surface with the properties that all incident light is reflected without loss (its reflectance is 100%) and that the light is uniformly diffused over a hemisphere according to *Lambert*'s law of diffusion. This latter property means that its radiance or luminance (in common parlance, its brightness) is independent of the angle of viewing. More recently, pressings of very pure barium sulphate have come into use as reference standards: these have the advantage that unlike magnesium oxide they do not go yellower and darker after a day or so. Working standards for industrial laboratories need to be durable, and polished plaques of special Russian opal MS-20 have been the most successful calibrated transfer standards.

In 1971, the CIE recommended that all reflection measurements should be "absolute," that is, referred to the perfect reflecting diffuser. The definition of reflectance was unaffected (the ratio of the light reflected over all angles to the light incident), but the definition of radiance factor was altered, becoming the ratio of the radiance of the sample under the stated geometry conditions to that of the perfect reflecting diffuser. This action by CIE presupposed that it was possible for national standardising laboratories to make available stable standards of reflectance or radiance factors that were calibrated on the "absolute" scale of reflection. Unfortunately, the absolute accuracy with which this is possible is still not good enough for the most exacting applications of colorimetry: an uncertainty of $\pm 0.3\%$ at the 50% confidence level is all that can be achieved at present.

Methods of Colorimetry

There are three basic methods of colorimetry: (1) matching the test sample against standardised and finely graded reference samples organised as in a colour atlas and interpolating to find the best estimate of the colour specification; (2) measuring the colour specification directly by means of a tristimulus colorimeter; and (3) measuring the spectrophotometric characteristic of the sample and calculating the tristimulus values. In principle, all three methods could be implemented by visual or by photoelectric means. The use of a colour atlas is too slow and inaccurate for normal industrial use; the inaccuracies arise mainly from metamerism (see page 474) and difficulty of keeping the reference samples clean, undamaged, and within calibration. Visual tristimulus colorimetry is slower and less precise than photoelectric methods, but is reliable. The most widely used types of visual colorimeter are made by The Tintometer Ltd. and make use of sets of graded coloured glass transmission standards as described by *Chamberlin & Chamberlin* (1980) and by *Judd* and *Wyszecki* (1975). The user finds the combination of the glass standards in the instrument that produces the closest colour match to the sample. For these instruments, charts are used to derive (X, Y, Z) values from the glass scale values.

Photoelectric Tristimulus Colorimeters

In order to measure a light source directly in terms of the CIE (X, Y, Z) System of colorimetry, all that is necessary in principle is to take three measurements using photocell-filter combinations of which the spectral responsivities are respectively proportional to $\bar{x}(\lambda)$, $\bar{y}(\lambda)$ and $\bar{z}(\lambda)$. In practice, a reference measurement would also need to be made on a standard source in order to scale or normalise the readings on the unknown source.

As explained earlier, in order to measure a surface colour, use must be made of one or more CIE Standard Illuminants, the geometry of illumination and view must be one of those recommended by CIE, and a reflection standard will need to be employed. As far as the spectral responsivities of the three photocell-filter combinations are concerned, the overall response must be made equal to $P(\lambda).\bar{x}(\lambda)$, $P(\lambda).\bar{y}(\lambda)$ and $P(\lambda).\bar{z}(\lambda)$ respectively (or a known linear transformation thereof), where $P(\lambda)$ is the spectral power distribution of the Standard Illuminant. If the instrument lamp has a spectral distribution $E(\lambda)$ and the photocell has a spectral response $S(\lambda)$, then the X, Y, Z filters should have an overall spectral transmittance of

$$\text{l. } \frac{\bar{x}(\lambda).P(\lambda)}{E(\lambda).S(\lambda)}, \quad \text{m. } \frac{\bar{y}(\lambda).P(\lambda)}{E(\lambda).S(\lambda)}, \quad \text{n. } \frac{\bar{z}(\lambda).P(\lambda)}{E(\lambda).S(\lambda)}$$

respectively,

where l, m, n are constants that are taken care of when the normalizing readings are taken on the white reference standard. At present, Illuminant C is in most common use as reference illuminant $P(\lambda)$, but new instruments are increasingly attempting to simulate a response involving Illuminant D_{65}. Commercially made colorimeters are described by *Wright* (1969), *Judd* and *Wyszecki* (1975), *Grum* and *Bartleson* (1980) and *Billmeyer* and *Salzman* (1981), as well as by their manufacturers, and only the principles governing their function are described here.

The main limitations of accuracy with photoelectric tristimulus colorimeters are the difficulty in realising the required spectral responses and the imperfections in the geometrical conformity to CIE Recommendations governing the conditions of illumination and viewing of the samples. Concerning the problem of spectral response, instrument makers need to design multi-component optical filters to correct the spectral response according to the expressions given above, or some known linear transformation thereof. Splitting the X response between two filters, because of the awkward two-lobed distribution of $\bar{x}(\lambda)$ (see Fig. 3), and using separate Y and Z filters to make a total of four filters, X_1, X_2, Y, Z, is a common device. Some makers use the Z filter for measuring X_2 (the shortwave lobe of the $\bar{x}(\lambda)$ distribution) and have only three: X_1, Y, Z, with $X = k_1.X_1 + k_2.Z$.

There are three basic ways in which the correction filters can be fitted in the optical system: either between source and sample (Fig. 7a), between sample and detector (Fig. 7b), or partially placed in both sections of the optical system so as to give the reference illuminant $P(\lambda)$ at the sample and the net responses $\bar{x}(\lambda)$, $\bar{y}(\lambda)$, $\bar{z}(\lambda)$ for light collected from the sample. As explained later in Section 7, only the last arrangement is valid for fluorescent samples, but few instruments provide it. Considering here simply the colorimetry of nonfluorescent samples, the overall spectral responses of commercially available instruments are not very close simulations of $P(\lambda).\bar{x}(\lambda), P(\lambda).\bar{y}(\lambda), P(\lambda).\bar{z}(\lambda)$ and hence they cannot be used accurately for direct measurement of X, Y, Z values. However, many industrial checks on production colours require the speed of a photoelectric tristimulus colorimeter, and differences of colour rather than the actual colour specifications are what count: thus most use of tristimulus colorimeters is in differential colorimetry. This is likely to be true of dental requirements.

The implementation of the CIE recommended geometries of illumination and view in commercial tristimulus colorimeters is imperfect, due to a number of reasons. This is also true of reflection spectrophotometers used for colorimetry, and the comments here apply to both classes of instrument. For the 0°/45° and 45°/0° geometries, the principal ray of the nominally 45° optical system needs to be set accurately to 45°±1° and the angular distribution of light in that system should be narrow and symmetrically disposed about the 45° direction. This avoids systematic errors since obliquity effects change rapidly with angle at around 45°. The tolerance on angle and range of angles is much less restricting

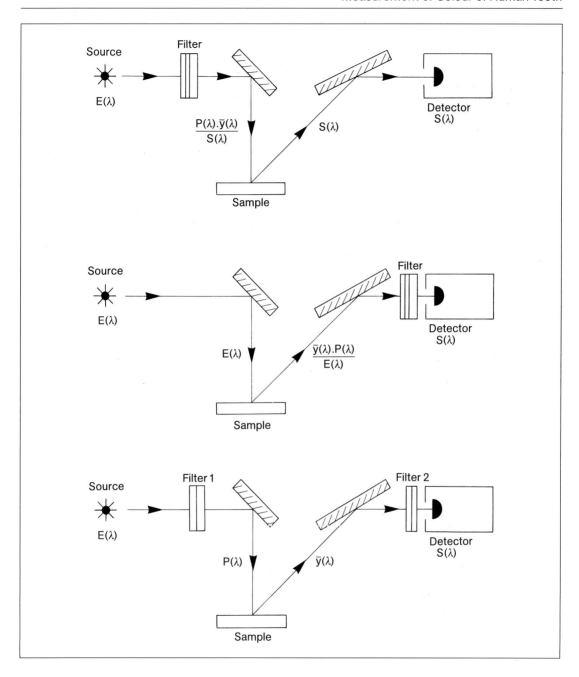

Fig. 7　Filtering arrangements in a tristimulus colorimeter (only the Y filter shown in each case).
(a) All filtering placed between source and sample.
(b) All filtering placed between sample and detector.
(c) Separate filtering to correct source to Standard Illuminant and to correct detector to Standard Observer. Only this arrangement is valid for fluorescent samples.

469

for the optical system nominally perpendicular to the sample, as changes with angle are much smaller in this case. Some instruments have the 45° system in the form of an annular cone of, say, 45° ± 5° rather than arranged as a directional beam. This has two main advantages, for the amount of light collected is much greater (improving sensitivity) and when inhomogeneous or directionally structured samples like textiles are measured, the values obtained are a good average of values obtained with directional 45° collection when the sample is turned through various orientations. Hardly any commercial 0°/45° or 45°/0° instruments have an optical diffuser in front of the photodetector: this is desirable to ensure that all parts of the solid angle of collection of light from the sample have an equal or nearly equal detection efficiency. In the case of double beam instruments it also helps to ensure that the beam balance is stable.

Integrating sphere instruments should have a screen between the sample and detection porthole in the case of 0°/d geometry: this is shown in Figure 6. Its purpose is to prevent the reflected light that would otherwise go straight from the sample to the detector port from being overweighted with respect to the light reflected in all other directions, which would suffer attenuation at each of the multiple reflections at the sphere wall before some component of it reaches the detector port. Double-beam optical systems are necessary to avoid a different error, namely that the average reflectance (and hence collection efficiency) of the sphere is slightly altered by the presence of the sample: this makes a single-beam integrating sphere reflectometer nonlinear in its response. The double-beam arrangement compensates for this effect because the comparison beam response is similarly altered, resulting in the sample beam to comparison beam reading ratio being properly proportional to the sample reflectance (assuming that the photodetector system is adequately linear in its response). In order to fully compensate the effect of sample reflectance on the sphere efficiency and to preserve beam-balance over the whole spectrum, it is good practice to make the sphere symmetrical by having a screen for the comparison beam matching that described above for the sample beam.

The samples needed for general purpose colorimeters and spectrophotometers are generally at least 25 mm across, and in some cases they need to be 50 or even 100 mm across. The textile industry is one where large sampled areas are advantageous in averaging out the effect of woven or knitted structure or colour patterning. It is assumed by manufacturers that samples are flat and nonrecessed, opaque, and uniform (or if with a structure or pattern they are assumed to be uniform over repetitions of the structure or pattern). Microcolorimeters and microspectrophotometers, based on microscope technology using annular oblique illumination and near-normal viewing of a spot a fraction of a millimetre across, have been devised for reflection measurements, but these are only valid for measuring very densely scattering surfaces that are opaque within 0.1 mm of depth, such as paint films or opaque ceramic glazes. With opal glass or other translucent material, they give erroneously low reflection values, due to the back scattered light being laterally diffused too far and escaping from the optical system.

Spectrophotometric Colorimetry

Spectrophotometers are instruments that measure, wavelength by wavelength, the spectral variation of transmittance or reflectance of a sample. Whereas a pen recorder can give a graphic representation of the spectral profile for easy comprehension, this is inconvenient for colorimetry as the computations mentioned on page 458 require a table of numerical values. For cost-effective use of manpower, these values should be transferred by an interface from the spectrophotometer directly to a computer in order to avoid laborious reading off and entry of data via a keyboard. Modern instrumentation has increasingly gone in this direction, and many current spectrophotometers have a microprocessor within them for normalising the spectral data and for colorimetric and other computation. As mentioned on page 466, spectrophotometers share with tristimulus colorimeters the problems of implementing the CIE recommended geometries of illumination and view, and these were discussed there. A general discussion of the errors in spectrophotometry and the means by which these can be determined in order to achieve known absolute accuracies has been given by *Clarke* (1972).

The measurement of a spectral profile could imply a continuous measurement process, with a monochromator scanning continuously through the spectrum while photometric data are output at suitable wavelength intervals. (A monochromator is an optical system based on a dispersing prism or a diffraction grating for isolating any chosen narrow band of wavelengths within the spectral range covered). When analytical research spectrophotometers are used for colour measurement, this is the mode they traditionally work in. Some modern analytical spectrophotometers use a stepper-motor to increment the wavelength setting in steps between the taking of measurements, but are otherwise very similar in function to the traditional types. These instruments allow great versatility in their scanning speed, increments of wavelength for data output, spectral range covered (often ultraviolet and near infrared, as well as the visible region), and choice of illuminating and viewing geometries: the greatest absolute accuracy can be obtained from such instruments, but at the price of a slow measurement process (scans plus computation using spectral values for anything from 31 to 80 wavelengths and taking several minutes per scan). Analytical research spectrophotometers are usually arranged as regular transmittance instruments in their basic form, with purchasable reflectance accessories: integrating sphere for 0°/diffuse or diffuse/0° geometry, and annular ring-mirror collector device for 0°/45° geometry.

For routine industrial colorimetry, faster and more ergonomic instruments are needed. These have traditionally been *abridged spectrophotometers,* which have the scanning monochromator of a true spectrophotometer (or the correction filters of a tristimulus colorimeter) replaced by a wheel of narrow passband interference filters. They can present a predetermined succession of filter transmitting wavebands at typically 10 nm or 20 nm intervals in the visible region, and achieve a colour measurement in perhaps a couple of minutes using anything from 16 to 40 wavebands. The method is intermediate in accuracy and speed between a traditional spectrophotometer and a tristimulus colorimeter. The main limitations of accuracy lie in the coarse intervals between wavelengths when 20 nm intervals are used, the difficulty in calibrating and selecting the filters for their correct effective wavelengths, and in the poor long-term stability of interference filters.

Recently a new generation of special-purpose fast-reading colorimetric spectrophotometers has been devised. Some instruments have *simultaneous* multi-wavelength readout, achieved by focusing a complete spectrum formed from a diffraction grating on to a multi-element semiconductor photodiode array. The number of elements, and hence wavelengths of measurement, varies from 16 to 512 in different instruments. Other designs use very fast scans from some kind of monochromator, the better ones from a grating, the poorer ones from an interference wedge. All these instruments have microprocessors to give properly normalised spectral and colorimetric data, and total measurement time

is typically a fraction of a minute. The accuracy of measurement achieved is usually less than by the more traditional methods, but speed is more important for many industrial applications. Descriptions of various types of commercial spectrophotometer are given by *Wright* (1969), *Judd* and *Wyszecki* (1975), *Grum* and *Bartleson* (1980) and *Billmeyer* and *Salzman* (1981).

Four Great Problems in Colorimetry

Fluorescent Samples

Certain substances exhibit the phenomenon of *photoluminescence,* whereby radiant energy is absorbed in one part of the spectrum and re-emitted in another part of the spectrum. If the emission appears to be simultaneous with the absorption, the effect is commonly called *fluorescence,* although strictly speaking those emissions occurring after intervals longer than 10^{-8} sec should be called *phosphorescence.* Phosphorescence effects can be included with true fluorescence if the delay in emission is less than about a millisecond, since neither the eye nor normal photoelectric colour measuring instruments can distinguish the two. Most fluorescent substances (fluorophors), including all organic ones, have their emission spectra overlapping with their excitation spectra, but in all cases the maximum region of emission is at a longer wavelength than the maximum region of excitation: this is because energy is lost in the optical transition, and the energy of a photon (the elementary "particle" of light) is inversely proportional to its wavelength.

An opaque fluorescent sample seen by reflected light has its apparent diffuse reflectance factor (its *total radiance factor*) made up of two parts, the true reflective component where a fraction of the incident light at each wavelength is scattered back without change of wavelength (see page 448), and the fluorescent component where a fraction of the light incident at wavelengths in the excitation region is re-emitted in a waveband centred at a longer wavelength. Normal colorimetric instruments for surface colours are capable of handling correctly the ordinary reflected component of light, but not the fluorescent component. This is because the reflected light of each wavelength is only influenced by the incident light of the corresponding wavelength, so that each wavelength is independent of the others and it is simply the overall throughput of the complete optical system from source to detector that counts. That is why the arrangements of optical filtering in Figures 7a and 7b are just as good as that of Figure 7c, for non-fluorescent samples, and why for such samples the spectrophotometer arrangements of Figure 8 (1 and 2) are equivalent and valid, irrespective of the particular instrument source or photocell used.

The fluorescent component of the total radiance factor of a sample is, however, dependent on the relative spectral power distribution of the incident light, as shown by *Clarke* (1975), *Grum* and *Bartleson* (1980) and *Billmeyer* and *Salzman* (1981). This means that the correct admixture of reflective and fluorescent components of the colour can only be obtained for a stated reference illuminant by actually irradiating the sample with that reference illuminant during measurement. With a colorimeter, only the arrangement of Figure 7c is valid, and the colour specification cannot be calculated for any other illuminant than the one used for illuminating the sample. With a spectrophotometer, the arrangement of Figure 8 (1) is quite invalid, and the arrangement of Figure 8 (2) is only valid if the required illuminant can be simulated by filtering the instrument source. Unfortunately, illuminant D_{65} is the one most required nowadays, and it is not practicable to produce a good quality simulation due to the irregular shape of the spectral distribution required. When polychromatic irradiation and monochromatic viewing is used as the method of spectrophotometric colorimetry, as in Figure 8 (2), ordinary industrial laboratories have to rely on the quality of simulation provided by the instrument maker and use the measured results as they come. The rigorous methods of correction necessary to give the true colour specification under the reference illuminant described by *Clarke* (1975), *Burns, Clarke,* and *Verrill* (1980) and *Grum* and *Bartleson* (1980) are too difficult to implement in such laboratories. Less accurate methods also described by *Grum* and *Bartleson* (1980) are possible but still inconvenient for an industrial laboratory. Only specially equipped laboratories can use the most

473

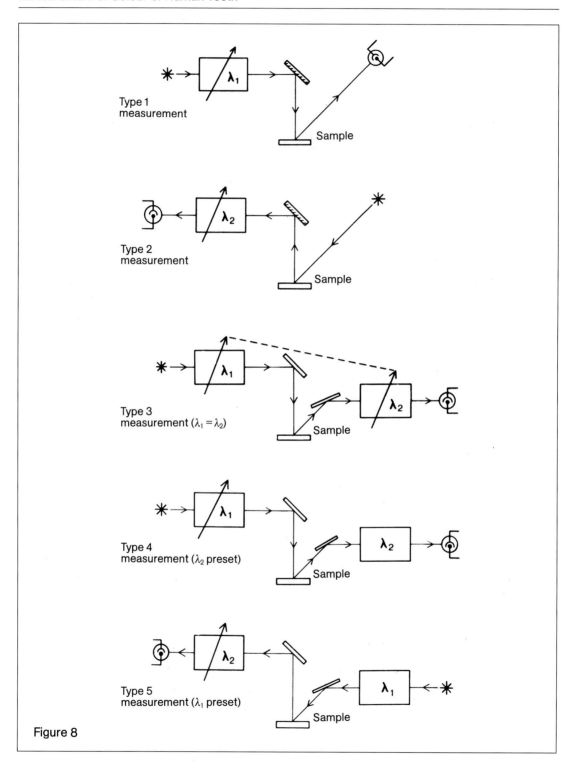

Figure 8

accurate methods of correction, which make use of measurements with a *spectrofluorimeter* fitted with an integrating sphere or 0°/45° annular ring collector reflectance accessory. Such equipment cannot yet be purchased commercially, and special optical modifications need to be made to achieve it (*Clarke* 1975).

A spectrofluorimeter has two independently settable or scannable monochromators, one between source and sample and one between sample and detector, so that it is logically an extended spectrophotometer. There are three additional modes of measurement that can be made with such an instrument, and these are shown in Figure 8 (3–5). In Figure 8 (3), the two monochromators are shown coupled together so that they can scan in synchronism, with both set to the same wavelength at any instant. This measures the true reflective component of radiance factor. In Figure 8 (4), the detecting monochromator is shown pre-set to a certain wavelength (usually chosen to be near the emission peak of the fluorophor), while the irradiating monochromator scans through the spectrum. This measures the *excitation spectrum,* and, after certain calibration and calculation procedures, allows the external spectral quantum efficiency to be calculated. In Figure 8 (5), the irradiating monochromator is pre-set to a certain wavelength (usually chosen to be near the excitation peak of the fluorophor), while the detecting monochromator scans through the spectrum. This measures the *emission spectrum.*

The measurements of Figure 8 (3–5) allow a complete physical description of the reflective and fluorescent components to be derived. This allows results under a reference illuminant to be predicted (provided nonlinear energy transfer effects are absent), or accurate corrections to be made to results obtained under an imperfect illuminant by the method of Figure 8 (2). The theory of the necessary procedures and calculations is given by *Clarke* (1975) and *Burns, Clarke,* and *Verrill* (1980), but is too involved to include here.

Fig. 8   Types of measurement possible with spectrophotometers and spectrofluorimeters:
(1) Monochromatic illumination and whole-spectrum detection: only valid for nonfluorescent samples.
(2) Whole-spectrum illumination and monochromatic detection: valid for any sample if the illumination is the required Standard Illuminant.
(3) Synchronous scanning, keeping the irradiating and detecting monochromators in step at the same wavelength setting: this measures the reflected component only.
(4) Pre-set detecting monochromator and scanning with the irradiating monochromator gives the excitation spectrum of the fluorescence.
(5) Pre-set irradiating monochromator and scanning with the detecting monochromator gives the emission spectrum.
(From *Clarke,* 1975)

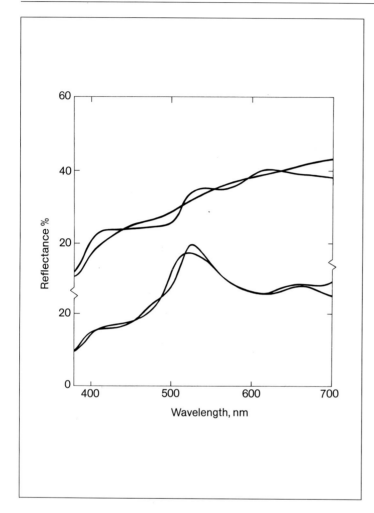

Fig. 9 Spectral reflection profiles of two pairs of metameric colours, which happen to match for no less than three illuminants but which do not match for others. Most metameric pairs of colours only match for one illuminant. (Adapted from *Longley,* 1976)

Metamerism

When two surfaces match or nearly match for colour under some illuminant, but mismatch under one or more other illuminants, they are said to be *metameric,* and their spectral reflection profiles will be found to be different (Fig. 9). For any colour, there are, in general, many possible spectral distributions, a fact that follows from the trivariance of human colour vision: any colour, regardless of spectral distribution, can be matched by a suitable mixture of any of many different possible sets of matching stimuli. Metamerism arises to some extent whenever a target colour sample is matched using different colorants, substrates, or kinds of material: it is never possible to duplicate exactly the target colour's spectral reflection profile when such changes of materials are involved.

The concept of metamerism can be extended to human observers as well; in this case it is termed *observer metamerism,* and arises because of the variation in colour matching found among the normal trichromatic observers making up the bulk of the population. Observer metamerism means that what is a colour match for one observer is not exactly so for another. Thus if there is a metameric colour match between two surfaces of different spectral reflectance profile, then for the Standard Observer they will match under a stated illuminant. For any other illuminant or with that illuminant for those real observers who differ from the Standard Observer, there will probably be some degree of mismatch. Some metameric matched surface colours have spectral differences such that they happen to match under two or even three illuminants, but not under other illuminants (Fig. 9).

Industrial colorimeters are often not accurate enough to give reliable absolute colour specifications, though they may be sensitive and consistent in measurement. For this reason, they should be used purely differentially: the target colour (or "standard" sample) must be made of the same materials and with a similar colorant formulation to the production items being measured. Again, if a stable reference standard is to be used for normalisation, of similar colour to the items to be measured, then metamerism should be minimised by selection of its spectral profile as well as its colour. Metamerism is a problem that restricts the accuracy with which colour atlases can be used for colour matching and specification: even with the correct and specified illuminant for the colour atlas, observer metamerism will, in general, cause some mismatches. In addition, the matches will not necessarily be valid under any other illuminant, since they will usually be metameric due to differences in the colouring materials.

Samples made of Translucent Material

It was explained on page 468 that samples measured by reflection colorimetry and spectrophotometry are assumed by instrument makers to be not made of translucent material. A sample that is fairly densely scattering but thin, such as a sheet of typical white paper, will not be opaque. Lack of opacity is, by itself, a problem that can be coped with. A representative measuring method can be specified, either by measuring the thin sheet backed by a neutral gray material of a stated reflectance or by packing together a stack of a sufficient number of the sheets such that the stack is opaque or nearly so and a limiting value of reflectance is achieved (the *reflectivity*). Some specifications for thin translucent sheets require one sheet to be measured both with a specified black or near-black backing and a specified near-white backing: this gives a measure of the translucency as well as the reflection properties.

A much more difficult problem arises with materials with low scattering coefficients, such as ordinary pot opal glass or milk white acrylic used for translucent lighting fittings, dental prosthetic materials, or fruit juices. The colorimetry of orange juice or lemon juice is a notoriously difficult problem. Ordinary general purpose colour measuring instruments are incapable of determining a colour specification that correlates with how the juice looks in typical containers as seen by consumers. The reason is that a restricted illuminating beam is diffused internally and sideways for a considerable distance, of order centimetres, and *all* the light that escapes back through the illuminated surface in the viewing direction needs to be collected and measured. This means that a large area needs to be viewed, much larger than the illuminated area. Alternatively, the illuminated area needs to be much larger than the area viewed. In both cases the margin of size around the smaller area as well as the thickness of sample needs to correspond to the maximum distance of significant lateral diffusion. Clearly, a small phial of the juice could not be used for instrumental measuring, nor indeed, visual appraisal, for it would measure or look darker and less colourful than the juice normally does in a larger volume.

could attempt to measure the average colour, and use a viewed patch that is large compared with the size of spatial variations.

When the lack of uniformity occurs in depth, it can be unstructured (randomly inhomogeneous) or structured (lamellar): the depth of penetration of light is all that we need consider here. With unstructured inhomogenity, a large sampled area is required to obtain a representative measurement. With a lamellar structure free of patchiness, it is possible to obtain a representative measurement with a small sampled area. However it is necessary to realise that the reflection properties depend markedly on the area and angle of illumination. If the object is translucent and lamellar in structure and is usually illuminated from a large range of angles, sometimes completely diffusely, as with a tooth, then the only way to get a representative measurement of colour is to light the object with hemispherical diffuse illumination. This would have the effect of averaging out the angular effects of selective lighting.

Inhomogeneous Samples

Inhomogeneity in a sample can take two main forms: lack of uniformity across its surface or in depth. The former arises with deliberately patterned or fortuitously patchy materials. In this case, one can attempt to measure the colour spot by spot to find its variation, using a viewed spot that is small compared with the size of spatial variations. Alternatively one

Measurement and Matching of Human Teeth

Dentistry is an occupation where aesthetics is of considerable importance, especially when patients are stage or public figures. However it is interesting to note that colour science has not so far been applied very successfully in dental shade matching to give quantitative

Plate 7 Fluorescence of human teeth when irradiated by the near-ultra-violet component of natural daylight, with the visible region filtered out. The true colour of the fluorescent emission is a bluish white. (From *Preston* and *Bergen,* 1980).

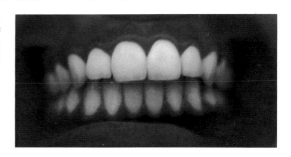

answers to the problems. There are very good reasons for this, which are discussed below. The needs, however, are clear enough and may be stated as the selection, colouring, and processing of the right dental prosthetic materials so as to produce a convincing match in appearance to the natural teeth of the patient. This is a much harder problem than those met with by the colour production industries, such as textiles, paints, and plastics, for reasons which will now be explained.

Teeth as Colorimetric Samples

The properties of samples presented for measurement with colorimeters and spectrophotometers that give rise to difficulties and systematic errors have been mentioned in previous sections: fluorescence, metamerism, non-uniformity across the surface, inhomogeneous internal structure in layers, translucency, small size, irregular shape, and surrounding projections which would prevent their close presentation against the instrument measuring port. The reasons why

these properties create difficulties have been briefly indicated earlier. Teeth must be just about the only objects to have *all* the properties at once and in abundant measure. The fluorescence is readily seen by illuminating with near-ultraviolet light (Plate 7), and its emission is a pale bluish-white in colour. As the near ultra-violet is present in natural daylight, it is likely that fluorescence influences the colour of teeth when illuminated by daylight. How much will be indicated later. It is worth noting that only a minority of dental prosthetic materials have the right colour of fluorescence, and few have the right amount as well. Metamerism is inevitable when synthetic materials such as coloured dental porcelains, cements, and polymers are matched against natural teeth.

However, it is the geometrical properties in the above list of awkward sample properties that make instrumental colorimetry unlikely to be fully successful. A cross-section through a human tooth is shown in Plate 8, which shows the three principal layers within it: enamel, dentine, and nutritional pulp. These layers have different scattering coefficients, and

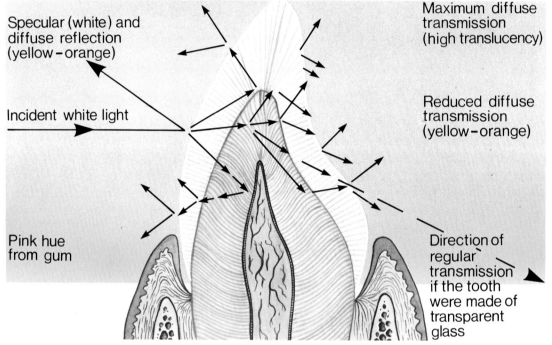

Specular (white) and diffuse reflection (yellow – orange)

Incident white light

Pink hue from gum

Maximum diffuse transmission (high translucency)

Reduced diffuse transmission (yellow – orange)

Direction of regular transmission if the tooth were made of transparent glass

Plate 8   Cross-section of a human tooth with arrows indicating an incident light ray and various resulting reflected, scattered, and transmitted components.
(Diagram produced by FJJ Clarke, Diana McLean and JW McLean)

hence different opacity and translucency properties. The spectral absorption property of the pulp is markedly different from that of the enamel and dentine, giving it the pinky red colour. The layers are not themselves homogeneous, even if we ignore fissures, due to the way the tooth grows and modifies with age, and an additional layer of secondary dentine usually forms between the dentine and pulp. The enamel and dentine are a yellowish white, but the enamel with about 97% hydroxyapatite content is more translucent than the dentine, which has about 70% hydroxyapatite content. Some teeth that are very translucent seem almost bluish-white in parts; this is probably due to the bluish Rayleigh scattering of small sub-wavelength particles, seen against the yellowish white of the more densely scattering parts where the shortwave absorption and natural yellowish colour predominates. All natural whites are slightly yellowish, and in the case of teeth the least yellow end of the tooth colour range is accepted as "white" even though by spectrophotometric measurement it is still yellowish (*Sproull,* 1973; *Clarke,* 1975). This arises because of residual shortwave absorption of the proteins present.

From the preceeding information it is clear that teeth are translucent and inhomogeneous in several different ways. This, combined with the small size and the geometrically complicated shape of a tooth and of its neighbouring teeth and gum tissue, means that a different fraction of an incident ray of illuminating light will be scattered back as reflected light for almost every angle of illumination, and with each given angle of illumination for almost every portion of a tooth illuminated. It follows that representative and reproducible measurements will not be possible with strongly directional illumination. The only way to try to even out the selective local and angular effects would be to use hemispherical, or nearly hemispherical, diffuse illumination of a tooth as well as its adjoining teeth and gum tissues. However, such illumination applied uniformly to the whole mouth would be preferable. Not only would such diffuse whole-mouth illumination give the most reproducible colour measurements; it would be the most natural illumination and allow the full range of tooth/gum/tongue/palate/lip interreflections. Hence, such measurements should correlate with the normal colour appearance.

In view of what has been mentioned earlier, it is clear that the general purpose commercial colorimetric instruments do not offer the possibility of measuring teeth *in vivo* satisfactorily. The area sampled by the viewing beam is normally far too large in relation to the size of a tooth, and is usually an appreciable fraction of the area illuminated in the case of the diffuse/0° geometry instruments required to deal with the fluorescence. The main requirement, therefore, is that the whole mouth should be diffusely and uniformly illuminated with only a small area viewed, of perhaps 3 or 4 mm across; this implies a large integrating sphere and hence a low overall optical efficiency, so that a high power lamp or lamps would be needed. Further, the large integrating sphere would need to be coupled to the mouth by means of a conical funnel just long enough to allow the nose to be outside the integrating sphere surface, and this funnel would need to be coated with a matte white material like the inside of the integrating sphere. In order to view a small patch on a tooth from a point on the far side of the integrating sphere, a small-angle viewing system is needed, such as would be used with a telephotometer, so that a telespectroradiometer or telecolorimeter (designed for measuring small or distant light sources) could usefully form part of the complete instrument.

There are instruments that can be applied locally to a tooth surface. Some colorimeters (photoelectric and visual) have a fibre-optic flexible measuring head with 45°/0° or 0°/45° illuminating and viewing geometry; however, the illuminated area is far too small and is directional, so that representative measurements are not likely to be made. The same applies to microcolorimeters or microspectrophotometers using the annular or split aperture dark ground mode of microscopy.

A feature of teeth that further complicates the issue is local staining, often confined to cracks or superficial fissures. Whereas the human observer can ignore this and concentrate on the main tooth body colour, photoelectric instruments cannot do anything but measure the average colour within the sampled area. A dentist needs to match the main body colour of the natural teeth and can apply artistic simulated stain markings afterwards to the selected prosthetic crown material. A uniform material of the average colour of the natural teeth would not look right, if the teeth have stain markings, a point discussed by *McLean* (1979) and *Preston* and *Bergen* (1980).

Measurements on Teeth at the National Physical Laboratory

In order to support a programme of work at British Ceramic Research Association on dental porcelains, the National Physical Laboratory made an investigation of the colour and fluorescence of teeth and of some dental porcelains (*Clarke*, 1975). Extracted teeth preserved in formalin solution were observed to be unnaturally dark and brownish, due to their being waterlogged because of the correct osmotic balance no longer being maintained. Attempts at drying them led to the measured colour being progressively lighter and lighter with no stable endpoint; after a while they looked unnaturally light and started to craze, eventually falling to pieces. Because of this it was decided that no credible colorimetry could be carried out on extracted teeth, even when stored under idealized conditions, and that measurements *in vivo* were necessary.

The methods of measurement used were those shown in Figure 8 (1 and 2), monochromatic directional illumination with diffuse whole-spectrum detection and diffuse whole-spectrum illumination with monochromatic directional detection. The NPL spectrofluorimeter facility was not yet developed, and the techniques used were those available from a versatile reversible-optics spectrophotometer such as a Cary 14. Plate 9 shows a meas-

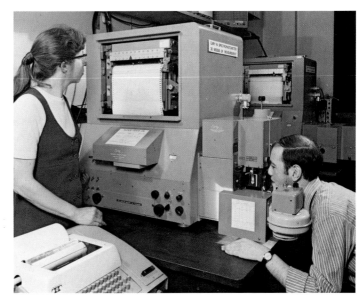

Plate 9 Spectrophotometric measurement of a tooth *in vivo* at the National Physical Laboratory, using a Cary 14 spectrophotometer with small integrating sphere. Illumination of the tooth is diffuse and with simulated daylight in this case, and the reflected light is analysed monochromatically. (From *Clarke*, 1975)

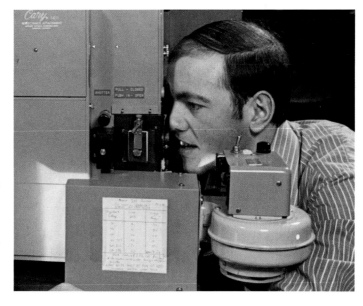

Plate 10 Close-up of the subject during the measurements of Plate 8. A small funnel attached to the normal sphere port forms a very small stand-off sample port, against which the tooth can be pressed. The illuminated tooth can be seen to emit internally scattered light sideways: even more escapes from the rear surface. (From *Clarke*, 1975)

urement in progress with polychromatic (whole-spectrum) illumination of a front upper incisor from a small integrating sphere, while Plate 10 shows a close-up of the subject, with the lateral translucency of the illuminated tooth clearly visible. In this case the illumination was from a tungsten-halogen lamp filtered selectively with a two-component glass filter so as to simulate CIE Illuminant D_{65} representing daylight. The other kind of measurement using monochromatic illumination had to take place in a totally darkened laboratory, due to the translucency and curved surface of a tooth, which would otherwise let in ambient light to the sensitive detector measuring the reflected light via the integrating sphere. To clear the nose and lips, the tooth was pressed against a stand-off miniature porthole on a conical funnel attached temporarily to the sphere port. This meant that the diffuse measurement was not over a complete hemisphere but over a range of angles from $0°$ to roughly $60°$. The type of result from the two modes of measurement is shown in Fig. 10, using hypothetical data to illustrate the problem of interpretation where the fluorescent and reflected components need to be separated. Organic fluorophors always have an overlap of excitation and emission spectra, and in this region it is difficult to separate the fluorescent and reflected components from the total spectral radiance factor. Actual results from a tooth are shown in Figure 11, and the data are not free of systematic error in the region of overlap at the blue end of the spectrum. Calculations showed that the fluorescence does produce a notice-

able effect in reducing the inherent yellowness of teeth when seen in daylight. It should be noted that although diffuse illumination was used, this was only applied to about half of the tooth being measured. Nevertheless, these are as accurate as any other measurements so far reported.

The implication of this work is that dental prosthetic materials should not only match the natural teeth in the visible region of the spectrum, but their fluorescence should roughly match as well. In the case of show-business and other patients who are public figures, the fluorescence needs to match quite well, to cover public appearances in discos, theatres, or other places with ornamental ultraviolet illumination.

Colour Matching of Dental Prosthetic Materials

It has become clear from previous sections and subsections that the widely used general-purpose colorimetric instruments are unsuitable for dental problems, due to size of the measured area, and that the special-purpose instruments with small measured areas have completely unsuitable means of illuminating the whole mouth (or at least part of the mouth to include the tooth and all neighbouring structures and tissues). It was suggested on page 480 that a suitable instrument might be developed with a large integrating sphere for illumination: it would need to be 0.5 m to 1 m in diameter, have a coupling funnel to the

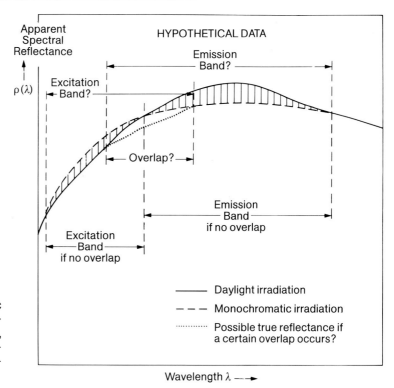

Fig. 10 Spectrophotometric measurements by the techniques of Fig. 8/1 and 8/2, showing the problem of interpretation in the region of overlap. (From *Clarke*, 1975)

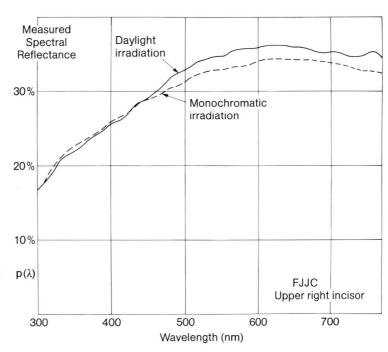

Fig. 11 Results for a tooth *in vivo* with the techniques of Fig. 8/1 and 8/2, using a simulation of CIE Illuminant D_{65} in the latter case. (From *Clarke*, 1975)

485

mouth and very small-angle detecting optics for the spectrophotometer.

In the absence of this special dental spectrophotometer, visual methods will have to be relied on for some time to come. However, the problem is that dental prosthetic materials are not normally available to the dentist in the right form. They should be fabricated as tooth-shaped samples forming a *dental colour atlas,* that is, a shade guide constructed to show the three-dimensional variation of colour found in natural teeth, with the variations being systematic and uniformly graded according to some stated criteria. The materials should be selected to give minimal metamerism with natural teeth, this also applying to the fluorescence seen under near-ultraviolet irradiation. The samples should be removable, so that they can be placed in a patient's mouth. *Lemire* and *Burk* (1975) show that J. M. Ney Co. have made some promising moves in this direction.

One problem is how the colour atlas should be organised. Clearly, to cover a three-dimensional section of colour space, a number of two-dimensional arrays of samples are needed. The Munsell system, and indeed most colour atlases, have a fundamental weakness in their cylindrical structure around a central vertical grey scale with radial sections on each page or card; this leads to the samples of a given lightness (value) and saturation (chroma) of two stated neighbouring hues being much closer in colour difference at low saturations than at higher saturations. A system with equal colour differences between all neighbouring samples would have to have a

Cartesian rather than a cylindrical radial structure of axes and units. It could be constructed effectively by having all samples of a given lightness L* on one card showing graded samples at regular intervals of the rectangular axes (a*, b*) of the CIELAB or Adams-Nickerson System, and a series of cards for the different lightness L* values. The CIE (L*, a*, b*) System is certainly uniform enough for dental purposes, in view of the limitations of accuracy inherent in this field, which I have endeavoured to explain in this contribution. Plate 11 shows the CIELAB colour solid viewed from above.

The practical arrangement could be in the form of clear acrylic trays, each carrying the samples of a given L* value, which slide into a box-frame so that when all trays are in position, the samples are seen correctly located in the colour solid with their separations in all three dimensions proportional to their colour differences

$$\Delta E = \sqrt{(\Delta L^*)^2 + (\Delta a^*)^2 + (\Delta b^*)^2}$$

For ease of matching the natural teeth in a mouth, one or more trays of about the correct L* value could be slid out so that appropriate (a*, b*) samples could be removed and tested at the patient's mouth.

Implementation should be organised via an international committee, not by one organization, so that the leading suppliers of materials can all use a common system of display in a common dental colour atlas system, but realised in their

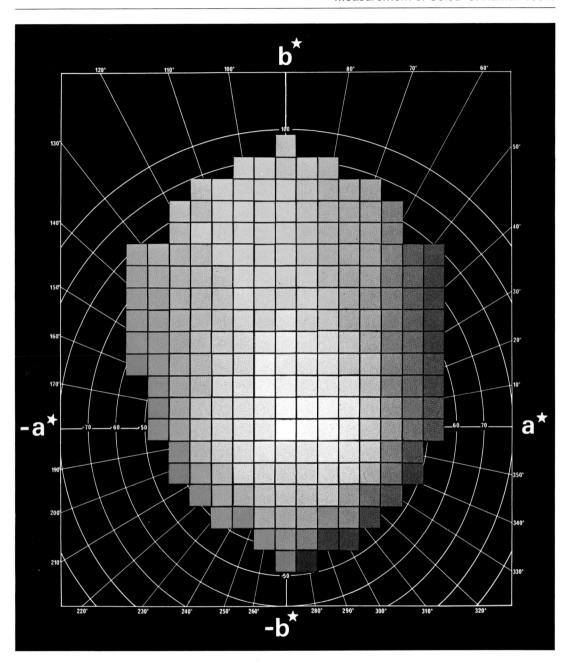

Plate 11   The CIE (L*, a*, b*) colour solid, with the realisable surface colours represented in coarse cubic steps. This is a view looking down along the L* lightness axis, showing the distribution of the lightest realisable surface colours for different locations in the chromatic coordinates (a*, b*). Also shown are radial lines of constant hue angle and circles of constant metric chroma. (Adapted from an original of *K. McLaren*)

own materials. This last arises because of translucency or metameric differences between shade samples from different suppliers or in different materials. The first step is to organise measurements of teeth and of dental materials, these to be definitive and by an agreed technique.

The second step is to define a family of spectrophotometric curves to avoid problems of metamerism and fluorescence. I leave it to the dental profession to suggest the remaining steps in such an endeavour.

References

Billmeyer, F. W., and Salzman, M. (1981): Principles of color technology. New York: Wiley.

Burns, R. A., Clarke, F. J. J., and Verrill, J. F. (1980): Measurement of fluorescent radiation from opaque surfaces. Proc. Soc. Photo-opt. Instrum. Engs. 234: 48.

Chamberlin, G. J., and Chamberlin, D. G. (1980): Colour: its measurement, computation and application. London: Heyden.

C.I.E. (1931): Compte Rendu des Séances, 19. Paris: Commission Internationale de l'Eclairage.

C.I.E. (1964): Compte Rendu des Séances, A: 35. Paris: Commission Internationale de l'Eclairage.

Clark, E. B. (1933): The Clark tooth colour system, parts I and II. Dent. Mag. Oral Top. 50: 139.

Clarke, F. J. J. (1972): High accuracy spectrophotometry at the National Physical Laboratory. J. Res. N.B.S. 76 A: 375.

Clarke, F. J. J. (1975): Problems of spectrofluorimetric standards for reflection and colorimetric use. NPL Report MOM 12 (National Physical Laboratory, Teddington).

Colorizer Associates. (1947): The Colorizer. Salt Lake City: Colorizer Associates.

Container Corp. of America. (1948): Color Harmony Manual. Third edition. Chicago: Container Corp. of America.

Davidson, H. R., Godlove, M. N., and Hemmendinger, H. (1957): A Munsell book in high-gloss colors. J. Opt. Soc. Amer. 47: 336.

Grum, F., and Bartleson, C. J., eds. (1980): Optical radiation measurements. Vol 2, Color measurement. New York: Academic Press.

Hård, A. (1970): The Natural Colour System. Proc. Int. Colour Assoc. Meeting Color 69, 1: 351. Göttingen: Musterschmidt.

Henderson, S. T. (1977): Daylight and its spectrum. Second edition. Bristol: Adam Hilger.

Imperial Chemical Industries, Ltd. (1969): The ICI Colour Atlas. London: Butterworths.

Judd, D. B., and Wyszecki, G. (1975): Color in Business, Science and Industry. Third edition. New York: Wiley.

Lemire, P. A., and Burk, A. A. S. (1975): Color in Dentistry. Hartford: J. M. Ney Co.

Longley, W. V. (1976): A visual approach to controlling metamerism. Color Res. Appl. 1: 43.

Maerz, A., and Paul, M. R. (1950): A Dictionary of Color. Second edition. New York: McGraw.

Martin Senour, Co. (1946): Nu-hue Custom Color System. Chicago: Martin Senour Co.

McLean, J. W. (1979): The Science and Art of Dental Ceramics. Vol. 1: The nature of dental ceramics and their clinical use. Chicago: Quintessence Publishing Co., Inc..

Munsell Color Co. (1929, 1943): The Munsell Book of Color. Vol. I, 1929; Vol. II, 1943. Baltimore: Munsell Color Co.

Pantone Inc. (1963, Rev. 1974): The Pantone matching system. Moonachie, N. J.: Pantone Inc.

Plochere, G., and Plochere, G. (1948): Plochere Color System. Los Angeles: G & G Plochere.

Preston, J. D., and Bergen, S. F. (1980): Color science and dental art, a self-teaching program. St. Louis: C. V. Mosby.

Ridgway, R. (1912): Color standards and color nomenclature. Baltimore: A Hoen & Co.

Sproull, R. C. (1973): Colour matching in dentistry, Part II. J. Prosthet. Dent. 29: 556.

Villalobos, R. (1947): Villalobos Colour Atlas. Buenos Aires & New York: Stechert-Hafner.

Wright, W. D. (1969): The Measurement of Colour. Third edition. Bristol: Adam Hilger.

The Elements of Esthetics – Application of Color Science

Jack Preston

Introduction

History has recorded mankind's interest in his personal appearance and the effect that self image has on confidence, performance, and social intercourse. Dental esthetics has figured prominently in this role of self image and various ethnic groups have adorned and altered their dentitions in diverse manners. Whether these modifications have been attractive or repulsive is largely subjective, and evaluation is subject to ethnic, geographic, and social bias.

Similarly, any treatise on esthetics is subject to individual interpretation. Agreement or disagreement with the concepts presented neither affirms nor denies their validity, for in the final analysis the judgment of whether or not a restoration is esthetic, be it a single tooth or a complete dentition, lies with the patient. The dentist must, therefore, attempt to use the technical and conceptual ability to develop for the patient a restoration that best meets the patient's psychological and biological needs and desires. It is wrong only when it contributes to the further deterioration of the tissues, inhibits function, or is psychologically traumatic to the patient. In this context, it can be seen that not only are restorations that are ill-conceived or poorly fabricated capable of iatrogenic physical degeneration, but also of psychologic iatrogenic failure.

Esthetic excellence is largely an art with primarily subjective interpretation; not enough has been done to effectively analyze and formulate it. Certainly some of the great artists – Michaelangelo, Da Vinci, Van Gogh, Seurat – incorporated scientific elements in their works using linear perspective, shadow, logical color, and individual formulae to breathe life into their work. It will be the purpose of this chapter to pursue some of the definable elements of dental esthetics. Although a consideration of color and shade matching will receive major emphasis, the relative role of this element must be placed in context.

The Elements of Esthetics

Esthetic elements can be approached from a number of different viewpoints and any approach to taxonomy or grouping results in some redundancy and inadequacy.

I have frequently tried to simplistically confine the elements of esthetics within the heading of "form, texture and color." This attempt has proven rather crude and incomplete. For want of a better system I shall herein approach the dissection of components of esthetics into "spatial," "optical," and "biological" considerations.

Spatial

Spatial components are those factors which apply to tridimensional form and the relation of the teeth to one another as well as to the approximating or enclosing elements. Among the tangible components are physical dimension, embrasures, long axes, transitional line angles, contact areas, diastemata, arch position and surface contour. There are also perceptual elements, which include linear harmony, perspective of view, and orientation to the soft tissue. The latter aspect could probably just as well be considered tangible, depending upon the particular situation. These elements individually and in concert deliver the greatest impact to the viewer. However, they are not the sole elements involved and alone they would not be able to convey an acceptable impression. Additionally, the actual and finite may not be as important as the effect perceived. Illusion is a most significant entity, for sometimes the true form desired may not be obtainable. Later in this chapter, the spatial elements will be related to one another and to the optical and biological considerations.

Optical

Anyone who has tried to match teeth with a restorative material recognizes that the procedure is complex. The optical appearance is not merely one of "color," as great a concern as that phenomenon is, but also involves light and shadow, surface texture, translucency, and opacity. The interaction of the elements not only occurs on the surface but within the body of both the natural tooth and its simulation. Although the topic of color will be the prime consideration of this chapter, it is convenient to first pursue the third category of esthetic elements.

Biologic

The biologic elements include those vital factors which separate the dynamic and physiologic from the static and lifeless. These are the elements that are largely absent on a stone cast and must be understood by and communicated to the technician if the restoration is to nestle harmlessly and esthetically into its biological residence. Included within this domain are the movable oral frame, facial relationship, gingival tissues, residual ridge elements, phonetics, and those needs forced by function and parafunction.

Analytical Problems

When all of these considerations are expanded into their subordinate components it is little wonder that obtaining esthetic excellence has presented some analytical problems. As with most problems, the solution often comes not by attacking the entire entity all at once, but by breaking it down into its components and assessing each one in turn with its co-acting elements. When success is obtained it will always have a dynamic coherence … what has been called "dynamic unity" as opposed to static, and therefore lifeless, unity. This is further reason why final evaluation must be done with the patient "wrapped around the restoration" and why the dentist has the primary and continuing responsibility to initially ascertain what the esthetic potential is and how it may be best achieved. This may be simply stated by noting that the dentist must (a) understand what the patient wants (psychologic), (b) what the patient needs (physiologic), and (c) of what dental science, especially as expressed by the dental team rendering the specific service, is capable (technical). Unless the psychologic, physiologic, and technical elements can be brought into consonance, therapy should not be initiated.

Pre-Treatment Planning

It is not my purpose here to review techniques that have been previously well explained and with which, it is hoped, the reader is familiar. The needs for adequate radiographs, intraoral and extraoral examination, appraisal of soft and hard tissues, and evaluation of the functional adequacy of the stomatognathic system are essential prerequisites for any therapy. The complexities presented by the partially edentulous patient are usually greater than those of the patient who has not lost any teeth. The lack of adequate residual ridge tissues may call for augmentation or graft procedures or necessitate the use of a removable or fixed-removable prosthesis, which can supply the tissue component as well as the teeth. Other complicating factors such as unfavorable maxillomandibular relations, excessive vertical or horizontal overlap, anterior open bite, lost vertical dimension of occlusion, version or tipping, malformation, or congenital anomalies mitigate against obtaining the degree of success desirable. All esthetic results must be calculated from "what is" to "what can be." The need for referral to another specialist can range from the dental specialties (orthodontics, oral surgery, periodontics, etc.) to medical consultations with a plastic surgeon or psychiatrist or even a cosmetologist. The importance of the patient interview and pretreatment planning cannot be overstressed and recognition of the need to consult with other disciplines can enhance patient satisfaction.

Essential to the planning of a restoration

or prosthesis is an adequate set of diagnostic casts that reproduce the patient's soft and hard tissues with fidelity. It is advisable to make a duplicate set of casts to provide a baseline record that will have both therapeutic and legal value. Such casts should usually be mounted, although simpler procedures can be accomplished on unmounted casts.

Diagnostic Waxing

Modification to meet both esthetic and functional needs can best be planned for through the use of a diagnostic waxing procedure. In this manner, problems and potential solutions can be ascertained in advance of any irreversible procedure. Although the diagnostic waxing procedure is limited by the inanimate properties of the cast, it nonetheless can reveal many of the features that may indicate or limit success. Together with clinical judgment developed from observing the lip lines, phonetics, and information gleaned from the patient interview, a precursor of the final restoration can be developed. When this prototype is combined with a prepreparation trial restoration and the provisional restoration (*Preston,* 1976) a definitive restoration with the desired dynamic unity can be developed. Furthermore, the patient becomes a participant in defining the esthetic result. This incorporation of the patient's desires enhances acceptance and greatly reduces the possibility of dissatisfaction or disappointment at the time of placement of the completed restoration (*Hirsch,*

Levin, and *Tiber,* 1973; *Rosenthal* et al, 1964).

It is essential to ascertain the desired esthetic result for metal ceramic units in advance in order to allow waxing a framework that provides proper metal support, yet does not interfere with translucency and color nor infringe upon the adjacent tissues.

Not enough emphasis has been placed upon understanding the limitations imposed by the materials employed in either the metal ceramic restoration or the all-ceramic unit. Porcelain is a material that has intrinsic limitations that must be recognized and for which accommodations must be made. The marriage of metal to porcelain in the metal ceramic restoration is an attempt to take advantage of the strength of metal and the beauty of porcelain. Similarly, the all ceramic restoration employing an aluminous core (either brush-applied or pressed) is a procedure that enhances success through dispersion strengthening (*McLean* and *Hughes,* 1965). Porcelain fails in either system when there is excess bulk or, to phrase it in the negative, inadequate support. Therefore, the strengthening support system (either metal or alumina) must be developed to allow as little of the esthetic veneering glass as possible (to allow for strength), yet leave sufficient bulk to cover the substructure and develop the esthetic optical properties desired. Such an accomplishment requires knowledge and planning. The desired result must be preestablished if both optimum strength and esthetic excellence are to be obtained.

An observation of esthetically appealing natural dentitions will confirm that a pattern emerges that can serve as a matrix to develop pleasing restorations. Certainly these are not rules, but rather guides that make dissection of the whole into component parts possible. The division of the total esthetic composite into its elements simplifies understanding and makes detection of any flaws in a completed restoration easier. It is frequently difficult to recognize why a prosthesis or restoration does not achieve the desired effect until it's component parts are analyzed. It is helpful, then, to consider the elements previously mentioned in greater detail and relate them to one another. This analysis will not be complete but will serve only to stimulate the reader to initiate further study.

Implied Gender

It may be well, initially, to dispense with a myth that has evolved regarding the illusion of the masculinity or femininity of a dentition (*Frush* and *Fisher,* 1956). Anthropologically, there is no sexual dimorphism of human teeth. Whereas it has been convenient to consider the male form as one that is more cuboidal (robust) and the feminine as being more rounded (gracile), attempts to verify this have failed (*Abrams,* 1978). As the dentition wears as a result of function or parafunction, the more juvenile incisal edge contours are lost, and the rounded form evolves into one that is more angular. Thus, it appears that wear and aging have been translated into "masculine," while

the more youthful or unaltered form is thought of as "feminine." Even though the genesis of the concept may be false, the interpretation of the more rounded and fluid form as being feminine seems to persist and is used when such an illusion is desirable.

Although it is not the purpose of this treatise to explore in detail the relationships of the elements of esthetics, it is desirable to point out some of the major factors that are essential to esthetic success.

Embrasures

All of the four embrasure spaces (incisal, cervical, labial, and lingual) are important, but often the first perception of form is the silhouette of the teeth against the dark background of the oral cavity. This silhouette is generated by the incisal embrasures and the connecting incisal edges. There is, obviously, an interface between the incisal and cervical embrasures, which forms the inciso-gingival contact area. This contact area generally lies in the incisal two thirds between the maxillary central incisors, the middle third of the maxillary lateral and central incisors and the middle to cervical third of the maxillary lateral incisor and canine. Sometimes actual contact may not be present: contact is only implied. This is the illusion created by the perspective given when the mouth is seen in a frontal view. Then the contact area is not seen at all but rather the distal transitional line angle. The "contact" is hidden in the depths of the labial embrasure. It is only when the view is changed to a lateral

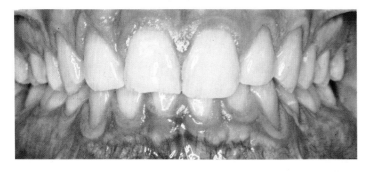

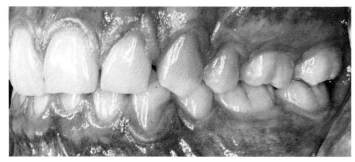

Fig. 1a and b   A frontal view of anterior teeth. The transitional line angles obscure the presence of diastemas which are seen in the lateral view.

angle that the diastema is then seen (see Fig. 1a and b). This ever-changing view is the embodiment of dynamic unity.

Once the inciso-gingival and mesio-distal dimension is determined, real or illusionary contours may be established. Either the space available (for pontics or crowns) or the contralateral form that is to be replicated will impose the demands for tooth dimension. If this essential dimension is unsatisfactory, then illusions must be created to imply something that is more acceptable. This may be done by lapping to create the illusion of greater space, by moving the position of the contact area and transitional line angles, by altering the labial surface, and by the use of color to produce shadows and highlights, which create or enhance the illusion of form (*Pincus,* 1967). It must

be pointed out, however, that illusions are only illusions and may lose their effect when the angle of view is changed or lighting conditions vary.

To create the impression of a narrower tooth, the proximal contacts are moved further to the lingual and the transitional line angles are moved further toward the center of the tooth: This increases the size of the labial embrasure. The incisal edge is usually narrowed by rounding the incisal corners–which is to say that the incisal embrasures are increased. To further enhance the illusion of narrowness, the labial surface may be more convex and may be given more labial texturing, which reduces the amount of light reflectance (Fig. 2a and b). Color may be applied to enhance shadows and highlights. Widening, the reverse of narrowing, is

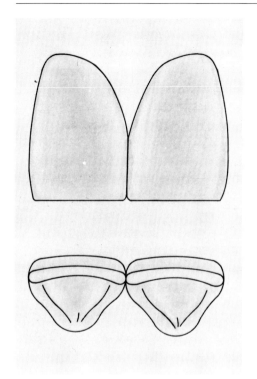
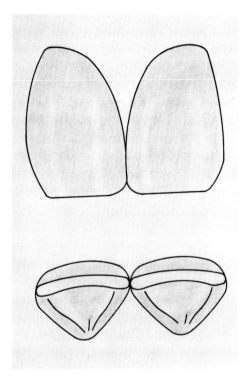

Fig. 2a and b   Although the pairs of teeth illustrated occupy the same physical dimension (b) is made to appear more narrow and delicate than (a) by increasing the size of the incisal embrasures, thus altering the contact areas. The transitional line angles have been moved toward the center of the tooth and the contact area placed further toward the lingual, both altering the labial embrasure. The labial surface has been rounded reducing the amount of light reflected directly toward the viewer enhancing the illusion of narrowness.

accomplIshed by reversing all of the above illusions. Incisal embrasures are less severely carved, leaving the incisal edges broad; the labial embrasures are reduced, moving the contact area further labially. The transitional line angles are moved further apart and the labial surface flattened. The surface is made more smooth for greater light reflection. The principles employed are simple and by no means exhaust the interrelationships of the "spatial, optical and biologic complex." When a restoration has been placed that somehow just "doesn't look right" an analysis of the individual elements will help to solve esthetic problems. Often it is no more than a recarving of the embrasure that is necessary. Creating proper embrasure form is an exercise in developing the positive form by carving the negative. Once the embrasures are correct, the outline is established.

For multiple units, be they fixed restorations, individual units, or artificial teeth on a removable partial or complete denture,

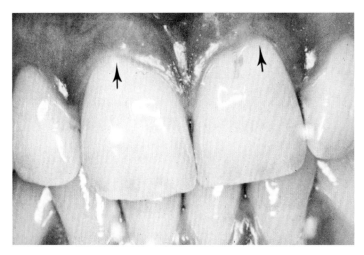

Fig. 3 The apical crest of the soft tissue will be determined largely by the morphology of the underlying structure (see text).

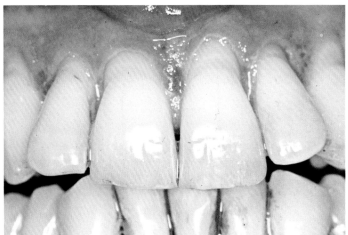

Fig. 4 These lateral incisor axes incline mesioapically, rather than the more typical distoapical direction. Note the absence of one mandibular anterior tooth, which has altered occlusal contacts.

attention to the long axes is essential. The intention is to deceive the observer into believing that the artificial tooth is actually growing in place. This implies an unseen root beneath the visible crown. The long axis is a factor that is developed by an interaction of the transitional line angles, heights of contour of the crown and/or root, the incisal edge, and the gingiva or residual ridge. This gingival contour is essential and must be realis-

tically developed, even though it is usually a subliminal factor. The apical crest of the soft tissue is found in the distal third of the cervical portion (*Stein,* 1978). This has frequently been pointed out, but the underlying cause has generally escaped attention. The position of the crest is determined by the labial prominence of the underlying tooth structure (Fig. 3). Thus the position and direction of the unseen tooth structure becomes mani-

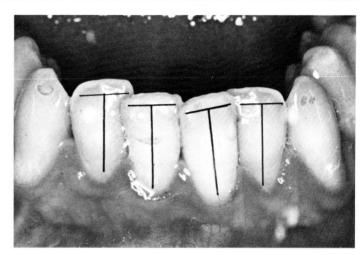

Fig. 5 The incisal edges generally form a visual line perpendicular to the long axis. This relationship may be conveyed by line drawing (Figure 3).

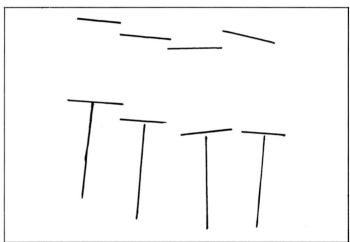

Figure 6

fest in the contour of the soft tissue and gives an indication of the long axis. Generally, the maxillary central incisors have a long axis that slightly diverges distoapically from vertical, the lateral incisors diverge more so, and the canines appear to be almost vertical when viewed from the front. A lateral view will usually demonstrate that the canines actually have a distoapical inclination. The lateral incisor axis is the most frequently im-

properly placed in fixed restorations, and may be made to incline mesioapically. It is true that such axes are seen in natural dentitions but are atypical and usually a functional modification (Fig. 4). An altered vertical dimension with lost posterior support may cause facial migration, altering the long axis, or similar interarch relationships may be the cause. Whatever the cause, the result is rarely esthetically pleasing. The long axis is generally at right angles (or a visual right angle) to the incisal edge. The incisal edge then becomes an indicator of the long axis and the shaping of this line is important to esthetics (Fig. 5). This interaction is demonstrable in the lower anterior teeth, where the indiscriminate leveling of the incisal surfaces is rarely acceptable esthetically. When a tooth is lapped over or under another tooth, the long axis is altered and the incisal edge must be carved to be coherent with the long axis, which is implied. The desired edge-long axis relationship is easily communicated to the technician by simple line drawings (*Shelby,* 1976; Fig. 6).

While considering the lower anterior teeth it is appropriate to note that the form of the lingual incisal one-third merits attention, for it is frequently in the "esthetic zone" and not infrequently mishandled during restoration. The lingual fossae are concave and if the teeth are lapped, three dimensions must be created. Too often fixed prostheses only give the impression of lapping when viewed from the labial, but the lapping is not carried out on the lingual surfaces as well. The lingual fossae must flow into the transitional line angles and the lingual embrasures must be carved, not implied.

It is frequently difficult to ascertain just what area comprises the so-called "esthetic zone." It may not be as important to know what actually is in this area, but rather what the patient thinks the area is. Even though the patient has a fairly long and flaccid maxillary lip and small oral orifice, that person may be concerned with all that is seen when the lips are manually reflected. There is, there-fore, a functional esthetic zone that may differ from the patient's "psychological esthetic area." A discerning interview to ascertain the patient's desires must precede any attempt at esthetic restoration.

The interaction of the spatial elements with the biologic elements is quite apparent. The gingival tissue form defines the visible crown. The morphology of the tooth helps establish the tissue contour. The mobility of the oral frame alters the amount and direction of light on the area viewed and thus interacts with all the optical elements. The functions that are performed by the dentition and the soft tissues impose great limitations, yet they also give excellent clues for proper placement of the anterior teeth (*Pound,* 1966; *Murrell,* 1974). The correctness of incisal edge position can be verified by the competent phonation of sibilant and fricative sounds. This has been well documented in the literature on complete denture prosthodontics but applies to multiple fixed restorations as well. The mandibular movements may dictate the lingual form of maxillary anteriors, and this again demonstrates the harmonious coexistence of form and function. The curve of the mandibular lip during smiling ("smile line") is a very effective beginning for determining the length of the maxillary anterior teeth, and is generally found to be in concert with the phonetic and functional determinants.

In all the effort to obtain correct individual tooth form, the relationship of the dentition to the patient must not be lost. The dental midline is best determined by the patient's facial midline (*Lombardi,* 1973).

Fig. 7a to d The "Dentindex" (Howmedica, Chicago Ill.) is a pliable wax form that may be placed in the patients mouth to record midline, horizontal plane and soft tissue landmarks (Figs. 7b and c). This is then sent to the laboratory to aid in mounting casts and conveying physiologic details not otherwise available (Fig. 7d).

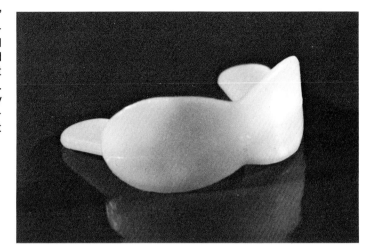

Figure 7a

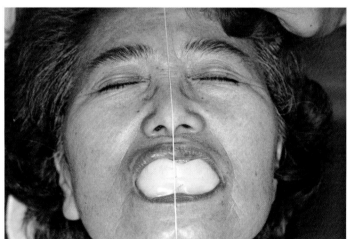

Figure 7b

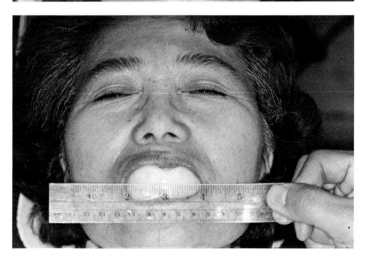

Figure 7c

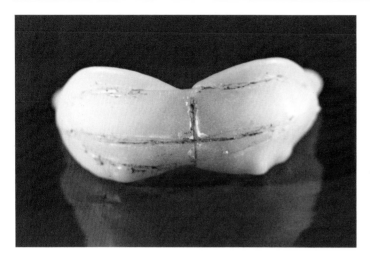

Figure 7 d

This is the line from the point of the hairline through the tip of the nose (which may be misleading) to the midpoint of the prominence of the chin. A piece of dental floss joining these points makes a good visual indicator for defining this midline. The horizontal plane must also be established and communicated to the laboratory whenever either significant tooth loss or tooth reduction during preparation has obliterated the horizontal orientation. Either the maxillary cast must be properly transferred with a face bow registering the patient's horizontal plane (which may not be done with a kinematic facebow transfer; *Preston,* 1979), or another method must be used. A simple device (Figs. 7 a to d) made of wax allows the marking of facial relationships as well as the high lip line and the curve of the lower lip.*

* Dentindex-Howmedica, Chicago, IL

Optical Elements

The intricate interaction of all the components of the esthetic complex should be easily apparent. These interrelationships are limitless and much controlled study must be given to substantiate some of the apparent correlations that clinical observations have implied. There are many voids in the knowledge of esthetic formulation, but some of these are slowly being filled. Certainly the transfer of knowledge from the physical sciences into the understanding of dental esthetics is most obvious in understanding color. The study of color in dentistry must include translucency, opacity, and the effect of light and shadow.

Indeed, it must be recognized that color and light are a single entity with different manifestations. One cannot study color without studying light, a fact ascertained by *Newton* (1966) over three hundred years ago. Unfortunately, the development of restorative material shading systems and procedures seems to have circumvented logic and a review of some well established facts is an essential prerequisite to any study of dental color.

As Dr. *Bruce Clark* noted almost 50 years ago (1933), "Color—like form—has three dimensions." These three dimensions form the cornerstone of the logical approach to clinical shade matching. Color is a complex phenomenon and its recognition involves a physical stimulus, a psycho-physical interchange between the stimulus and the receptor cells of the eye, and the subjective response by the brain to the information transmitted from the receptor organ. It becomes important, therefore, to understand all three levels of this stimulus/receptor/interpretation chain, for distortion at any of the three levels will result in an incorrect or inappropriate understanding of the "real" (physical) situation. Color must be perceived, not merely seen.

Just as dental esthetics must be dissected into its component parts to be comprehended, so "color" must be dissected into its three dimensions if it is to be "seen" and shade comparisons made. When a shade guide and a tooth do not match, it is not enough to note that a "match" is lacking, but deviations in each of the three dimensions must be noted. This requires a basic and clear understanding of those three dimensions.

Hue

The first dimension, hue, is usually defined as "the name of the color." This is an inadequate definition because it fails to recognize that hue names are very imprecise. There are many different reds, oranges, greens, etc. A slightly better definition would be "the name given to a hue family." Hue is generated by the wavelength of the stimulus. Energy of the electromagnetic spectrum is manifest in widely varying phenomena such as cosmic rays, X-rays, television, radio, and electricity. The only things that differentiate between these forms of energy are wavelength and frequency. Visible light is composed of waves of between 380 and 760 nanometers. The shortest waves are seen as violet, while the longest are red. The physical sequence, dictated by wavelength, is violet, blue, green, yellow, orange, and red. This is rather a convenient, though incomplete, series of hue names, for it must be recognized that there is a constant subtle change from one hue to the next. Green, for example does not suddenly become yellow, it becomes "less green" and then "more yellow," progressing to "less yellow," "and more orange," and so on.

It may, then, be said, "Hue is the quality of color designated by a convenient family name, and determined by the wavelength of the stimulus."

Value

The second dimension, value, is merely the quality of blackness or whiteness. It is the equation of the color to a gray scale. Hue and value are independent, for value can exist without hue (the converse is not true), as anyone who has watched black and white television or seen black and white photographs knows. These are merely one-dimensional renditions (value without hue or chroma) of a three-dimensional (colored) object. Because the human observer is so very sensitive to slight differences in value, it is this dimension that is most important in dentistry.

Chroma (Saturation)

Although value exists in the absence of hue, chroma is only present when there is hue. Chroma is merely the intensity, concentration, or strength of the hue. Any one of the three dimensions may be varied independent of the others, but in dentistry this rarely happens. For instance, if one merely wanted to change the hue of a color, it would require that the proper colorant of the same value be added to the color and added in the correct quantity so as to make the hue shift without varying chroma. Because the range of dental colorants (metal oxides) is so limited, color modifications most probably will involve all three dimensions.

Color Ordering

Many systems have been devised to interrelate the various colors possible by changing hue, value, and chroma. Some are best suited to measurement by colorimeters or spectrophotometers. The one best suited for visual examination (a psychological system) is that devised by *A. H. Munsell* (1936). *Munsell* merely related hue, value, and chroma in the same manner that length, width, and depth are related. The hues were made a continuum by taking advantage of the fact that the shortest wavelengths (violet) contained visual elements of the next shortest (blue) and the longest (red). Therefore, a visual circle could be made with violet as the connecting link. Using the six hues previously named, this circle would read "violet, blue, green, yellow, orange, red, violet, blue, etc." *Munsell*, however, assigned the less arbitrary names of purple-blue, blue, blue-green, green, yellow-green, yellow, red-yellow, red, red-purple, purple. *Munsell* then established a value scale of 0 (black) to 10 (white). Hues can be related to values much the same way a wheel is related to an axle. Hues of a low value appear dull, those of high value, bright. Chroma, the third dimension, would be analogous to the spokes of a wheel and represents the intensity of the color at any hue or value (see Plate 3 on page 447 and Plate 4 on page 448).

This ordered color system makes possible the expression of all colors in terms of hue, value, and chroma. Such a standardization is universal and can be numerically expressed. Levels of discrimination can be established to any degree and color chips of the precise shade can be obtained from commercial sources. Color matching can be done from a standard and interpolation between available color chips can be made in hue, value, and chroma.

Contrast this ordered logic with the procedures now used in dentistry. No shading system has both logical order and adequate distribution; most have neither. Work done by *Clark* (1931), *Sproull* (1973), *Lemire* and *Burk* (1975), and *Miller* (1981) has documented the lack of correlation between the hue, value, and chroma of natural teeth and that of available shade guides.

The enormity of the problem is made even greater when one recognizes that nearly all available spectrophotometric data on natural teeth comes from measurements made on extracted teeth. The data from *Sproull's* original work and the much more exhaustive new studies by *Miller* demonstrate that the available shades do not extend far enough into the yellow-red hues but are too yellow. This deficiency will only be amplified when intraoral measurements are done, for the surrounding tissues and vital dental pulp can only shift apparent tooth color further into the red range. Generally, shade guides do not include enough low value and higher chroma samples. A conservative estimate had been made that less than fifty percent of the population may be satisfactorily matched by dental shade guides. The requirement for adequate distribution has never been met. Even the relatively few samples that are available are not logically ordered. In fact, there is no apparent unifying concept that would have led to the development of current guides.

Should one be fortunate enough to find a shade tab that apparently satisfies the patient's needs, the problem is not solved. Metamerism is a continually perplexing factor, since the spectral curves of porcelain do not match those of natural teeth. As a result, the "match" that is apparent in the clinical environment may not be present in other areas of illumination. (This problem of light and lighting will be discussed later). Metamerism in shade matching has evolved from more areas than just the discrepancy of spectral curves of natural teeth and porcelain (or resins). In most instances the porcelain used in the shade guide is not even the same material employed in the fabrication of the restoration, nor is the shade guide fabricated in the same manner as the restoration. There are only a very few shade guides that are used for porcelain matching although many companies manufacture porcelain systems that are based on these guides. The dentist who uses a guide from manufacturer B and whose technician uses porcelain from manufacturer C has an even greater gap in the logical chain of shade determination—restoration—fabrication. Still another problem exists: the porcelain-to-metal restoration requires an opaque porcelain to mask the metal and a body porcelain to develop contours. One might assume that the body and opaque materials would be the same color, but again such reasoning seems to have eluded the manufacturers. Opaque and body porcelains, as shown by the work recently done by *Miller* and *Hemmendinger,* have quite different hue, value, and chroma plots. This means that the opaque is applied to mask the metal and then the body porcelain must be applied in a quantity great enough to mask the opaque.

When this complex series of inaccuracies is considered, the recurring problem of mismatched shades is not surprising. Acceptance of a shade is an individual factor and no absolute parameters are definable. Unfortunately, the fewer the number of teeth restored, the greater the problem and the less the remuneration for the more difficult service. Thus the restoration of a single central incisor continues to be the greatest challenge for the least compensation.

Imposing Logic on an Illogical System

The absence of a shade guide with logical order and adequate distribution does not detract from the need to intimately understand hue, value, and chroma, for with this knowledge logic can be introduced to the shade matching procedure at chairside and in the laboratory. The comparison between the teeth to be matched and the shade guide is made and an assessment of "difference" or "no difference" is then necessary. If the difference exceeds the acceptable level, a description of that difference is needed so that modification may be made to correct the deviation. Three questions will make that description possible.

1. *"Is the shade guide of a higher or lower value than the tooth being matched?"* The value difference is most important and is sometimes difficult to separate from chroma. The rods of the retina do not see hue but are entirely monitors of brightness. They outnumber the hue receptors (cones) and are found most-

ly peripheral to the focal center, where vision is most acute. When one squints, the amount of light admitted is decreased and the vision is less central and more peripheral—hence more rods and fewer cones are used. If the difference between the shade guides is greater when squinting, then a difference in value exists. This does not mean that there is no difference in the other two dimensions. This use of visual physiology can be very helpful in discerning differences in value levels.

2. *"Is the shade guide yellower than or redder than the tooth being matched?"* This question deals with the dimension of hue and acknowledges that since teeth are only in the yellow to yellow-red range, no other hue error can be present.

3. *"Is the shade guide hue more saturated or less saturated than that of the tooth being matched?"* Again, this may be difficult to separate from value, and either value, saturation, or both deviations may be present.

These three questions will help define the difference between a shade guide tooth and the tooth to be replicated. If no satisfactory match is available, a guide tooth that is higher in value and lower in chroma should be selected. A higher value shade can be rather easily lowered without loss of translucency by the use of the complementary color externally or gray or complementary modifiers internally. Some mention should be made here also about the use of the color brown. When the ten hues *Munsell* named were given, nothing was said of "brown," for brown is not a hue, it is a color. Brown is a low value of several hues, but for our purposes in dentistry, the browns are low value yellow-reds. The addition of brown to a shade effectively lowers value while holding chroma, and is useful for both intrinsic or extrinsic modification. Small quantities are quite effective.

Even though the initial selection is high in value and low in chroma with the intention to make changes, the final restoration at the time of insertion should not be of higher value. If any deviation is made it should be toward the lower value area, since such errors are less quickly noticeable.

Shade Guide Use

It is helpful for the dentist who offers porcelain restorations to patients to have a knowledge of how such units are fabricated. Unfortunately, many practitioners have never had the opportunity to manipulate porcelain and lack basic understanding of the procedure. Such instruction is not the purpose of this writing, but the reader is encouraged to take courses in porcelain fabrication through commercial course offerings or continuing education facilities. Even though there is no intention of actually doing one's own laboratory work, the knowledge can greatly improve dentist–technician communication and appreciation.

Suffice it to say that porcelain is built up in layers using opaque, body, and incisal porcelains. Each of these contributes to the final optical effect and each may be modified with colorants to create desired effects. Shade guides frequently have characterized areas that may or may not be appropriate to the teeth being matched. For this reason, at least three of each of the shade guides used should be available to the dentist. The first is an unmodified guide: this guide may (and probably does) have a cervical area that is different from the standard body shade. The second guide should have this cervical section, composed of "special effect" porcelain, removed. The third guide should have the glaze removed (with stones, discs, or abrasive spray) for modification with ceramic colorants. (This procedure will be described later under the heading "Extrinsic Modification.") A fourth guide with both cervical and incisal areas removed may be desirable, also.

The overlay of the enamel portion on the body may be done in different quantities and at different angles and may not be at all like the standard guide. A sagittal drawing (Fig. 8) can be very helpful to indicate the layering desired. The "optical" elements of translucency and opacity can be as important as "color" in developing an esthetically acceptable restoration, but tangible means of measuring or communicating them are largely lacking. Most porcelain systems have a series of different incisal porcelains that may be used, though most dentists are unaware of their importance.

The shade guide tab should be held in the same position as that to be occupied by the restoration being fabricated. This is easier to do for a pontic than for a crown.

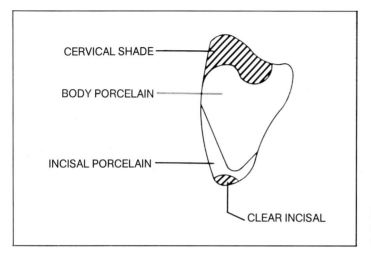

CERVICAL SHADE

BODY PORCELAIN

INCISAL PORCELAIN

CLEAR INCISAL

Fig. 8   A sagittal line drawing can communicate the layering of cervical, body and incisal porcelains.

The gingival area of the shade guide should approximate the gingival portion of the tooth being matched, and the incisal edge of the guide should be in the same position as that of the natural tooth. The goal is to have the light to be incident on the guide the same way the intended restoration will receive and reflect light. Frequently the remaining teeth will exhibit different shades and the goal must be not to match any particular one but to achieve an acceptable blend.

The position of teeth in the arch alters light reflection and sometimes accommodations must be made. For example, if there is crowding in the arch the two maxillary central incisors may not occupy the same relative position—one may be lingual to the other. The one that is the more labial will appear brighter (higher in value). The tooth that is more prominent is more likely to require restoration (because it is more subject to traumatic damage). When the restoration is planned, a shade that is slightly lower in value

might be selected in order to blend with the adjacent central incisor, which, being in the shadow of the approximating more labial teeth, reflects less light. The logic of such a modification is easily applicable to similar situations.

Surface Texture

Since color is entirely a result of light, the manner in which the light is reflected is important. The surface topography of both the shade guide and the tooth may alter the quantity and quality of light. The replication of surface morphology is important in order to effectively produce natural tooth appearances. This is done by proper carving of the surface and obtaining the correct degree of glaze (see section on glazing technique). Not only does surface texture affect the apparent value of a restoration, but there are indications that it also affects hue (*Obregon,* et al., 1981). To help offset the difference between a shade guide tooth and the natural tooth, both should be viewed after moistening to fill surface differences without introducing a variable.

Controlled Environment

It has been repeatedly stated in this chapter that the light incident to and reflected from an object entirely controls color. The object has the ability to absorb or reflect certain spectra of light. If it absorbs all light, it is seen as black; if it reflects all light, it is seen as white, provided a full spectral light is incident upon it. When the object reflects some rays and absorbs others, the nature of the reflected rays determines the stimulus to the eye to receive and the brain to perceive "color." If the dental shade matching procedure is to be controlled, then the incident light must also be controlled. There are three areas that require attention if environmental control is to be effective. First, the light radiated must be complete spectrum lighting, at least as complete as is reasonably possible. This is accomplished by selecting an illuminant that produces consistently acceptable illumination and that negates the use of daylight. Daylight changes hour to hour, day to day, and season to season. It varies in intensity and in quality. The use of a proper color-corrected fluorescent source is this author's preference. To ensure that the tubes selected are acceptable, three criteria should be met. First, the tube should have a correlated color temperature similar to that of standard daylight. (Standard daylight is defined in the U.S. as that light available in Washington, D.C. during the month of June between the hours of 12:00 and 1:00 o'clock, with a slightly overcast sky). This temperature is approximately 5,500° Kelvin. Second, the spectral curve of the light source should be similar to that of this same "standard daylight." Finally, the illuminant should have a color rendering index (C.R.I.) of 90 or greater. The manufacturers of such fluorescent tubes readily make such data available, and if the illuminant in question does not offer the desired data it probably does not possess the qualities desired.

The quantity of light required is mediated by many factors, but to greatly simplify matters, a 10′ x 10′ room with an 8′ ceiling should be illuminated by twelve 4′ color-corrected tubes (*Preston* et al., 1978). Once the quantity and quality of light have been achieved, attention must be given to several factors to preserve both. In order to maintain the spectral quality and brightness, no intense colors or dark surfaces should be used in the room. Remember that when light hits a body, some rays are absorbed and some are reflected. The darker that body, the fewer are the rays reflected. The more highly colored the body, the more the hue will be reflected and the less spectrally pure will be the light in the environment. Every colored object alters the light that is incident upon it. Therefore, the larger the surface (such as walls or cabinet fronts) or the closer it is to the critical color matching area–the patient's mouth (for example, the patient's bib or the dental assistant's dress)–the more influence that surface will exert on the matching process. A third factor, after the light source and reflecting surfaces, is the acuity of the vision of the observer making the evaluation. This acuity can be diminished by sustained viewing, and the evaluation period should be limited to five seconds. After the shade guide-tooth comparison, the viewer should avoid hue adaptation by looking at a medium blue or gray card (this writer prefers the blue) before making another comparison.

The control of light source, room features, and viewer perception is essential to effective color matching.

Modification of Restorations

Color Systems–Additive, Subtractive, and Partitive

When Sir *Isaac Newton* determined that "white light" is composed of different colored rays he, in effect, described what has come to be knowns as "the additive color system." Notable uses of this system, which is composed of three specific primary hues–red, green, and blue–are theatric lighting and colorimeters. The three combinations of two light primaries are the secondary hues of cyan (blue-green), magenta (blue-red), and yellow (red-green). When light is taken away from a source or surface, the reverse of the same system is found. The subtractive color system has as its primary colors cyan, magenta, and yellow. The secondary colors result when the red of the magenta blocks (or absorbs) the green of the cyan to yield blue, the yellow blocks the blue of the magenta to produce red, and yellow also blocks the blue of the cyan to yield green. Thus red, green, and blue are the subtractive secondary colors. The interaction of all three subtractive primaries prevents all light from passing and results in black.

In some situations, neither a pure additive nor a pure subtractive system can be said to be present. Sometimes the subtractive primary hues can be used to give additive results. Common examples of this phenomenon are mosaic tile murals, halftone color printing, and pointilistic oil paintings. Several names are given to this system: "mosaic fusion," "spatial fusion" or "partitive color system" (*Gerritsen,* 1975). In partitive situations, colors do not act either additively nor subtractively, but produce hues, values, and chromas that are averages of the colorants involved. Since porcelain colorants are opaque metal oxides dispersed through the porcelain matrix, they are subject to some of the reactions of the partitive dictates, even though they are most frequently thought of as obeying subtractive principles.

Complementary Colors

When a primary hue is combined with the secondary hue formed by the other two primary hues, the result is the same as all three primaries–white for the additive system, black for the subtractive. This use of "complementary colors" is very important for shade modification procedures.

Glazes and Glazing

When a dental glass (porcelain) is carried to a temperature where the surface vitrifies and exhibits a typical glossy appearance, it is said to be glazed. A glaze can be obtained "naturally" by allowing the restoration to form its own glossy surface, or a lower fusing glass may be applied to the surface and fired. The latter process is usually referred to as "over-glazing." Unless specifically stated otherwise, in this chapter the term "glaze" will always refer to a natural glaze.

The glazing procedure is simple. The goal is to cycle the restoration through a porcelain furnace at a time/temperature schedule that achieves the proper surface quality without causing any functional or esthetic damage. If the surface is underfired it will not have the vitality or optical quality desired. If it is overfired it will be too glossy, and surface morphology can be lost and edges rounded. The actual temperature may vary with any number of factors, including the brand of porcelain employed, the type of furnace used, and the number and temperature of previous firings. The communication of this information from the ceramic technician to the dentist can be very helpful. Visual appraisal of the fired unit is the only accurate analysis; however, the unit should be carefully removed from the furnace a short distance, rotated slightly to change the angle of incident light, and either reinserted to achieve a glossier surface, or removed to cool. (Firing cycles vary, but rise from approximately 1200° to 1750° F [650°–955° C] at 100° F per minute). The furnace used need not be complex but should have an automatic pyrometer and an alarm to signal the arrival at the desired temperature. The additional cost of these features is easily justified by the prevention of the disaster encountered when a unit is forgotten and irretrievably overfired.

Clinical Procedures

When a restoration is received from the laboratory, it may be either in a glazed or unglazed condition, although metal-ceramic porcelains are always carried to maturity (glazed) and then shaped prior to final glazing. At the try-in of the restoration, the modifications of form are made first (assuming that the fit and marginal adaptation are acceptable). The principles for this procedure have been discussed at length previously. Next, the proper surface texture is achieved using diamond stones, disks, or other instruments.

In the process of reshaping, the glaze may be removed in some areas and not in others. The glaze should be removed from all surfaces with the possible exception of tissue surfaces of pontics or non-visible areas such as the lingual aspect. The glaze is best removed with an abrasive spray, but if this is not possible emery disks or fine diamond stones may be used. Removing the glaze from all surfaces allows homogenous reglazing rather than having surfaces with different degrees of glaze on various areas of the restoration.

If colorants are to be added to the surfaces, they will be fired at the same time the restoration is reglazed. The ability to reglaze in the office is valuable, requires a rather small financial commitment, and greatly increases the versatility of techniques to achieve a better result. Furthermore, it often permits completing the restoration satisfactorily rather than having to return it to the laboratory for modification. This is both psychologically beneficial to patient management and economically advantageous, since it precludes another office visit.

It is important to achieve proper surface texture first. Since surface topography is not reproduced in detail by the cast, this is best done at chairside. The restoration is then cleaned, either with steam, distilled water in an ultrasonic cleaner, or by simply scrubbing with a clean brush under running water. The restoration is then ready for reglazing, or the addition of surface colorants.

Color Modifications

When any shade other than a basic shade guide color is indicated, the color modification may be either intrinsic, i.e., added into the porcelain at the time of fabrication, or extrinsic, i.e., applied to the surface after firing. The same is true with characterizations. Both procedures have advantages and disadvantages.

Intrinsic additions offer the broadest range of shade alteration, are most like natural teeth in that the color is "built in," are the most durable, and have excellent optical properties. Internal modification, however, requires skill, is reversible only

by removal of the porcelain itself, and cannot be previewed prior to firing. The addition of color to the surface is limited in the degree to which shades may be altered, it lacks true depth and is lost if the glaze is abraded. However, surface colorants are easily applied or removed, look very much the same before firing as after, and do offer a simple manner of making final shade corrections and adding characterizations.

It is best to make all changes possible intrinsically and reserve extrinsic modification for needed final minor adjustments. All porcelain systems have modifiers for both opaque and body powers. For more intense effects, the more concentrated colors called "stains" can be added to either the basic porcelain or modifiers. These stains are metal oxides in a fluxed porcelain base. The need for a colorant that can survive the firing temperatures of ceramic fabrication limits the range of colors to those formed by the various oxides of metal. Metal oxides are opaque and must be dispersed through the glass matrix to give the desired optical effect. The opaque porcelain powders may be more intensely colored without any detrimental effects, since they are, by necessity, already opaque. Conversely, surface modifications are limited in the degree of saturation possible, since the translucency of the restoration may be lost as concentration increases.

Extrinsic Modification

To understand the effect of modifiers on porcelain color it is necessary to recog-

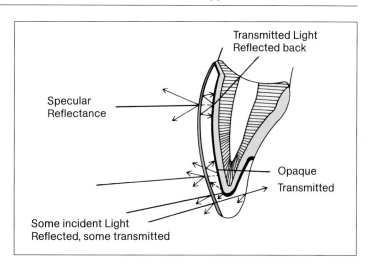

Fig. 9 Color is generated and modified at many levels. Specular reflectance may be altered by surface texture, and the opaque extrinsic colorant particles may alter light incident upon the surface or reflected from underlying areas. Light is transmitted–reflected and scattered according to the colorants, opacifiers and density found in the various parts of the restorations.

nize the many elements that enter into the generation of color in a restoration. As light falls upon the unit, some of the light is reflected from the surface–specular reflectance–and some passes through that surface and is transmitted into the porcelain. The body and incisal porcelain contains opacifiers, colorants, and voids that all scatter, reflect, and transmit light. Whatever light is not reflected back from the body porcelain is eventually reflected or absorbed at the opaque area. This may be either the opaque porcelain that was applied to the metal to mask metal reflectance, or the opaque aluminous core of a jacket. At each interface, some light energy is absorbed and some is reflected. The more light that is absorbed, the lower the value will be. Thus the final appearance of color is generated at many levels (Fig. 9).

Since extrinsic colors (stains) are applied to the surface, they produce their effect differently than do intensic color modifiers. Much of the effect is the result of specular reflectance. The more heavily the surface stain is applied, the greater will be the specular reflectance and the less will the color be generated from within. The cause of this is twofold. First, less incident light will pass through the surface modifiers, since they are opaque, and will be directly reflected from them. Second, some of the light that did pass through the surface layer to the underlying porcelain will be reflected from the undersurface of the extrinsic stains back into the restoration. At each interface of all these elements there will be some absorbtion, reflectance, and scattering.

In spite of the limitations of extrinsic modification, the procedure has many applications that can enhance the esthetic acceptability of a restoration and should be in the armamentarium of every restorative dentist.

An essential prerequisite to effective extrinsic modification is the mixing of the colorant powders with the liquid medium to achieve a suitable consistency. Vari-

513

ous media are used, but all have a higher viscosity than water to reduce flow. Propylene glycol is often used. The consistency should be such that the mixture flows easily onto the restoration but does not run, once placed.

If the modifications are to be made at chairside, the colorants should be mixed and applied to the restoration after it has been placed in the mouth. Once the proper effect has been achieved, the unit should be removed from the mouth and cleaned. This may be done most effectively with steam, but this facility is rarely available in a dental office. Either distilled water in an ultrasonic cleaner or vigorous brushing with a clean brush under running water will suffice. The restoration is then dried and the colorants reapplied. The need for this apparently repetitious procedure is to obviate contamination from saliva, crevicular fluid, or debris. Furthermore, it is not possible to place colorants interproximally on single restorations, beneath or approximating gingival tissue, nor on the apical surfaces of pontics or connectors. Once the desired colorants have been mixed and the effect visualized, it is a simple matter to reproduce the effect in the second application.

A further word about chairside procedures. It is best to refer to the act as "personalizing," "characterizing," or even just "modifying." The word "stain" or "staining" is not a word that conjures up a positive procedure in the mind of the patient.

One of the simplest shade modification procedures is increasing chroma. It was stated earlier that if no proper guide tooth was available, one that is higher in value and lower in chroma should be chosen. If the final restoration is low in chroma, the properly hued colorant is chosen. The colorant is rather generously applied with a sable brush (a 1–0 works well), and homogenously distributed. It may then be diluted as necessary by cleaning the brush with a tissue paper and then stroking off the superfluous material. Hue shifts are made in the same manner.

Decreasing value is similarly simple. The perception is often expressed as a need for "more gray." Gray stain, however, is not the colorant of choice. If the value decrease is to give the impression of greater translucency or neutralize hue, violet is the proper colorant. This use of a complementary color to achieve a lower value is one of the most common applications of extrinsic colorants. It is, however, limited in the degree to which it can be effective, and the colorant itself should not be seen, merely the effect.

The dental colorants do not meet the requirements of the subtractive color system. Instead of cyan (primary) and green (secondary), yellow and red, magenta and blue, cyan is omitted and orange is added. This perversion accommodates to available metal oxides and is more advantageous in the range of hues needed for tooth modification. It does, however, yield an imperfect complementary system. To be perfect, complements must follow the order of the true subtractive system and be of equal saturation. That the dental set of altered subtractive colors proves adequate for the needs of the profession is an indication that hue is not as well perceived as the other dimensions. For this reason, violet works for nearly all shades when an increase in apparent translucency is needed or value needs to be lowered moderately. Another property of metal oxides that prevents them from satisfying the requirements of the subtractive system is their opacity. This dispersion of opaque particles in the glassy medium makes surface colorants follow partitive color dictates more than it does subtractive principles.

Brown is most effective for more significant value decreases when chroma is being raised concomitantly. When brown is mixed with the colorant being used to increase chroma, the value lowering effect is much greater than when violet is used.

Extrinsic characterizations can also be effective. One of the most natural and simple is the addition of white to emulate hypocalcified areas. These areas are frequently found in varying intensities and shapes in natural dentitions. Use of white colorants is an effective way to break up the monotones of standard shades.

When actual form cannot be achieved, the addition of surface color can help create the illusion of the desired form. The illusion of narrower teeth is initiated by moving the contact area to the lingual, opening the labial embrasure, and moving the transitional line angles toward the center of the tooth. The effect can be enhanced by adding brown or orange-brown modifiers to create shadows. The same colorants can be used to simulate root surfaces and cervical lines, effectively "shortening" a clinical crown.

Many effects, from hyperchromatic areas, crack and stain lines, to enhancement of occlusal morphology are possible with superficial colorants. There are a number of different kits available from various manufacturers, representing a variety of different colors. The colorants will look very much the same before and after firing. This ability to preview the effect is a distinct advantage.

Another use of superficial colorants is the modification of the shade guide to predict the deviations from the standard guide and to communicate them to the fabricating ceramist. The shade guide that had the glaze removed is used for this purpose. Various colorants may be applied to the unglazed surface until experimentation produces the desired result. To communicate this effect to the laboratory, a vehicle made for the purpose* replaces the standard liquid medium when mixing the colorants. When the shade guide has been modified to emulate the natural teeth, the stains may be kept from smudging by drying the guide in front of a heat source such as a burner or a lightbulb. The guide will appear very chalky, but can be returned to its original appearance by adding another liquid in the laboratory.** This system can greatly aid in communicating the shades and characterizations desired.

Any stain product may be used with any porcelain system. Even though there may be variations in the coefficients of

---

*   Stain Set – Ceramco Division of Johnson & Johnson Dental Products, Windsor, NJ.

** Stain Wet – Ceramco Division of Johnson & Johnson Dental Products, Windsor, NJ.

thermal expansion, these have not proven to be a problem.

All the effects that may be accomplished with extrinsic colorants can be achieved with internal modifiers as well as many that are beyond the scope of extrinsic coloring. Instrinsic modification develops color more in the manner natural teeth do, from within. Shade alternations are more predictable when custom shade tabs made with dilutions of various modifiers are employed. Unfortunately, the batch-to-batch variations found in commercial porcelain fabrication makes such tabs imperfect, but they are still closer than the limited standard guide.

Many of the desired modifications of standard shades can only effectively be done intrinsically. Major shade alterations, development of color in thin sections, hyperpigmented areas, crack simulations, opalescence, and similar effects may best be achieved by adding modifiers to the opaque, body, or incisal porcelains. It is not the purpose here to detail techniques that are described in other places (*Preston* and *Bergen,* 1980; *McLean,* 1980) but rather to relate generally to the procedure. There are some inherent precautions necessary with internal modification. The addition of modifiers for either shade alteration or characterization requires skill development to learn just how much change a certain modifier will make in the porcelain to which it is added. Experimentation and experience are essential to predictable success. Characterization employing wedge techniques or layering requires deft handling of the porcelain to ensure coalesence of the added colorants with the

matrix porcelain. If the wetting is inadequate, cracking can result, yet if the addition is too moist, the characterization may be indistinct and flow where it is not wanted. As was previously stated, one of the few limitations of internal modification is the need for a greater degree of technical skill. The resulting effects, however, are most gratifying and merit the effort involved.

Fluoresence

Another factor that has been the subject of great concern and frequent consternation to those manufacturing dental porcelain is that of fluoresence. Fluoresence is a form of luminesence wherein a stimulus below the visible spectrum (ultraviolet) causes a body to emit light within the visible spectrum. Since daylight and many artificial light sources have a u.v. component, such stimulation-emmission occurs along with visible light illumination. The degree to which the combination visible/u.v. illumination affects "vitality" is only conjecture. When u.v. (black light) is the primary source, the difference between natural teeth and most restorations is gross. Some recent fluoresence formulas* have been innovatively successful in achieving excitation–emission properties similar to natural teeth, yet some porcelains lack any significant fluoresence.

Another manufacturer** has overcome

---

* Crystar–Shofu Dental Manufacturing Company
** Microbond porcelain, Howmedica Inc. Chicago, Illinois.

the problem of obtaining fluoresence in opaque porcelain. Heretofore, in areas where body porcelain was thin, the absence of fluoresence in the opaque porcelain layer always resulted in gray, nonfluorescing spots that were unnatural and unesthetic when viewed under ultra violet illumination. The use of fluorescent opaque produces acceptable fluoresence regardless of the thickness of the body porcelain layer.

Other Optimal Properties

The replication of anomalous teeth with porcelain can still be frustrating. Color is not the only variable that requires adjustment: relative translucency and opacity must also be considered. Some teeth actually may be seen to become more opaque as they dry, and each shade comparison is different. In these situations, I have found the application of a material such as glycerine or liquid medium for stains to be useful in keeping the surface moist. Some teeth exhibit a "pearlescent" effect and are most difficult to simulate. Much of the final success comes only with patience and skilled artistry, and sometimes success is simply not obtained to the degree desired.

Time spent in advance of irreversible procedures may preclude the unfortunate consequences, including litigation, which may attend the initiation of therapy without pre-established, well-defined goals. The patient interview, diagnostic waxing, rational mouth and tooth preparation, a provisional restoration that is the prototype of the finished unit, knowledgeable use of materials, capable communication with talented technicians, and patient chairside modification all are necessary to achieve the optimal result.

The author is well aware that this chapter gives only a moderate amount of definitive information and leaves to the reader's enthusiasm and desire for excellence the pursuit of more sources of information. That only a very small portion of the dentists and technicians who provide ceramic restorative services to the public shall ever take the time to seek such information is a rather depressing fact.

What Lies Ahead?

The advent of an era in dentistry when porcelain is the focus of so much attention should not be perceived as an indication that this is the ultimate material. Porcelain has excellent esthetic properties and the fabrication procedures, while not entirely simple, allow the production of a significant percentage of the restorative materials in use. Porcelain by itself, lacks tensile strength and failures are not uncommon. When bonded to metal to achieve greater strength, a hostile environment for the framework is established. The abrasiveness of porcelain against natural teeth creates a rather destructive occlusal problem in some situations. The firing temperatures preclude the use of organic pigments limiting the procedures available for color control.

It seems likely, with the increased capabilities of resin polymer technology, that at some point in the future porcelain may well lose its preeminence as a restorative material. Resin polymers can be bonded to metal oxides just as glass polymers can. Grafting procedures seem to make virtually any property possible. It seems probable that resins without metal support can be developed for dental use. In fact, if one sets down the physical and biologic requirements for an esthetic dental restorative material, there is nothing that precludes the eventual development of a more universal restorative material–except, possibly, finances.

For the present, however, some interesting modifications of current techniques are at hand.

Simpler procedures for porcelain labial margins will make this approach increasingly attractive. *Prince* (1981) describes the addition of wax as a vehicle to carry porcelain to place and facilitates margins that are both esthetically excellent and biologically acceptable. The substitution of wax for the usual liquid does not affect density nor detract from esthetics. Higher-firing porcelains are being introduced to enhance stability during firing*. Glasses that are fabricated in a manner previously considered atypical or even impossible are now being researched and marketed. One process makes use of an epoxy resin die material that has controlled and reliable expansion.** Upon such a die a coping is waxed, invested in plaster, the wax eliminated, and a porcelain/resin coping pressure-formed on the die. This high alumina core is then fired with an extended (12-hour) firing cycle, during which dimension is closely controlled. The core can range from no expansion to approximately 3% enlargement. The high alumina content gives much greater strength upon which to bake a very esthetic boro-silicate glass. The accuracy has proven quite remarkable and heralds a new era for porcelain restorations.

Regardless of the materials employed, the development of esthetically satisfying restorations will always require artistic skills from concerned and conscientious dentists and technicians. These subjective skills must be more effectively taught and the inclusion of classes in esthetics in at least two dental schools (University of Southern California, Los Angeles, CA, and Emory University, Atlanta, GA) is an encouraging development.

Public recognition of the need for more esthetic dental restorations will only increase, as will demand. The skillful dentist will always find a need for personal improvement and a marketplace for the talents developed.

---

* Shofu Dental Manufacturing Company, Menlo Park, CA
** Cerestore Coors Biomedical, Lakewood, CO.

Summation of Technique

The pursuit of excellence holds it own compensation. The development of increased skill is sometimes visible only in retrospect and there seems to be a perpetual dissatisfaction with one's present talent. I have attempted to communicate some of the factors that I have found helpful in my own progressive learning endeavors. If there is one word that holds the best advice for improved esthetics it would be "observe." It is the natural, pleasing dental composition we seek to emulate and it is the human dentition and its associated tissues that become the textbook of study. Goethe stated, "What we know, we see." It is essential that we not only look, but must study and perceive.

A second word for success is "plan." The result should be envisioned before definitive therapy is intiated. This anticipated "result" must be the same in the mind of the patient as it is in the mind of the dentist if dissatisfaction and iatrogenic esthetic failure are to be avoided.

References

Abrams, Leonard (1978): Person Communication, Colorado Springs, August.

Clark, E., Bruce (1931): An analysis of tooth color. JADA 18: 2093–2103.

Clark, E., Bruce (1933): Tooth color selection. JADA 20: 1065–1073.

Frush, John P., and Fisher, Roland, D., (1956): How dentogenic restorations interpret the sex factor. J. Prosthet. Dent. 6: 160–172.

Gerritsen, Frans (1975): Theory & Practice of Color. New York: Van Nostrand Reinhold, division of Litton Educational Publishing.

Goldstein, Ronald (1976): Esthetics in Dentistry. Lippincott.

Hirsch, B., Levin, B., and Tiber N. (1973): Effect of dentist authoritarianism on patient evaluation of dentures. J. Prosthet. Dent. 30: 745–748.

Lemire P.A., and Burk, B. (1975): Color in Dentistry. Bloomfield. J. M. Ney Company.

Lombardi, R. E. (1973): The principles of visual perception and their clinical perception and their clinical application to denture esthetics. J. Prosthet. Dent. 29: 358.

McLean, J. W. and Hughes, T. H. (1965): The reinforcement of dental porcelain with ceramic oxides. Brit. Dent. J. 119: 251–267.

McLean, John W. (1980): The Science and Art of Dental Ceramics. Vol. II Chicago: Quintessence Publishing Company, Inc.

Miller, Lloyd (1981): Personal Communication, Lecture before American Academy of Denture Prosthetics. Seattle, Washington, May.

Munsell, A. H. (1936): A Color Notation. Baltimore: Munsell Color Co.

Murrell, George (1974): Phonetics, function and anterior occlusion. J. Prosthet. Dent. 32: 23–31.

Newton, Isaac (1966): Optiks New York: Dover Publications (Based on ed. 4, 1730).

Obregon, Alejandro, Goodkind, R. J, Schwabacher, Wm. B. (1981): Effects of opaque and porcelain surface texture on the color of ceramometal restorations. J. Prosthet. Dent. 46: 330–340.

Pincus, Charles (1967): Cosmetics: the psychologic fourth dimension in full mouth rehabilitation. DCNA, 71–88, March.

Pound, Earl (1966): The mandibular movements of speech and their seven related values. J. So. Calif. St. Dent. Assoc. 4: 435–441.

Preston, J. D. (1976): A systematic approach to the control of esthetic form. J. Prosthet. Dent. 35: 393–402.

Preston, J. D. (1979): A reassessment of the mandibular transverse horizontal axis theory. J. Prosthet. Dent. 41: 605–613.

Preston, J. D., Ward, Leo, C., and Bobrick, M. (1978): Light and lighting in the dental office. D. C. N. A. 23: 431–451.

Prince, Jonathan (1981): Personal Communication. Los Angeles: USC School of Dentistry.

Rosenthal, L. E., Pleasure, M. A., and Lefer, L. (1964): Patient reaction to denture esthetics. J. Dental Medicine 19: 103–110.

Shelby, David (1976): Anterior Restoration Fixed Bridgework and Esthetics. p. 201. Springfield: Charles C. Thomas.

Sproull, Robert (1973): Color matching in dentistry Pt. II "Practical applications of the organization of color". J. Prosthet. Dent. 29: 556–566, May.

Stein, R. S. (1979): Lecture, Academy of Crown and Bridge Prosthodontics Chicago, Feb.

Panel of Experts: Dr. *Frank Clarke,* Dr. *Lloyd Miller,* Dr. *Jack D. Preston,*
Dr. *David E. Simmons*

Chairman: Dr. *J. W. McLean*

Prof. McLean

The first question is from Dr. *Miller* to Dr. *Clarke:* How significant is the difference
between whole mouth and single tooth illumination for *in vivo* color measurement of teeth? Can you relate this visually?

Dr. Clarke

I have not been able to make measurements with whole mouth illumination and
compare them with single tooth illumination, so the answer is that no one knows
quantitatively what the difference is. But from the basic fundamentals, there
must be a significant difference and, it seems to me that we are in a fortunate
position, because we have no established instrumentation in widespread use.
There are no dental instruments available yet that will function correctly. I have
already proposed that the ideal dental instrument would have a fairly large integrating sphere, at least 0.5 m in diameter. It should have a little funnel so that the
measuring area could come in close proximity with the oral cavity. You could
illuminate the whole mouth in a natural way with diffuse illumination. A fiber
sensor is unsuitable because it will obstruct the tooth that you are trying to
measure.
The best method is to use a telephotometer system, that is, a telescopic optical
system. On the far side of the integrating sphere, which is a white-coated sphere
containing a light source, there is a small hole through which an optical system
may view a sightable area. In fact, the optical system must have a photoelectric
spectrophotometer to do the measurement, and a beam splitter with an eye-
piece is needed so that the dentist can use cross-wires to actually aim the device
where measurements must be taken.
The whole mouth must be illuminated to simulate a natural situation. So the two
parts of the instrument would be the large integrating sphere with a typical

mouth-sized aperture opening out of the sphere for illuminating the mouth, and a very small angle system, which would view only part of the tooth. Generally, one wants to isolate different areas on a tooth, because of the areas of different morphology such as mamelons and vertical striation–cracks and fissures. In addition there is the thin, translucent incisal tip, and the deeper, more orange color near the gingiva. For this reason, a relatively small viewing area is needed but it has to be remote and that means a very small angle telescopic system. Cost? Industrial instruments in the color industry typically cost $ 10,000 to $ 20,000, depending how much computational effort is provided. Dentists will have enough computation with a little microprocessor to convert to a good system. A small scanning spectrophotometer and the integrating sphere cannot be purchased for less than $ 10,000. It would be unrealistic to think otherwise. In order for such systems to achieve worldwide acceptance, it inevitably means guidelines from an international committee.

Participant

Why didn't you give us some results of your work on *in vivo* colour measurement?

Dr. Clarke

That particular work was sponsored by another organization. However, the British Ceramic Research Association will make the report available to you.

Participant

Dr. *Preston,* as the shade guides are so inadequate, what are your thoughts on the use of individual tabs of the fired single powders, which some manufacturers supply? They seem more accurate than the shade guide per se.

Dr. Preston

Anything is more accurate than the shade guide per se. You would have to consider the dilutions to be used and permutations of the particular powders. The variables are going to be the color control-batch-to-batch variations which exist from one product to another and from one batch to another. There are no ADA standards on porcelain. The manufacturer has no limitations on deviations (e.g., differences in coefficient of thermal expansion, etc.). There have never been any standards set up for porcelain. The individual shade guide fabrication is a step in the right direction. I think that when *Lloyd Miller's* data are available, you will be very surprised at the amount of work he has done in specialized shade guide production. He has shown the effect of adding oranges, because this brings us toward the red range. He noted recently one particular portion that is so yellow, it is almost green. We are on that end of the spectrum with our porcelains; the addition of the oranges and reds to push them toward natural tooth color is certainly an advantage.

Dr. *Clarke,* when we measure teeth *in vivo* and then create a restoration outside the mouth, I wonder if it might be too red when inserted in the mouth?

Dr. Clarke

The idea has occurred to me that someone might like to make an oral model (on a large scale). This artificial mouth would have all the various tissues correctly colored with correct spectrophotometric curves. Again, this means measurements that will be made on gingiva, etc. If such measurements can be made on teeth, they certainly can be made on gingiva, tongue, and palate. This artificial mouth might be helpful to the technician.

Participant

Dr. *Miller,* would you describe briefly your recent research on color and any clinically pertinent conclusions that would be of interest to a practicing dentist or technician?

Dr. Miller

We borrowed *Bob Sproul's* work, which coordinates very nicely with the work done by *Lemire* and *Burke, Hayashi* and *Bruce Clark.* All came out with similar numbers for hue, value and chroma of natural teeth. We plotted these on a graph, as we showed today, and then we had *Hemmendinger* read out all the shade guides. We fired sample tabs from all of the systems I have in the office and submitted them to him for analysis. That was transferred into hue, value and chroma numbers and plotted. What you find is similar to what we have been saying today. Unfortunately, the present systems are old. Originally, a series of shades, based on what were pleasing colors that were thought to cover the colour space was developed by some "expert". So we find that presently available shade guides do not represent natural colors of enough teeth, just a few. Yet spectrophotometrically analyzed, most "average" shades are on the yellow side of the spectrum with very little orange. We have an illogical distribution. We also find that another key factor is not chroma, but value. The values are too high for the important colors of porcelain, and the important colors are the shades such as A2, A3, B2, and B3 in this area of prettiness. There is no problem in making dark, ugly shades, A4, C4, who cares what the difference is between C4 and A4 or B4? But the difference between A2 and A3 is important and the difference in lightness and darkness of these is critical. Flexibility is needed in changing the value of certain key shades. We still need high value in A1 and B1. We still need a very white, bright tooth. We do not need any more dark ugly teeth. But for the ones in the middle, which cover the greater part of the population, we need flexibility by changing that most critical perceptive mechanism – value – and the spectrophotometer is a useful and predictable device for measuring the changes that are needed in the porcelain we use.

What we find, as Dr. *Preston* has shown, is that the opaques do not match the body porcelain in the most critical dimension-value. Technicians learned a long time ago how to change that. For example, when A3 porcelain is used and a slightly lower value is desired, the opaque of C3 can be substituted. Or as *Paul Muia* showed in his four-dimensional system, the value is altered by changing the enamel on the surface, providing a filter mechanism for reducing light reflection. The spectrophotometric studies show how we can dovetail what are called hue changes with value changes.

Why do we use brown so much? Because brown is a good filter system, and it selectively absorbs and filters out certain kinds of brightness in color. Therefore, when you see reflected light, it is lower in value.

You don't have to ask the manufacturers. Ask patients what is wrong with the crowns they see in people's mouths. They are too bright and too big. However, until a spectrophotometric system enjoys widespread use, that's as far as we are going until we set standards. Yet, I do not see any solution, despite all our recommendations for setting standards. I believe marketing decisions cominate and control any important changes that could be made.

Prof. McLean

Dr. *Miller,* I have been involved in the manufacture of porcelain. To be fair to manufacturers, it is a formidable task. One of the problems is that we use dental porcelain in varying thicknesses. Although you could probably come much closer to the values on which we all agree, the difficulties in producing porcelains commercially, to achieve ideal value and chroma in thin sections, are such that a thin section looks washed out and too low in chroma and value, whereas a thick section may look too bright. A compromise has to be reached.

Dr. Miller

The manufacturers know what the trouble is. They have been changing the shade guides. If you have any old shade guides, throw them away; they are different from the new ones. Today, the spectrophotometer can show me rather clearly that the shade guides made in the mid-1970s are very different from the ones made now. The differences, particularly in lightness and darkness, are recognizable and improvements are being made. What we need are hues with flexibility in brightness levels. We need an A3, for example, that has a value of 7.5 and 7 and 6.5, but we do not need another hue halfway between A3 and A4. In order to increase the shades in that system, a whole new system must be devised and that costs money. Manufacturers are beginning to understand how they can make improvements to their marketing advantage, but they are not trying hard enough.

Dr. Preston

There are only two manufacturers of shade guides in the U.S., and eight companies emulate them. While the manufacturers of shade guides may have changed the guides, the people who are making porcelains may still be using old shade guides as models.

Prof. McLean

Dr. *Clarke,* please comment about reducing value by using dentinoenamels.

Dr. Clarke

I was very impressed with what I saw Mr. *Kedge* doing in London on the layering of porcelain. Large discontinuities of light diffusion, in which the first layer over the metal has to be extremely opaque, and suddenly another porcelain simulating natural dentin is introduced, and then a further porcelain layer is added to simulate natural enamel, these very sharp boundaries are a source of potential trouble. Therefore, the kind of system with a more graded structure has much to commend it. Thinking of the point that Dr. *Miller* made about the difficulty of introducing an improved system into the marketplace, I think that if we could get a proper dental color atlas—and I use that word deliberately to mean a logically constructed one—such a system could be introduced by publishing the findings of an authoritative, international committee such as the International Standards Organization. However, a proper dental color atlas is something that will not happen overnight. Organizations like the American Dental Association and others throughout the world will need to support it. What is important, though, is that it be set up in the right way. Good measurements must be made at the start —and this means using an instrument that does not yet exist to take valid measurements *in vivo.*

Prof. McLean

How practical do you think it is for manufacturers to make opaques that are within the hue and chroma value of dentin body porcelains? Could they achieve a more balanced color by making neutral tone opaques that do not affect the color of the veneer porcelain? Is this feasible?

Dr. Clarke

It makes no sense to have an opaque that is incompatible in its spectral values and its color coordinates. It should be possible to make opaques that have the right spectral character and pseudo dentins, pseudo enamels, and the dentino-enamels and possible dentino-opaques might also be produced. All of them ought to belong to a common family of spectrophotometric curves. Variations should suit the individual patient, but they should all be in conformity with naturally occurring spectral curves to avoid metamerism. It seems to me that there is enough freedom in the available tolerance to allow this; it is merely a question of proper selection. I think that it is possible to do this. Of course, the real absurdity is that historically we have measured extracted teeth, and they are too yellowish and not orange enough.

Dr. Miller

If all surface stains are opaque, why is the opacity of white surface stains so different from the other colors?

Dr. Preston

I am not sure I can answer absolutely—perhaps Dr. *Clarke* will correct me if I am wrong. Consider particle size and reflectance. I assume that the whites of which you speak are of a particle size that provides opacity and scattering. There is no white that is not opaque. The relative degree of saturation of that powder in the metal ceramic flux is going to give the appearance of white, as found in various kits. However, I assume that any of the whites are white because of the scattering effect, and that they have a fairly flat spectral curve. I do not think that they are metameric whites; they are whites, and appear different because whites are always opaque. All other colors are relatively translucent. The other color—more properly stain—which is less translucent, is the grey and for the same reason. It is just a lower value of the same thing.

Dr. Clarke

It is worth noting that staining is mainly caused by absorption, rather than by scattering. Staining by nicotine or beverages, etc., unless it is contained within a fissure, acts as a foreign substance that is attached to or adsorbed onto the tooth surface. This surface stain is not so much altering the scattering, but is selectively absorbing in the short-wave end of the spectrum, which is why it appears brownish or yellowish. Therefore, pigment or stain that you add to simulate this effect should have a similar characteristic, that is, it should be applied in the surface layer and should not be so much a scatterer as an absorber.

Dr. Preston

Why are whites unique as compared to the rest of the stains?

Dr. Clarke

If you want a white it has to be a scatterer. Otherwise it can't be a white; it just becomes transparent. Are white surface markings, in fact, placed?

Prof. McLean

Well, they are, but I'm rather inclined to think they are better built in.

Dr. Clarke

True whites are not natural, since in nature, there are no white surfaces.

Prof. McLean

No, and I am delighted to see that dentistry is moving away from surface staining. I have not liked it for a very long time. We have always built our color in layers and it is interesting to note that people are now recognizing, as a study in Canada shows, that surface stains are even being removed by toothbrushing with fluoride toothpaste.

Dr. Simmons

If we are going to build color from within the tooth, the technician has to know at the start the size, shape, and position of that tooth in the final outcome. Today we are lucky to have provisional materials in which adequate thickness of porcelain and adequate tooth reduction can be checked at the provisional stage to see if we have sufficient depth of material. We should plan so that we know where we are going to end up before we begin. As Dr. *Miller* said, when you take away the tooth, you can't put it back so easily. If initial planning is poor, a tooth might be indexed, but if there is a change in the position of that tooth in any manner or size, the indexing is lost. Planning must be complete.

I would like to see ceramics instruction move away from the ceramic try in, involving grinding and shaping at the chairside, to a provisional restoration, which is anatomically accurate and reduces grinding and shaping of the final porcelain restoration, thereby preserving fine detail and layering of colors. How do you produce hue, chroma, and value when you layer? You change the value as you layer the porcelain and this is a very complicated process. We owe the technician better guidelines. Technicians do not have biological considerations at the bench, whereas we do, and I would like to see more communication via anatomically accurate provisionals and study casts.

Dr. Miller

I'd like to reply to Dr. *McLean's* use of internal staining and coloring in his laboratory. For average dentists who do not have an in-house laboratory or who do not have the expertise to put it on themselves, surface staining is a means of teaching dentists how to do something about color: how to sit at the chair and put color on without a lot of numbers and a lot of formulas. To put it on, see that it's wrong, take it off, put it on, and get an improved, logical system out of the present illogical mess. I will defend the use of color surface stains for years based on that. When the color is put underneath, that is a total commitment. Nothing can be done about too much color in that case. For the average dentist, this means taking the porcelain off and putting it on again and that costs money. So I defend surface stains on the basis that it has some significance for a lot of people, despite the fact that there is some evidence available now to show that low pH materials will dissolve surface colorants and that vigorous toothbrushing for a period of 8–10 years will remove some of the surface color. A crown does not last forever; the color will be pretty good for 10 years and then it will change. But that is better than starting with nothing and ending up with worse.

Prof. McLean

It may be an advantage because, as patients age, their crowns whiten and they think they are definitely improving and getting younger!

Dr. Preston

I would also defend and support Dr. *Miller*. Once dentists begin to use surface stains they are more prone to learn to use intrinsic stains.

Prof. McLean

There seems to be controversy about cooling of the finished ceramic. Some advise slow cooling, some advise immediate removal from the furnace, and others cool the work with compressed air.
Ian Sced and I worked at the NPL on dynamic air cooling, and even helium air cooling, which was really dynamic. We checked bond strengths with a slow furnace cool of the crown and with a cool in which the crown was cooled at the muffle entrance. Using our conical shear test for bond strength, we found that cooling at the muffle entrance produced the best bond strengths, with low standard deviations. I think that use of compressed air, which is really a dynamic air cool, is an absolute disaster. With slow cooling, if it is too slow, you run into the problem of the metal and porcelain losing heat at different rates and producing different thermal gradients.

Dr. Preston

Cooling is one way of dynamically affecting the coefficient of thermal expansion. The coefficient of thermal expansion is a volatile number; it is a variable number. It may be decided by the fabricating ceramist or by the manufacturer to accomplish a certain purpose, but it changes in the manner of fabrication. The cooling curve is changed; the cooling approach is changed. You change the coefficient of thermal expansion. This is very valuable as long as it is recognized and controlled, to adapt different ceramics to different alloys. A ceramic with a coefficient matched to a particular alloy under slow cooling may be cooled rapidly so that its coefficient now matches adequately for use of the alloy system. Cooling should be controlled so that it is replicable for the system that works. The idea of rapid cooling, that is, flushing with air, evolves from the optical industry, in which it is used to age (harden) glasses. It is strictly a glass system; it is not a metal-glass system. Once that disparity in cooling exists, it is entirely disastrous. Probably no single system is correct. It depends entirely upon the alloy-porcelain system being used and the effect on coefficient matching.

Prof. McLean—written question

Dr. *Clarke,* would you comment on *Land's* theory of color vision, according to which the rods participate in color vision by mediating the quantity of light, (luminosity) at each wave length, linking centrally with cone information to give a composite (hue-chroma value) impression of light (color).

Dr. Clarke

There are two issues here. The rods are involved in peri foveal and peripheral vision, not in central vision, and you can never get close enough to a tooth to get to what we call large field color matching, in which the rods may play a role. We are always in the fovea for normal distance viewing of teeth. There is a large field CIE color matching system as well as a small one. The textile industry likes the large field, because large rolls of cloth and large areas are being viewed, but this, of course, is totally irrelevant to teeth. For the normal two degree standard observer, the normal CIE system is relevant to the viewing of teeth and rods do not come into it at all, because there are no rods in the fovea. *Land's* theories of color vision caused some slight stir when he first proposed them, but they were refuted by *Judd,* of the National Bureau of Standards, and *McAdam,* the two greatest American color scientists at the time. In fact, *Land* merely rediscovered *Goethe's* colored shadows. The German philosopher, *Goethe,* discovered that effect and made some interesting comments on it. The illustration, incidentally, of stage lighting shown by Dr. *Preston* with two different lights falling onto an object at different angles depicts what is known as *Goethe's* colored shadows. I do not think one needs to worry too much about *Land's* ideas.

Participant

As a ceramist, I am very much interested in the weeping of dentists about the quality of porcelain. In fact, what is important is the quality of the technician's skills and the knowledge to use the materials in a very difficult situation. The juxtaposition of color, the lip creating a shadow, the dark oral cavity, the relationship of one tooth to another; it's a very complex problem, and technicians must understand the theory of color, their material, and the situation in which it is made.

Prof. McLean

Yes, I absolutely support you. This is one of the reasons why we are making an attempt to form an International Society for Dental Ceramics specifically directed to technicians. I am trying to encourage technicians to do much more teaching. One of the biggest problems is that the top technicians often guard much of their technology.

No matter what color systems we evolve, if we cannot train the technicians to lay in this color—and this is the vital issue—we cannot develop color and depth of translucency where we are restricted in color space by limitations of thickness. The cause of high value, to be fair to the manufacturer, is that often one is almost certain to produce high value in a 1 mm section of porcelain on metal. My technicians admit they simply cannot produce esthetic, low value anterior crowns on metal if they are limited to 0.8 mm of porcelain thickness. Inevitably, the crowns look bright and lack depth of translucency

Dr. Miller

Despite all the number systems and the scientific approach that has been discussed, the spectrophotometer leaves out the dimension of translucency. Today, one can make samples of opaque paper with *Munsell's* system which match natural teeth. However, these are two different materials—a tooth and paper—and one lacks a certain property: translucency. Translucency is critical for light refraction. Opacity does not have that capacity. So when one finally comes down to all the numbers and the machines, one must consider the artistic ability to handle the material.

Prof. McLean

One of the dangers today is that many drawings are being made of cross-sections of crowns in which not only is the thickness of the metal reduced but also the thickness of the opaque, the dentin and the enamel. And the claim is made that a beautiful translucent tooth can be made in this way. I can assure you that I have looked at work done by most of the internationally famous technicians and not one of them can produce translucent metal-ceramic crowns when they use less than a millimeter's thickness of porcelain. I have taken a lot of pictures *in vivo* and have yet to see such a crown.

Dr. Clarke

In the paper industry, and one or two others, the standard method of gauging translucency is to take a sample of a known thickness, maybe a millimeter would be useful, and simply measure the sample over a white and over a near-black background of known reflectance and observe the difference between the two readings. Simple conventions exist for dealing with this problem. Stable near-blacks and stable near-whites are available, and the British Ceramic Research Association will be very happy to provide standard near-white and standard near-black backgrounds.

Participant

In terms of the communication of color, I think dentists have to be willing to look in the mouth and give technicians information, for example, the difference between the cervical and the gingival. *Muia's* new book, *The Four-Dimensional Tooth Color System,* provides relevant information. My clients use the colors that I am able to make, so we can reproduce the tooth if we have adequate reduction of tooth structure.

Prof. McLean

We have every intention at the next International Ceramics Symposium of placing strong emphasis on dental technology. As one who began as a dental technician, I have a great interest in this side of our profession.

Participant

Many dentists use an acrylic shade guide to determine the so-called value. Two very interesting things about acrylic are its edge-lighting factors and optical factors. The translucent areas, particularly mesially and distally, which give a translucent or edge-lighting factor, are critical if we are to make teeth that blend harmoniously.

Prof. McLean

Actually, you can make a much easier match with acrylic simply because it is translucent and absorbs a lot of the color that surrounds it. In the case of porcelain, particularly when applied to metal on the anterior teeth, one must rely almost entirely on an illusion in order to create the translucency.

Participant

How helpful would instant color pictures be in supplying information to the dental ceramist?

Participant

It helps in terms of color distribution, but not in terms of accuracy of color.

Prof. McLean

Yes, that is what our technicians find. You can use Polaroid film to determine areas of translucency, internal stains, and crack lines, and this is quite helpful, but it does not give an accurate representation of color.

Dr. Clarke

If you analyze all the color films on the market, from all the principal makers in America, Germany, Japan, etc. you will find that the spectral responses of those color films are quite different from human spectral responses. Adding non-standard lighting that is not one of the preferred CIE sources such as fluorescent lamps with their own emission lines, for example, you will obtain gross color distortions. You will see differences, but the actual color rendering will be wrong. Any metamerism between synthetic and natural dentine will be particularly liable to give a misleading effect.

Closing Remarks

John W. McLean

In closing this Conference, I would like, first of all, to thank Mr. *Haase* and Miss *Tsuchiya* of Quintessence, who have given such strong support to this first Symposium, and for their continuing interest in furthering the knowledge of dental ceramics and technology all around the world. In addition, we are all very grateful to Dr. *Jack Rayson,* Dean of Louisiana State University Dental School, for his enthusiasm and support for this program. In particular, I would also like to thank Dr. *Bruggers* and Dr. *Jeansonne* who have done an enormous amount of work to put this Conference together. Their auxiliary team – including all the technicians – deserve special mention because they have put in many hours of effort on our behalf.

Finally, to our panel of experts, we owe a great debt. They have certainly lived up to their reputations and enhanced the whole of the proceedings of this meeting. I thank the audience as well, for staying with us to the end. This has encouraged us to set up future international meetings to further the education of both dentists and technicians. The enthusiasm you have shown in the past three days has been a fitting reward to the organizers of the Conference.

Subject Index

Quintessential to dentistry.....

John W. McLean, O.B.E., D.Sc., M.D.S. (University of London), L.D.S.R.C.S. (England)

The Science and Art of Dental Ceramics

Volume I: The Nature of Dental Ceramics and their Clinical Use

The ever increasing demands of patients for better esthetics in dental restorations today provide more problems for the dentist than ever before. The publication of these monographs by Dr. John McLean therefore is timely. Not only are the fundamentals of ceramics, from applications in jacket crowns to combinations with cast restorations, discussed, but the therepeutic alternatives for the attainment of better, esthetically more satisfactory results are described for those cases in which conventional methods are simply insufficient to provide optimal results.

The dentist is shown how to use the possibilities provided by ceramics in a more differentiated, problem-oriented way than has been suggested in the past.

The practice-oriented dentist and the dental technician interested in ceramics will find a variety of information, useful not only at the chairside, but also in the dental laboratory. The book stimulates the interested reader while it teaches him. The monographs will have great value as well for dental students and for dental materials researchers.

Volume II: Bridge Design and Laboratory Procedures in Dental Ceramics

"... an exhaustive and fully documented text covering all aspects of dental ceramics ... the color photographs ... demonstrate the author's ability to reproduce the vital characteristics of the natural dentition in dental ceramic restorations with natural morphology and color."

Journal of Prosthetic Dentistry

"An excellent book that should be in the hands of every dentist and technician whose practice includes the restoration of the dentition with porcelain restorations."   *British Dental Journal*

The second volume of Professor McLean's *The Science and Art of Dental Ceramics* is the most comprehensive book ever published on ceramic technology. Detailed techniques for making metal, ceramic, or alumina reinforced crowns and bridges are fully illustrated with color photographs and diagrams. A complete chapter is devoted to producing "Special Effects" in dental porcelain.

Coping and bridge design, the fitting of precision attachments, casting techniques, and surface finishing of metal are examined critically in light of current research. The building of occlusion in dental porcelain is given considerable prominence, and a number of clinical cases are presented to show how to develop occlusion in difficult situations.

Techniques described represent years of research. Both the novice and expert ceramist will have the opportunity to use well-proven laboratory and clinical methods. In combining the science and art of dental technology, the dentist and ceramist will have a clearer understanding of their success or failure.

Volume I: 336 pages, over 300 illustrations, linenbound with gold stamping
ISBN 0-931386-04-7   Order 1501/0047

Volume II: 512 pages, 820 illustrations (680 in color), linenbound with gold stamping
ISBN 0-931386-11-X   Order 1506/011X

quintessence books

**Quintessence Publishing Co. Inc.
8 South Michigan Avenue, Suite 2301
Chicago, Illinois 60603**

Quintessential to dentistry.....

Paul Muia

The Four Dimensional Tooth Color System

New techniques in dental ceramics are combining science with art to produce ceramic restorations that are not only more accurate than in the past but also more aesthetically pleasing. Here, the author's original technique for detection, measurement, and duplication of composite tooth color is introduced.

Four color dimensions are assigned to the tooth—hue to dentin; chroma, a further refinement of hue; maverick color to any other color in the dentin not directly responsible for hue; and value (defined as brightness) to enamel. Fabrication of a customized tooth color guide for measuring the four tooth color dimensions is discussed in depth, as is its practical use. Over 400 accurate color illustrations vividly depict actual case studies—from chairside, through laboratory procedures, to completed ceramic restorations.

This new text offers you technical solutions—eliminating guesswork—to those pressing aesthetic problems that you encounter daily. The book that you have needed for a long time is now available.

281 pages, 420 colored illustrations, ISBN 0-931386-53-5

quintessence
books

Order 1606/0535

Quintessence Publishing Co. Inc.
8 South Michigan Avenue, Suite 2301
Chicago, Illinois 60603